W0050357

SURGERY IN GYNECOLOGICAL ONCOLOGY

DEVELOPMENTS IN ONCOLOGY

F.J. Cleton and J.W.I.M. Simons, eds., Genetic Origins of Tumour Cells
ISBN 90-247-2272-1

J. Aisner and P. Chang, eds., Cancer Treatment Research
ISBN 90-247-2358-2

B.W. Ongerboer de Visser, D.A. Bosch and W.M.H. van Woerkom-Eykenbook, eds.,
Neuro-oncology: Clinical and Experimental Aspects
ISBN 90-247-2421-X

K. Hellmann, P. Hilgard and S. Eccles, eds., Metastasis: Clinical and Experimental Aspects
ISBN 90-247-2424-4

H.F. Seigler, ed., Clinical Management of Melanoma
ISBN 90-247-2584-4

P. Correa and W. Haenszel, eds., Epidemiology of Cancer of the Digestive Tract
ISBN 90-247-2601-8

L.A. Liotta and I.R. Hart, eds., Tumour Invasion and Metastasis
ISBN 90-247-2611-5

J. Bánóczy, ed., Oral Leukoplakia
ISBN 90-247-2655-7

C. Tijssen, M. Halprin and L. Endtz, eds., Familial Brain Tumours
ISBN 90-247-2691-3

F.M. Muggia, C.W. Young and S.K. Carter, eds., Anthracycline Antibiotics in Cancer
ISBN 90-247-2711-1

B.W. Hancock, ed., Assessment of Tumour Response
ISBN 90-247-2712-X

D.E. Peterson, ed., Oral Complications of Cancer Chemotherapy
ISBN 0-89838-563-6

R. Mastrangelo, D.G. Poplack and R. Riccardi, eds., Central Nervous System Leukemia.
Prevention and Treatment
ISBN 0-89838-570-9

SURGERY IN GYNECOLOGICAL ONCOLOGY

edited by

A. PETER M. HEINTZ, MD
University of Leiden Medical Centre, Leiden

C. THOMAS GRIFFITHS, MD
Brigham and Womens Hospital
Harvard Medical School, Boston

J. BAPTIST TRIMBOS, MD
University of Leiden Medical Centre, Leiden

1984 **MARTINUS NIJHOFF PUBLISHERS**
a member of the KLUWER ACADEMIC PUBLISHERS GROUP
BOSTON / THE HAGUE / DORDRECHT / LANCASTER

This publication is based upon a Boerhaave course organized by
the Faculty of Medicine, University of Leiden

Distributors

for the United States and Canada: Kluwer Boston, Inc., 190 Old Derby Street,
Hingham, MA 02043, USA
for all other countries: Kluwer Academic Publishers Group, Distribution Center,
P.O.Box 322, 3300 AH Dordrecht, The Netherlands

Library of Congress Cataloging in Publication Data

Main entry under title:

Surgery in gynecological oncology.

   (Developments in oncology)
   Includes index.
   1. Generative organs, Female--Cancer--Surgery.
2. Gynecology, Operative. I. Heintz, A. Peter M.
II. Griffiths, C. Thomas. III. Trimbos, J. Baptist.
IV. Series. [DNLM: 1. Genital neoplasms, Female--
Surgery. W1 DE998N v. 16 / WP 145 S961]
RG104.6.S9 1983   616.99'465059   83-17424
ISBN-13:978-94-009-6752-6   e-ISBN-13:978-94-009-6750-2
DOI: 10.1007/978-94-009-6750-2

ISBN-13:978-94-009-6752-6

Copyright

© 1984 by Martinus Nijhoff Publishers, The Hague.
Softcover reprint of the hardcover 1st edition 1984

All rights reserved. No part of this publication may be reproduced, stored in a
retrieval system, or transmitted in any form or by any means, mechanical,
photocopying, recording, or otherwise, without the prior written permission of
the publishers,
Martinus Nijhoff Publishers, P.O. Box 566, 2501 CN The Hague,
The Netherlands.

INTRODUCTION

Gynecological oncology surgery has shown substantial progress in recent years. Most of the advances come from gynecologists with full time commitments to gynecological oncology.
It is important for the general obstetrician-gynecologist to be informed about the possibilities offered by modern gyneco-logical oncology. Thus he or she may acquire new techniques which can be used in general gynecological practice. On the other hand it is essential to know what his or her colleagues, specialised in gynecological oncology can offer in oncology centres.
The chapters in this book are based on a post-graduate course organised by the Boerhaave Committee for post-graduate medical education of the medical faculty of the University of Leiden, in the Netherlands. In view of the considerable interest shown by many highly qualified specialists we are extremely grateful to our contributors who were prepared to lucidly present their knowledge and expertise within the covers of the present book.
One of the conclusion of this book must be that the special surgical skills needed for adequate treatment of gynecological cancer cannot be developed within general residency programs.
Thus European gynecologists should examine whether and to what extent additional training as usual in the U.S.A. is necessary.
The editors want to thank the Royal College of Obstericians and Gynecologists for their kind permission to reproduce the contribution of J.A. Jordan (chapter 7) from "pre-clinical neoplasia of the cervix" (London, 1982).

A.P.M. Heintz, M.D.
C.Th.Griffiths, M.D.
J.B. Trimbos , M.D.

CONTRIBUTORS

M. Asmussen M.D. , Gynecologist, Århus Amtssygehus, Tage Hansen-
gade 23[4], 8000 Århus C, Danmark

O.P. Bleeker M.D. , Gynecologist, University of Amsterdam, Womens
Department, 1e Helmerstraat 104, 1054 EG Amsterdam, The Netherlands

G. Bos, Psychologist, Psychotherapist, Department of Obstetrics
and Gynecology, State University of Leiden, Rijnsburgerweg 10,
2333 AA Leiden, The Netherlands

I.D. Duncan M.D. , Gynecologist, Senior Lecturer, Department of
Obstetrics and Gynecology, University of Dundee, Medical School,
Ninewells Hospital, Dundee, Scotland

H. Fox M.D. , F.R.C. Path., Professor of Reproductive Pathology,
Department of Pathology, University of Manchester, Oxford Road,
M13 9PT Manchester, England

C.T. Griffiths M.D., Ass. Professor of Gynecology, Harvard Medi-
cal School, Ass. Chief on Gynecologic Oncology, Brigham and
Womens Hospital and Sydney Farber Cancer Institute, 75 Francis
Street, Boston, Massachusetts 02115, U.S.A.

A.P.M. Heintz M.D., Gynecologist, Section of Gynecologic Oncology,
Department of Obstetrics and Gynecology, State University of
Leiden, Rijnsburgerweg 10, 2333 AA Leiden, The Netherlands

J.A. Jordan M.D. , F.R. C.O.G., Gynecologist, The Birmingham Ma-
ternity Hospital, Queen Elisabeth Medical Centre, Edgbaston
Birmingham, B15 2TG England

B.W. Ketting M.D., Gynecologist, University of Amsterdam, Womens
Department, 1e Helmerstraat 104, 1054 EG Amsterdam, The Netherlands

E. van Kleef, Social Worker, University of Amsterdam, Womens
Department, 1e Helmerstraat 104, 1054 EG Amsterdam, The Netherlands

R.C. Knapp M.D. , Professor of Gynecology, Director of Gynecological Oncology, Harvard Medical School, Brigham and Woman's Hospital, 75 Francis Street, Boston, Massachusetts 02115, U.S.A.

K.E. Kjørstad M.D., The Norwegian Radium Hospital, Department of Gynecological Oncology, Montebello - Oslo 3, Norway

Tj. Kuipers M.D., Executive gynecologic therapist, the Rotterdam Radiation Therapy Institute, Dr. Daniël den Hoed Clinic, Groene Hilledijk 301, 3075 EA Rotterdam, The Netherlands

L.D. Lagasse M.D., Director Gynecologic Oncology, U.C.L.A. Center for Health Sciences, Los Angeles, California 90024, U.S.A.

F.B. Lammes M.D. , Director of Obstetrics and Gynecology, Zuiderziekenhuis, Groene Hilledijk 315, 3075 EA Rotterdam, Director of Gynecologic Oncology, Dr. Daniël den Hoed Clinic, Groene Hilledijk 301, 3075 EA Rotterdam, The Netherlands

M. van Lent M.D. , Gynecologist, Department of Obstetrics and Gynecology, Zuiderziekenhuis, Rotterdam, Dr. Daniël den Hoed Clinic, Groene Hilledijk 301, 3075 EA Rotterdam, The Netherlands

A.C.M. van Lindert M.D. , Gynecologist, Department of Gynecologic Oncology, State University of Utrecht, Catharijnesingel 101, 3583 CP Utrecht, The Netherlands

K.J. Lohe , Professor of Gynecology, University of Munich Womens Department and School of Midwifery, Maistrasse 11, 8000 Munich 2, West Germany

G.W. Morley M.D. , Director of Gynecology Oncology, University of Michigan Medical School, Ann Arbor, Michigan 48104, U.S.A.

J. Mylotte M.D. , Gynecologist, Department of Obstetrics and Gynecology, Regional Hospital, Galway, Irish Republic

N.B. Rosenshein M.D. , Director of Gynecologic Oncology, The John Hopkins Hospital, 600 North Wolfe Street, Baltimore, Maryland 21205, U.S.A.

K. Sekiba M.D., Professor of Gynecology, Okayama University Medical School, Okayama, Japan

J.B. Trimbos M.D., Gynecologist, Department of Obstetrics and Gynecology, State University of Leiden, Rijnsburgerweg 10, 2333 AA Leiden, The Netherlands

J.A. Wijnen M.D., Gynecologist, Department of Gynecological Oncology, University of Rotterdam, Dr. Molewaterplein 40, 3015 GD Rotterdam, The Netherlands

TABLE OF CONTENTS

X

1. CONSERVATIVE MANAGEMENT OF VAGINAL AND VULVAL INTRAEPITHE- LIAL NEOPLASIA

J.A. Jordan

Vaginal intraepithelial neoplasia (VAIN)

Unfortunately, this condition is more common than many gynae- cologists believe, and is regularly seen by those clinicians who run a colposcopy clinic. Neoplastic lesions of the vagina account for 1 to 4% of a-1 gynaecologic malignancies and re- cently there appears to have been an increasing incidence of intraepithelial lesions in the vagina, particularly after hysterectomy (17). Often, VAIN co-exists with CIN and it has been estimated that CIN extends to involve the vagina in 3 to 4% of patients.

Detection of VAIN

Because VAIN is asymptomatic its presence can only be suspec- ted by cytology or colposcopy. Since, in most countries, col- poscopy is not used as a routine screening procedure, it fol- lows that cytology is the means by which a lesion is usually detected. To some extent there are two problems in management. Namely the patient who still has a uterus and the patient who has had a hysterectomy. When the uterus is present VAIN is usually found by the colposcopist as an incidental finding to CIN. The vaginal lesion has the same characteristics as CIN, namely aceto-white, with punctation or mosaic, and is Schiller positive, and when present in conjunction with CIN it is easy to detect. However, when it is present following hysterectomy it may not be easy to localise because it is usually found in the vaginal angles at 3 o'clock and 9 o'clock, and since there are often "pockets of tissue" in the angles it may be diffi- cult to assess the full extent of the lesion: the colposcopist

will find iris hooks very helpful in assessing the extent of
the lesion. Also, if the lesion is multi-focal then there may
be difficulty unless the colposcopist assesses with great care
the whole length of the vagina. Finally, if the colposcopist
is dealing with what appears to be multi-focal VAIN then he
must be aware of the possibility that he is dealing with a
warty atypia and not VAIN.

Treatment

For many years VAIN has been treated by partial or total vaginectomy or irradiation (4-9). The advent of colposcopy and
new modalities of treatment have allowed a change in management, the treatment depending on the colposcopic findings. Current methods and use are summarised in Table 1.

Table 1.   Vaginal intraepithelial neoplasia: therapeutic modalitie

1.	Out-patient biopsy excision
2.	Intravaginal 5FU
3.	Cyrosurgery
4.	CO_2 laser
5.	Electrocautery
6.	Intravaginal or oral oestrogen
7.	Local excision
8.	Partial vaginectomy
9.	Total vaginectomy with graft
10.	Combined CO_2 laser and surgical excision
11.	Radiation
12.	Observation without treatment

---

1. Out-patient biopsy excision

By this is meant removal of one or two small areas of
VAIN by biopsy forceps in the out-patient clinic without anaesthesia.

2. *Intravaginal 5FU*

Woodruff (19) treated 9 patients with VAIN with 5-fluo-
rouracil (5FU) and reported a complete response in 8. It
can only be used if the lesion is not hyperkeratotic and
if the colposcopist is certain that the lesion is pre-
invasive. It is used as follows.

The patient inserts 5 gm of five per cent of 5FU into the
vagina and is reviewed four days later by colposcopy. If
the lesion has altered it is deemed sensitive and she
is instructed to insert a further 5 gm each night for
five nights. The patient is then assessed six and twelve
weeks later to determine the degree of side effects and
the stage of healing. The mechanism of action involves
a necrosing effect on the vaginal epithelium after which
re-epithelialisation takes several weeks. If the examination at twelve weeks suggests that there is still persistent disease an additional course using 5 gm of five
per cent 5FU at night for five nights is prescribed. If
the repeat course is also ineffective in eradicating the
disease another method of therapy such as excision is
suggested. In some patients no sloughing of the vaginal
lesion will be seen after the test dose and the lesion
is then deemed resistant - these patients are instructed
to use 5 gm intravaginally morning and night for five
days following which the same follow-up regimen as for
sensitive lesions is followed. In post-menopausal patients
the tissues are unusually sensitive and therapy is continued for only four days.

Contamination of the vulva produces an acute chemical in-
flammation and care must be taken to avoid this.

3. *Destruction by cryosurgery, CO_2 laser and electrocautery*

These methods have a place in the management of small
lesions and should only be carried out under colposcopic
control. If using cryocautery it is imperative to be a-
ware of the proximity of the urethra, bladder and rectum
and if the epithelium is atrophic in the post-menopausal

woman there is the possibility that a fistula may develop. If the epithelium is deemed atrophic then it is as well to give a six-week course of oestrogen before treatment is carried out. The CO_2 laser can destroy tissue with greater precision than cryocautery and Stafl et al (16) reported complete resolution in five of six patients with VAIN lesions treated by CO_2 laser. Electrocautery has very little part to play in the treatment of these lesions, partly because its depth of destruction is more difficult to ascertain but more important is the fibrosis which follows the healing process, particularly if the lesion destroyed has been extensive.

4. Intravaginal or oral oestrogen

In the post-menopausal patient with vaginal atrophy the colposcopist occasionally sees lesions which are suspicious of VAIN but which are simply due to atrophy. A six-week course of oestrogen, preferably by mouth, will allow a more accurate assessment and the gynaecologist is often pleasantly surprised to find that such lesions occasionally resolve and are found to be insignificant.

5. Surgical excision (local excision, partial vaginectomy and total vaginectomy

The amount of tissue to be removed will depend on the site and extent of the lesion and the presence or absence of the uterus. If the uterus is present and the lesion involves a small part of the vaginal vault then most surgeons find that a hysterectomy with an adequate cuff of the vagina is good treatment. If the uterus has been removed then excision of the VAIN will depend on the size of the lesion. Small lesions can be removed by local excision, lesions involving most of the vaginal vault will require partial vaginectomy and lesions involving most or all of the vagina will require total vaginectomy with or without a graft.

A special word must be made about the treatment of post-hysterectomy VAIN which involves the vaginal angles. This area of tissue is notoriously difficult to excise and it was thought that the CO_2 laser would be the answer to the problem. However, experience in our own clinic has shown that approximately half of our patients treated by laser have persistent disease requiring further treatment and it is my opinion that the majority of these lesions are best dealt with by surgical excision rather than destruction.

6. *Combined CO_2 laser and surgical excision*

If the patient presents with abnormal cytology and colposcopy shows that she has CIN with associated VAIN then an alternative to hysterectomy with cuff of vagina is to combine CO_2 laser vapourisation with surgical excision. If the lesion involves the ectocervix and vagina then it can be treated completely by laser vapourisation. If the lesion involves part of the endocervical canal then the vaginal and ectocervical lesion can be vapourised with CO_2 laser and the endocervical canal removed by cone biopsy or hysterectomy.

7. *Radiation Therapy*

Radiation will certainly eradicate the disease but the complications of treatment, particularly in the post-menopausal woman, may be severe, Radiation does however have a place, 6000 rads being delivered to the tumour site. One of the difficulties the radiotherapist will experience is in getting a good application of radium to the vaginal angels and he may have to make a special mould to suit the particular vagina he is dealing with.

Vulval intraepithelial neoplasia (VIN)

The international Society for the Study of Vulvar Disease is a multi-disciplinary group of gynaecologists, pathologists and dermatologists. The Society has tried to clarify the confusing nomenclature relating to pre-malignant disease of the vulva and in 1976 published the following definition: Squamous cell carcinoma in situ of the vulva is defined as: "characterized by disorientation and a loss of epithelial architecture which extends throughout the full thickness of the epithelium (not including the most superficial layers in tissue from keratinized surfaces). Giant cells, multinucleated cells, abnormalities of nuclear/cytoplasmic ration, dyskeratosis, individual cell keratinization, corps rond formation, abnormal mitoses, mitotic figures above the basal layer, and an increased density of cell population may all be seen in varying degrees. Less commonly, full thickness change is not present, but intraepithelial squamous "pearls" are present at the rete pegs, associated with loss or normal basal cell layer". (11)

A. *Diagnosis*

It is not possible to detect VIN by cytology in the same way that CIN and VAIN can be detected. The disease is uncommon and the third National Cancer Survey in the United States estimated that the incidence rate for in situ squamous cell carcinoma of the vulva was 0.53 cases per 100,000 women (10). It tends to occur in a slightly older age group than CIN and Friedrich et al (8) estimated that the average age was 38 years and that other reports confirm that it is a disease which now occurs primarily in the third and fourth decades of life. There is a definite association between VIN and other malignancies, particularly CIN (Table 2).

Table 2. Percent of cases of carcinoma in situ of the vulva
          (VIN) associated with other antecedent or concomi-
          tant malignancy (from Friedrich, 1981)

Author	Other malignancy all sites %	Carcinoma in situ of cervix %
Rutledge and Sinclair (1968)	30	11
Collins et al (1955)	25	12
Boutselis (1972)	29	17
Franklin and Rutledge (1972)	46	23
Woodruff et al (1973)	18	11
Kunschner et al (1978)	21	5
Friedrich et al (1980)	30	20
Average	28	14

There is also a correlation between sexually transmitted disease (Table 3).

Table 3. Percent of cases of carcinoma in situ of the vulva
          (VIN) with sexually transmitted disease by history
          or examination (from Friedrich, 1981)

Author	Sexually transmitted disease - all types %	Condylomata accuminata %
Collins et al (1955)	22	-
Franklin & Rutledge (1972)	--	7
Woodruff et al (1973)	20	9
Josey et al (1976)	--	22.5
Forney et al (1977)	38	31
Friedrich et al (1980)	60	26

There is increasing interest in the role of human papilloma
virus in the development of cervical and vaginal and vulval
lesions and there are now many case reports of patients with
vulval warts progressing to vulval carcinoma.

Clinical features of VIN

The lesions may be white, grey, pink, dull red or any shade
of brown. They may be small and sharply localised or may cover the entire vulva and spread to adjacent structures. Some
resemble condylomata accuminata. Despite this variation there
are certain distinctive features with most cases of VIN being
papular or raised above the level of the surrounding skin and
having a rough surface. Usually the lesions are multicentric,
making treatment more difficult.

Treatment

The methods of treatment are summarized in Table 4.

Table 4. Treatment of carcinoma in situ of the vulva (VIN)

Surgical excision
- Vulvectomy
- Vulvectomy preserving clitoris
- Skinning vulvectomy retaining clitoris
- Local excision

5FU

DNCB

Cryocautery

CO_2 laser

Surgical excision

For many years the standard treatment for VIN was wide local excision by vulvectomy. This removes the clitoris, usually rendering the patient anorgasmic. Occasionally there
is scarring around the meatus which may divert the stream,
but perhaps the greatest cost is incurred in emotional terms.
A number of patients treated with total vulvectomy come to
view the surgery as akin to mastectomy and once their relief as "escape from cancer" subsides they regret the loss
of the vulva and regard themselves as "disfigured". For
these reasons some surgeons perform a less wide excision

and preserve the clitoris. Others (15) devised a more shallow "skinning" procedure with partial amputation of the clitoris in selected patients. They follow their vulvectomy by a split thickness skin graft to the vulva from a donor site on the thigh. Recently, using colposcopy, there has been a move towards local excision of VIN lesions and recently Friedrich et al (8) reported the success of this treatment with only three recurrences in 17 patients.

5FU

The cream is massaged gently into the lesions twice daily for six weeks. At first there is little reaction but after two weeks there is erythema and irritation and after four weeks ulceration and sloughing. At this point the pain may be intense and most patients voluntarily discontinue the medication unless they are hospitalised and sedated for the rest of two weeks of treatment. The healing phase is usually associated with a great deal of discomfort and the total length of morbidity exceeds that of surgery. Nevertheless, the healed vulva is remarkably free of scarring and function is not usually impaired. The overall results however, are disappointing with an average of 50 per cent of patients showing a complete response.

DNCB

Weintraub and Lagasse (18) reported two cases which they treated successfully by sensitising the patient to 2, 4 dinitrochlorobenzene (DNCB). Sensitisation was accomplished by applying 2 mg of DNCB dissolved in 0.1 ml acetone under the skin of the arm. After two weeks a 0.1 per cent DNCB cream was applied to the vulval lesions and continued until the occurrence of ulceration was noted. Healing was similar to that seen using topical 5FU.

Cryosurgery

Cryosurgery offers some success when the lesions are small and the freezing applied under colposcopic control.

The CO_2 laser

If the local destruction is still employed then carbon dioxide laser is the treatment of choice. It is performed under colposcopic direction and tissue destroyed to a depth of about 4 mm. Quite large areas can be treated and indeed all of the vulval skin can be destroyed to a depth of 4 mm by a technique known as "skinning vulvectomy", a technique which is currently being used for vulval dystrophies. The long term results of this treatment are as yet unknown.

CONCLUSION

VIN and VAIN are being recognised with increasing frequency and as yet there is no ideal way of managing either lesion. All that can be said is that careful colposcopic assessment by an expert will help the gynaecologist to produce a treatment plan which is optimum for that particular patient and her lesion.

REFERENCES

1. Boutselis, J.G. 1972. Intraepithelial carcinoma of the vulva. Am. J. Obstet. Gynecol. 113, 733.
2. Collins, C.G., Kushner, J., Lewis, C.M. & LaPointe, R. 1955. Non-invasive malignancy of the vulva. Obstet. Gynecol. 6, 339.
3. Collins, C.G., Roman-Lopez, J.J. & Lee, F.Y.L. 1970. Intraepithelial carcinoma of the vulva. Am. J. Obstet. Gynecol. 108, 1187.
4. Ferguson, J.H. & Maclure, J.G. 1963. Intraepithelial carcinoma, dysplasia and exfoliation of cancer cells in the vaginal mucosa. Am. J. Obstet. Gunecol. 87, 326.
5. Forney, J.P., Morrow, C.P., Townsend, D.E. & Di Saia, P.J. 1977. Management of carcinoma in situ of the vulva. Am. J. Obstet. Gynecol. 127, 801.
6. Franklin, E.W. & Rutledge, F.D. 1972. Epidemiology of epidermoid carcinoma of the vulva. Obstet. Gynecol. 39, 165.
7. Friedrich, E.G. 1981. Intraepithelial neoplasia of vulva. Gynecol. Oncol. Ed. M. Coppleson, Churchill Livingstone, London, 303-319.
8. Friedrich, E.G., Wilkinson, E.J. & Fu, Y.S. 1980. Carcinoma in situ of the vulva: a continuing challenge. Am. J. Obstet. Gynecol. 136, 880.

9. Gallup, D.G. & Morley, G.W. 1975. Carcinoma in situ of the vagina. Obstet. Gynecol. 46, 334.

10. Hensen, D. & Tarone, R. 1977. An epidemiologic study of cancer of the cervix, vagina, and vulva based on third national cancer survey in the United States. Am. J. Obstet. Gynecol. 129, 525.

11. International Society for the Study of Vulvar Disease. 1976. New nomencalture for vulvar disease. Obstet. Gynecol. 47, 122.

12. Jordan, J.A. 1981. CO_2 laser therapy. Gynecologic Oncology. Ed. M. Coppleson, Churchill Livingstone, London, 816-820.

13. Josey, W.E., Nahmias, A.J. & Naib, Z.M. 1976. Viruses and cancer of the lower genital tract. Cancer 38, 526.

14. Kunschner, A., Kanbour, A.I. & David, B. 1978. Early vulvar carcinoma. Am. J. Obstet. Gynecol. 132, 599.

15. Rutledge, F. & Sinclair, M. 1968. Treatment of intraepithelial carcinoma of the vulva by skin excision and graft. Am. J. Obstet. Gynecol. 102, 806.

16. Stafl, Al, Wilkinson, E.J. & Mattingly, R. 1977. Laser treatment of cervical and vaginal neoplasia. Am. J. Obstet. Gynecol. 128, 128.

17. Townsend, D.E. 1981. Intraepithelial neoplasia of vagina. Gunecol. Oncol. Ed. M. Coppleson, Churchill Livingstone, London, 339-344.

18. Weintraub, I. & Lagasse, L.D. 1973. Reversability of vulvar atypia by DNCB-induced delayed hypersensitivity. Obstet. Gynecol. 41, 195.

19. Woodruff, J.D., Parmley, T.H. & Julian, C.G. 1975. Topical 5-fluorouracil in the treatment of vaginal carcinoma in situ. Gunecol. Oncol. 3, 124.

2. SURGICAL TREATMENT OF CANCER OF THE VULVA: SUPERFICIALLY INVASIVE VULVAR CANCER WITH NODAL METASTASES

L.D. Lagasse

Introduction

The role of radical vulvectomy and bilateral inguinal-femoral lymphadenectomy in the treatment of vulvar cancer has been well established though the operation is associated with considerable physical (1) and psychological (2) morbidity. Early vulvar cancer is increasing in frequency, and being seen more commonly in younger women (3), and some authorities have suggested modifying this radical surgical approach for such patients.

The concept of superficially invasive vulvar cancer was first introduced by Franklin and Rutledge in 1971 (4). They defined it as a lesion 2 cm or less in diameter with 5 mm or less of stromal invasion, a definition which most authors have subsequently used (5-8). Some have felt that stricter criteria should be applied, and have suggested excluding lesions with vascular space involvement (9, 10), diameters greater than 1 cm (11), or more than 3 mm of stromal invasion (10).

Optimal management for these superficially invasive vulvar cancers is controversial. Though some have felt that standard radical vulvectomy and bilateral inguinal lymphadenectomy remains the treatment of choice (10, 12), most agree that some modification of treatment may be appropriate.

Based on their experience with 25 patients, none of whom had lymph node metastases or subsequently developed recurrences, Wharton and colleagues (5) suggested that radical vulvectomy alone may be appropriate therapy. Parker (6) agreed with this approach provided the excisional biopsy of the tumor showed no evidence of anaplasia or vascular space involvement, while

Dean (8) reported that wide local excision or simple vulvectomy alone may be adequate.

Because of concern for the metastatic potential of these lesions, others have been reluctant to omit inguinal lymphadenectomy. DiSaia and colleagues (11) advocated wide local excision of the primary lesion, combined with bilateral superficial lymphadenectomy for lesions 1 cm or less in diameter.
They suggested that the superficial inguinal nodes (i.e.,
those above the cribriform fascia) could be regarded as sen-
tinal nodes, and more radical surgery performed only if these
were positive. Iverson (13) proposed hemivulvectomy and ipsilateral inguinal-femoral node dissection for stage I vulvar
cancer invasive to more than 1 mm. Magrina (7) suggested
omitting lymphadenectomy only if stromal invasion was less
than 2 mm.

In order to help identify patients at risk for lymph node
metastases, we have collected a group of 7 patients with
stage I squamous cell carcinoma of the vulva, stromal invasive of 5 mm or less, and metastases to regional lymph nodes
discovered either at the time of primary surgery, or during
subsequent follow-up.

Materials and Methods

A survey of members of the Western Association of Gynecologic
Oncologists yielded - patients with superficially invasive
vulvar cancer (less than 5 mm stromal invasion) and synchro-
nous or metachronous lymph node metastases. Four cases were
seen at UCLA, and one case each at the University of Washing-
ton (14), the Southern California Cancer Center (15), and the
University of California, San Diego.

The medical records of these patients were reviewed with particular reference to site and size of the primary lesion, and
method of treatment. Hematoxalin and eosin stained sections
from all excisional biopsies and operative specimens were
reviewed by one of us with particular reference to depth of
invasion, cellular differentiation, tumor pattern, multifoca-
lity, vascular space involvement, microscopic confluence, host

response, and associated vulvar pathology. From 9 to 26 sections were available for review from each case.

Only squamous cell carcinomas were included, and depth of invasion was calculated using a slide micrometer (A.O. CAT 1400), measuring the distance from the surface epithelium to the greatest depth of tumor, and subtracting the measured thickness of the intact epithelium adjacent to the micro-invasive focus. Confluence was defined as a compact mass of tumor occupying a 1 mm or greater field. Vascular space permeation was accepted only if tumor cells were present in a space containing a definable endothelial lining.

The World Health Organization (WHO) classification divides squamous cell carcinomas into 3 types: large cell keratinizing, large cell non-keratinizing and small cell (16). We combined the WHO classification with the Broder's grading system (17), which is based on the degree of cellular differentiation.

The patients ranged in age from 43 to 73 years, with a mean of 53 years. Parity ranged from 1 to 7 with a mean of 3.5. Three patients presented with vulvar itching, 2 with a vulvar lump, and 2 with a vulvar ulcer. Duration of symptoms ranged from 2 months to 5 years, but in 6 of the 7 patients, duration of symptoms was 12 months or less.

Pathology

The 7 tumors ranged from a predominantly poorly differentiated small cell type to a well differentiated large cell type. All lesions showed some variation in their degree of differentiation, although large cell keratinizing and non-keratinizing histologies predominated.

Five tumors invaded with a solid broad pushing front, and showed confluence of malignant nests. Two of the tumors were of the "spray" type as described by Crissman and Azoury (18). This pattern consisted of a few nests of well differentiated squamous cell carcinoma which evolved into ribbons, cords, and dissociated cells, as they invaded the underlying stroma. These two tumors alone elicited a prominent desmoplastic response from the host, and both had vascular space invasion.

Case 1 had 2 distinct patterns of neoplasia separated by a broad zone of carcinoma in situ. One focus revealed an endophytic papillary carcinoma of the large cell non-keratinizing type. Depth of invasion was 1.2 mm in the former focus, and 0.2 mm in the latter.

Case 6 revealed an unusual pseudoglandular pattern. Although keratin production was focally present, the majority of the tumor showed cell nests with central cell drop-out forming a glandular picture. The tumor expanded with a broad pushing front to a depth of 2.8 mm and elicited minimal lymphocytic response from the host.

Two of the cases ('s 4 and 7)exhibited normal surface squamous maturation in some foci, with the tumor arising from the basal keratinocytes and extending into the subjacent corium, as described by Schiller (19) for cervix cancer. Four of the 7 cases had multifocal areas of superficial invasion within the one gross lesion, and 5 cases showed areas of superficial invasion adjacent to unremarkable squamous epithelium. Whether carcinoma in situ was present prior to the stage of invasion in these cases could not be ascertained. Vascular space invasion was positively identified in 3 cases, although in others tumor was noted in close proximity to arteries and nerves.

Treatment

Four patients had standard treatment for vulvar cancer, 2 patients had radical vulvectomy alone, and 1 patient had wide local excision and bilateral superficial inguinal lymphadenectomy.

Lymph Node Status

Of the 4 patients having standard treatment, 2 patients had 1 positive inguinal node, 1 patient had 2 positive inguinal and 2 positive obturator nodes, and 1 patient, who had a periclitoral lesion, had 1 positive femoral node but negative inguinal nodes.

The 2 patients having radical vulvectomy alone developed lymph node metastases postoperatively at 3 and 17 months respectively. The patient who had bilateral inguinal lymphadenectomy without femoral lymphadenectomy (case 5) had negative inguinal nodes histologically, but developed a recurrence in a groin node 4 months postoperatively.

Outcome

Of the 4 patients who received standard treatment, 3 are alive and free of disease 18 months to 11 years postoperatively. The only death was the patient who had 4 positive nodes. The 3 patients in whom inguinal-femoral lymphadenectomy was either omitted or modified all died of disease 10 months to 22 months postoperatively. All recurred initially in the groin nodes, though 2 of the 3 had distant metastases at the time of death. The third has groin recurrence only, with erosion of the femoral artery.

Discussion

From a review of the literature, 9% of patients with superficially invasive vulvar cancer have lymph node metastases. Hence, identification of patients at risk for nodal disease is critical if omission of lymphadenectomy is contemplated. From this clinico-pathological review of 7 patients with superficially invasive disease and lymph node metastases, it would seem that prediction of nodal spread cannot be made reliably on the histopathologic findings in any individual case. Five of these tumors were of the moderate to well differentiated large cell type, with depth of invasion ranging from 1.2 mm to 3.5 mm. No patient with lymph node metastases had tumor invasion of 1 mm or less, an observation also reported by others (7).

The point of reference for measurement of depth of invasion has not been standardized. For this report, we measured from the basement membrane, which is the point of reference most authors have used (5, 6, 9, 11) though some have measured from the epithelial surface (7, 14). Recently Buscema et al

(21) reported 58 cases with depth of invasion measured from the base of the deepest rete peg.

Vascular space involvement was present in only 3 of the 7 cases, though it occurred in both cases of "spray" carcinomas, and these may represent a high risk group. The pseudoglandular or adenoid squamous cell carcinoma of the vulva may also represent a high risk (though uncommon) tumor. The histogenesis of this tumor has not yet been resolved. Underwood and colleagues (22) felt it arose from the cells of skin appendages, including mucin producing cells. Our case, like those studied by Lasser et al (23), did not show evidence of mucin production and is more consistent with an acantholytic variant of squamous cell carcinoma. This tumor has been shown to have a poorer survival and a higher rate of lymph node metastases than squamous cell vulvar carcinomas of corresponding stage (22).

The presence of associated carcinoma in situ of the vulva has been said to be associated with a good prognosis, and to be an indication for conservative surgery (9), but 5 of the 7 cases had associated carcinoma in situ in this series. Four of the cases were also associated with a hypertrophic vulvar dystrophy and 1 with lichen sclerosis. Hence, in any individual case, we do not feel that the presence of associated vulvar pathology is of prognostic significance.

In this series, all 3 patients in whom inguinal-femoral lymphadenectomy was omitted or modified because of N_o groin nodes died of disease. In our UCLA experience of 100 patients with stages I, II, or III vulvar cancer treated with radical vulvectomy and bilateral groin dissection, none of the 91 patients with less than 3 positive groin nodes died of disease (24). Hence, more stringent guidelines seem necessary for treatment modifications.

The standard treatment for vulvar cancer may be modified by limiting the vulvar resection and/or limiting the lymphadenectomy. Radical vulvectomy is usually recommended for the primary lesion, but this is associated with the distressing long term problems of disturbed sexual function and poor body

image (2). Thus if wide local excision does not compromise
survival, it would be a preferable mode of therapy.
DiSaia (11) reported 18 patients with negative nodes treated
with wide local excision of the primary tumor, and none had
evidence of recurrence 7 to 74 months later (mean 32 months).
Iverson (14) had one local recurrence among 6 patients treated with wide local excision. Parker (6) treated 4 patients
with wide local excision without invasive recurrence, whereas 4 of his 54 patients developed local recurrence after radical vulvectomy. We have treated 12 stage I patients with
wide local excision at UCLA, and 1 has developed a local recurrence. The patients have been followed from 14 months to
12 years with a mean follow-up of 5 years 2 months. Hence
wide local excision appears to provide good local control,
and radical vulvectomy does not protect against local recurrence. Should positive nodes be found at operation, radical
vulvectomy and bilateral inguinal-femoral lymphadenectomy
should be performed. In view of the 9% reported incidence of
lymph node metastases in patients with superficially invasive
vulvar cancer, and the inability to predict patients at risk
on the basis of the histopathology, routine omission of lymphadenectomy is inadvisable. However, since nodal metastases
have not been reported in lesions with less than 1 mm of invasion, it is reasonable to omit lymphadenectomy in such
cases. For more deeply invasive lesions, some type of inguinal
dissection seems essential, as groin recurrence carries a poor
prognosis.
One patient in this series (case 5) had negative nodes at
the time of superficial inguinal lymphadenectomy, but subsequently developed a palpable node in the groin and died with
disseminated disease (proven at autopsy) having refused further treatment. A second patient (case 3) with a periclitoral
lesion had negative inguinal nodes and a positive femoral node.
Parker (6) reported a patient with a lesion on the right la-
bium who had negative inguinal nodes and a positive Cloquet's
node.
Therefore, we recommend that standard inguinal-femoral lymph-

adenectomy be performed on the ipsilateral side for lateralized lesions, and bilaterally for midline lesions. Superficial inguinal lymphadenectomy should probably be performed
on the contralateral side for lateralized lesions, though
the risk for missing disease in an unresected contralateral
groin is only about 1% if the nodes are not suspicious to
palpation and the ipsilateral nodes are negative.

REFERENCES

1. Rutledge, F., Smith, J.P., Franklin E.W. 1970. Carcinoma
   of the vulva. Am. J. Obst. Gynec. 106:1117.
2. Sewell, H.H., Edwards, D.W. 1980. Pelvic genital cancer:
   Body image and sexuality. Frontiers of Rad. Ther. Onc.
   14:35.
3. Kunschner, A., Kanbour, A.I., David, B. 1978. Early vulvar
   carcinoma. Am. J. Obst. Gynec. 132:599.
4. Franklin, E.W., Rutledge, F.D. 1971. Prognostic factors
   in epidermoid carcinoma of the vulva. Obst. Gynec. 37:892.
5. Wharton, J.T., Gallager, S., Rutledge, F.M. 1974. Microinvasive carcinoma of the vulva. Am. J. Obst. Gynec. 118:
   159.
6. Parker, R.T., Duncan, I.,Rampone, J., Creasman, W. 1975.
   Operative Management of early invasive epidermoid carcinoma of the vulva. Am. J. Obst. Gynec. 123:349.
7. Magrina, J.F., Webb, M.J., Gaffey, T.A., Symmonds, R.E.
   1979. Stage I squamous cell cancer of the vulva. Am. J.
   Obst. Gynec. 143:453.
8. Dean, R.E., Taylor, E.S., Weisbrod, D.M., Martin, J.W.
   1974. The treatment of premalignant and malignant lesions
   of the vulva. Am. J. Obst. Gynec. 119:59.
9. Barnes, A.E., Crissman, J.D., Schellhas, H.F. Azoury, R.S.
   1980. Microinvasive carcinoma of the vulva: A clinicopathologic evaluation. Obst. Gynec. 56:234.
10. Jafari, K., Cartnick, E.M. 1976. Microinvasive squamous
    cell carcinoma of the vulva. Gynec. Onc. 4:158.
11. DiSaia, P.J., Creasman, W.T., Rich, W.M. 1979. An alter-
    native approach to early cancer of the vulva. Am. J. Ob-
    st. Gynec. 133:825.
12. Yazigi, R., Piver, S., Tsukada, Y. 1978. Microinvasive
    carcinoma of the vulva. Obst. Gynec. 51:368.
13. Iversen, T., Abeler, V., Aalders, J. 1981. Individualized
    treatment of stage I carcinoma of the vulva. Obst. Gynec.
    57:85.
14. Chu, J., Tamimi, H.K., Figge, D.C. 1981. Femoral node
    metastases with negative superficial inguinal nodes in
    early vulvar cancer. Am. J. Obst. Gynec. 140:337.
15. Nakao, C.Y., Nolan, J.F., DiSaia, P.J., Futoran, R. 1974.
    Microinvasive epidermoid carcinoma of the vulva with an
    unexpected natural history. Am. J. Obst. Gynec. 120:1122.

16. Poulsen, H., Taylor, C. 1975 Histologic typing of female genital tract tumors. No. 13, WHO.
17. Broders, A. 1925. The grading of carcinoma. Minn. Med. 8:726.
18. Crissman, J.D., Azoury, R.S. 1981. Microinvasive carcinoma of the vulva: A report of two cases with regional lymph node metastases. Dig. Gynec. Obst. 3:75.
19. Schiller, W., Darrow, A., Gollen, J., Primiano, P. 1953. Small preulcerative invasive carcinoma of the cervix: The spray carcinoma. Am. J. Obst. Gynec. 65:1088.
20. DiPaola, G.R., Gomez-Rueda, N., Arrighi, L. 1975. Relevance of microinvasion in carcinoma of the vulva. Obst. Gynec. 45:647.
21. Buscema, J., Stern, J.L., Woodruff, J.D. 1981. Early invasive carcinoma of the vulva. Am. J. Obst. Gynec. 140:563.
22. Underwood, J.W., Adcock, L.L., Okagaki, T. 1978. Adenosquamous carcinoma of skin appendages /adenoid squamous cell carcinoma, pseudo-glandular squamous cell carcinoma, adenocanthoma of sweat gland of Lever) of the vulva. Cancer, 42:1851.
23. Lasser, A., Cornog, J.L., Morris, J.M. 1974. Adenoid squamous cell carcinoma of the vulva. Cancer 33:224.
24. Hacker, N.F., Leuchter, R.S., Berek, J.S., et al. 1981. Radical vulvectomy and bilateral inguinal lymphadenectomy through separate incisions. Obst. Gynec. 58:574.

3. SURGICAL TREATMENT OF CANCER OF THE VULVA: RADICAL VULV-
ECTOMY AND BILATERAL LYMPHADENECTOMY THROUGH SEPARATE GROIN
INCISIONS

L.D. Lagasse

Introduction

Because of inadequate resection of the primary tumor and regional lymph nodes, early surgical attempts to treat vulvar
cancer proved disappointing (1, 2). Basset (3) was the first
to propose en bloc dissection of the vulva and inguinal-femoral
lymph nodes, and Taussig (4) and Way (5) subsequently demonstrated the value of a more radical surgical approach to this
disease. Although survival was improved by these techniques,
wound closure was often difficult and postoperative wound
breakdown common, frequently prolonging hospitalization (1,
6-8).

Various methods have been employed to improve wound healing
and decrease postoperative hospitalization. McGregor (9) reported the use of delayed skin grafting to shorten convales-
cence, and Daly and Pomerance (10) reported 13 patients in
whom the groin incisions were left open to granulate and heal
by secondary intention. In a study by Daly and Millon (11)
patients undergoing radical vulvectomy and bilateral inguinal
lymphadenectomy had an average postoperative hospital stay
of 34 days.

In a different approach to the same problem, Byron and colleagues (12) in 1962 described a technique for radical vulvectomy and bilateral groin dissection using three separate
incisions.

This report evaluates the technique of radical vulvectomy and
bilateral groin dissection through separate incisions in the
first 100 patients so treated.

Materials and Methods

The 100 cases were staged retrospectively according to the
criteria of the International Federation of Gynecology and
Obstetrics (FIGO). Information obtained from chart review
included site and size of the primary lesion, associated vulvar pathology, histology, status of regional lymph nodes, operative blood loss, postoperative morbidity, and pattern of
recurrence. Survival was calculated by using a standard actuarial life-table method (13) corrected for death from intercurrent disease.
There were 92 cases of squamous cell carcinoma, 6 of carcinoma
of Bartholin's gland (3 epidermoid, 1 adenosquamous, and 1
transitional cell), 2 of melanoma, and one of adenocarcinoma
underlying Paget's disease.

Operative Technique

The operation is performed with the patient in the "ski" position, and a 2-team approach reduces the operating time considerably. It is preferable to perform the vulvectomy first
so that the primary tumor has been removed should it become
medically necessary to curtail the surgery.
The operative technique has been described by Byron et al
(12). The vertical-type incision originally described has
been modified to an oblique incision parallel to and 1 cm
below the groin crease. If pelvic lymphadenectomy is to be
performed, the incision is carried vertically cephalad, and
an extra-peritoneal lymphadenectomy is performed as described
by Berman et al (14) (Fig. 1).
Following the groin dissection, 1 cm of skin margin is trimmed
from both medial and lateral flaps to decrease the risk of
necrosis. A Jackson-Pratt suction drain is placed in the femoral triangle and brought out through a separate stab wound
above the incision. This is left in place for about 10 days.
Patients are routinely given prophylactic low-dose heparin,
5000 units subcutaneously 2 hours postoperatively and 5000
units every 12 hours for at least 10 days. Prophylactic anti-

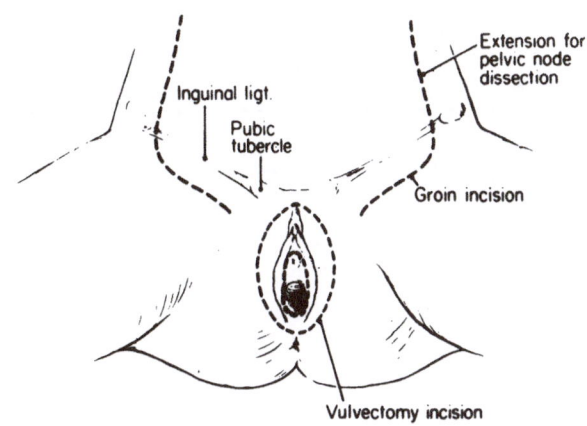

Fig. 1. Incisions used for radical vulvectomy and bilateral inguinal lymphadenectomy. Groin incisions are carried vertically cephalad if necessary to allow extraperitoneal pelvic lymphadenectomy.

biotics are given for 24 hours. In 7 patients, medical reasons necessitated performing the operation in 2 stages: the radical vulvectomy was performed initially and the groin dissections were done 6 to 8 weeks later.

Results

Blood loss ranged from 150 ml to 1900 ml, with a mean of 620 ml. Loss exceeded 1000 ml in 16 patients.

Seventy patients developed postoperative complications (Table I). Operative mortality was 1%, as one patient died on postoperative day 28 of halothane liver necrosis. Major breakdown of groin incisions occurred in only 14 patients (14%), unilaterally in 2 and bilaterally in 12. Minor breakdown of the groin incisions (less than half of the incision) occurred in 30 patients (30%), 14 unilaterally and 16 bilaterally. Primary healing of all incisions occurred in 38 patients, and of groin incisions in 56 patients. Only one patient required skin grafting. Twenty-five patients had inguinal lymph node involvement (Table II).

Table I

Acute Postoperative Complications (70 Patients)

Complication	No. of patients*
Groin complications	
Minor breakdown (N = 30)	
Unilateral	14
Bilateral	16
Major breakdown (N = 14)	
Unilateral	2
Bilateral	12
Cellulitis	9
Seroma	13
Vulvar complications	
Minor wound breakdown	28
Major wound breakdown	3
Systemic complications	
Urinary tract infection	6
Deep venous thrombosis	2
Pulmonary embolus	1
Myocardial infarction	1
Halothane liver necrosis	1

* Numbers also indicate percentage of total 100 patients in the study.

Table II

Incidence of Positive Inguinal Nodes

Stage	No. of patients	Positive nodes
I	49	5 (10.2%)
II	37	10 (27.0%)
III	14	10 (71.4%)
Total	100	25 (25.0%)

Recurrences

Nineteen patients developed recurrent disease; 3 had carcinoma in situ and 16 had invasive carcinoma. According to the
original pathology reports, margins of resection were free
of disease in all cases. The mean time to recurrence was 37
months for carcinoma in situ and 22 months for invasive carcinoma. Of the 4 patients developing recurrence in the vulva
alone, 1 died of myocardial infarction, and the other 3 were
alive after surgical resection at intervals from 2 years and
8 months to 13 years and 8 months. All other patients with
recurrent disease died, with a mean survival of 7.5 months
from the time of diagnosis of recurrence.
No patient developed an isolated groin recurrence. Two patients developed recurrence in the skin bridge between the
vulva and groin incisions in association with distant metastases.

Survival

Only one patient was lost to follow-up. She had a stage II
squamous cell carcinoma and was presumed dead of disease. The
overall survival at 5 years was 86%: 97.4% for stage I patients, 86% for stage II, and 49.2% for stage III. Fifty-one
patients were available for 10-year follow-up. The over-all
10-year survival was 82.3%: 97.4% for stage I patients, 75.5%
for stage II, and 49.2% for stage III.

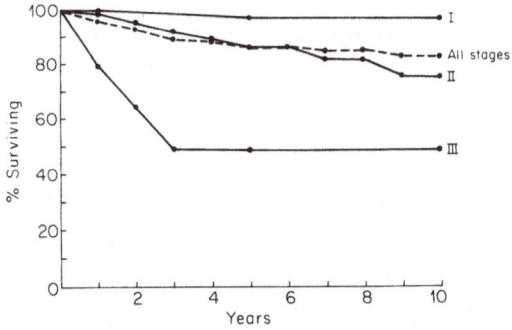

Table III. Actuarial survival for vulvar carcinoma by stage
of disease, corrected for death from intercurrent disease.

Patients with negative lymph nodes had a 5-year survival of
91.2%, whereas those with positive nodes had a 70.3% survival. Among patients with positive nodes, none with fewer than
three positive lymph nodes died of disease (Table III and IV).

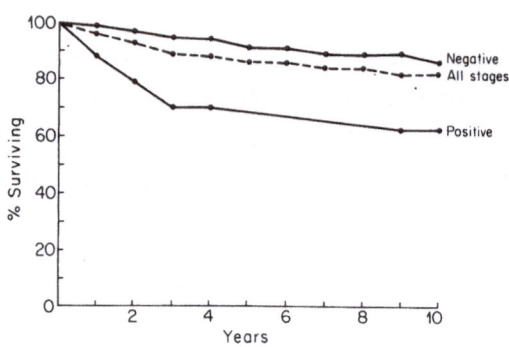

Table IV. Actuarial survival for vulvar carcinoma by status
of lymph nodes, corrected for death from intercurrent disease.

Discussion

The aim of surgery for vulvar cancer should be wide removal
of the primary lesion and excision of the regional lymph nodes.
Radical vulvectomy and bilateral inguinal lymphadenectomy
through separate incisions satisfy these requirements, but
leave a skin bridge between the primary tumor and the drain-
ing lymph nodes.
Taussig (4) reported no recurrences in the skin bridge; however, he did not state the number of operations he performed
using this technique.
With this method, primary wound closure is always possible
in the groins, and unless an unusually large vulvar tumor
requires resection, the vulvar incision can also be closed
primarily. Use of separate incisions for the groins in fact
facilitates the closure of large vulvar defects.
Primary healing of the groin incisions occurred in 56% of
the patients in this series, and many of the others had necrosis of only the central portion of the wound. Major wound

breakdown (i.e., more than half of the wound) was uncommon (14%). Only one patient required skin grafting because of extensive necrosis. The mean postoperative stay of only 19 days, the shortest yet of any major series, attests to the improved morbidity with this technique.

In attempting to achieve primary wound healing, to maintain skin vascularity it is important to leave an adequate thickness of subcutaneous fat when developing the superior and inferior skin flaps. The superficial inguinal lymph nodes are situated beneath the superficial fascia, and this layer should be identified by its fibrous, glistening appearance before developing the flaps. In obese patients, it may be 1.5 to 2 cm beneath the skin. Delicate handling of the tissues, resection of 1 cm of tissue from each skin edge before closure, and negative suction for a minimum of 10 postoperative days are also important in achieving healing. At present, the authors routinely give low-dose heparin, usually confine patients to bed for several days postoperatively, and encourage active leg exercises from the first postoperative day.

The operation is usually done with 2 teams operating simultaneously and may be done with 3 teams to shorten operating time further, an obvious advantage in elderly women. The mortality of 1% compares favorably with that of other reports in the literature (6-8).

Chronic postoperative morbidity continues to be of some concern, although the 20% incidence of leg edema compares favorably with the 32% reported by Rutledge et al (6) and the 65% reported by Calame (15). The lower incidence of chronic leg edema may be related to the improved healing of the inguinal incisions with this technique, In approximately one third of patients the edema is transient and can be controlled with elastic stockings until lymphatic channels regenerate (Table V).

Although none of the patients in this series developed isolated groin metastases, two patients developed recurrences in the skin bridge associated with metastases at other sites.

Table V

Chronic Postoperative Complications (35 Patients)

Complication	No.*
Leg edema	
Chronic	14
Temporary	6
Genital prolapse	16
Urinary stress incontinence	9
Temporary quadriceps femoris weakness	4
Introital stenosis	2
Recurrent erysipelas of legs	2
Pubic osteomyelitis	1
Rectoperineal fistula	1
Claudication of leg	1

* Numbers also indicate percentage of total 100 patients in
  the study.

Both patients had suspicious groin nodes and three or more
positive groin nodes on histologic sections. In such situations, retrograde permeation of lymphatic sections may occur,
and this surgical technique should probably not be used when
there is more than microscopic involvement of inguinal lymph
nodes. However, Frankling and Rutledge (16) reported that
even with en bloc dissections, 20% of their patients with
positive groin nodes developed recurrences in the skin surrounding the groin dissection. In all of their patients with
groin recurrences, the groin nodes were clinically suspicious
or positive postoperatively. One of the patients with occult
lymph node metastases developed a recurrence in the groin
after lymphadenectomy. Hence it seems that strong consideration should be given to the use of preoperative or postoperative irradiation in such patients, regardless of the
type of incision used.

With this surgical technique, improved wound healing and decreased postoperative hospitalization have been demonstrated.
With corrected actuarial 5-year survivals of 97.4% for stage I

and 86% for stage II patients, survival has not been compromised by deviating from the en bloc dissection. It would appear that this technique is apporpriate for patients with stage I and II carcinoma of the vulva.

REFERENCES

1. Way, S. 1948. The anatomy of the lymphatic drainage of the vulva and its influence on the radical operation for carcinoma. Ann. R. Coll. Surg. Engl. 3:187.
2. Blair Bell, W., Datnow, M.M. 1936. Primary malignant disease of the vulva, with special reference to treatment by operation. J. Obst. Gynaec. Br. Emp. 43:755.
3. Basset, A. 1912. Traitement chirurgical operatoire de l'epithelioma primitif du clitoris indications - technique - resultats. Rev. Chir. 46:546.
4. Taussig, F.J. 1940. Cancer of the vulva: An analysis of 155 cases (1911-1940). Am. J. Obst. Gynec. 40:764.
5. Way, S. 1960. Carcinoma of the vulva. Am. J. Obst. Gynec. 79:692.
6. Rutledge, F., Smith, J.P., Franklin, E.W. 1970. Carcinoma of the vulva. Am. J. Obst. Gynec. 106:1117.
7. Morley, G.W. 1976. Infiltrative carcinoma of the vulva: Results of surgical treatment. Am. J. Obst. Gynec. 124:874.
8. Green, T.H. 1978. Carcinoma of the vulva. A reassessment. Obst. Gynec. 52:462.
9. McGregor, I.A. 1966. Skin grafting after radical vulvectomy. J. Obst. Gynaec. Br. Commonw. 73:599.
10. Daly, J.W., Pomerance, A.J. 1979. Groin dissection with prevention of tissue loss and postoperative infection. Obst. Gynec. 53:395.
11. Daly, J.W., Millon, R.R. 1974. Radical vulvectomy combined with elective node irradiation for TxNo squamous carcinoma of the vulva. Cancer 34:161.
12. Byron, R.O., Lamb, E.J., Yonemoto, R.H., et al. 1962. Radical inguinal mode dissection in the treatment of cancer. Surg. Gynec. Obst. 114:401.
13. Cutler, S.J., Ederer, F. 1958. Maximum utilization of the life-table method in analysing survival J. Chronic. Dis. 8:699.
14. Berman, M.L. Lagasse, L.D. Watring, W.G., et al. 1977. The operative evaluation of patients with cervical carcinoma by an extraperitoneal approach. Obst. Gynec. 50:658.
15. Calame, R.J. 1980.Pelvic relaxation as a complication of the radical vulvectomy. Obst. Gynec. 55:716.
16. Franklin, E.W., Rutledge, F.D. 1971. Prognostic factors in epidermoid carcinoma of the vulva. Obst. Gynec. 37:892.

4. CARCINOMA OF THE VAGINA

Robert C. Knapp

Carcinoma of the vagina is defined as a malignant lesion in the vagina which does not involve the external os of the cervix superiorly, nor the vulva inferiorly. It accounts for about 2% of all gynecologic malignancies (1, 2). Herbst et al., in 1977 reported on the occurrence of clear cell adenocarcinoma of the vagina in women in their late teens and early twenties. This particular carcinoma was found to be related to the use of diethylstilbestrol (DES) by their mothers during pregnancy (3). In order to better delineate clear cell carcinoma, it will be described in a separate section in this chapter.

Carcinoma of the Vagina, other than Clear Cell

Primary vaginal carcinomas are generally squamous in origin. Most series reviewing genital carcinoma report a decrease in the incidence in recent years. This decrease may be due in part to close adherence to rigid staging criteria thereby eliminating cancers arising from the cervix or vulva or metastasis from endometrial carcinoma as well as early detection of pre-invasive lesions by cytology and colposcopy.

Epidemiology

There is no clear epidemiological predisposing factor to invasive squamous cell carcinoma of the vagina. Herbst et al., reviewing the literature for possible etiological factors of primary squamous cell carcinoma noted that the disease occurred primarily in the elderly population, but that no apparent etiology or associated factors were uncovered that predisposed

a patient to this malignancy (2). There are some reports that
implicate invasive squamous cell carcinoma of the vagina with
a prior history of radiation therapy to the pelvis. Pride et
al., noted that 9 of 43 patients (20.9%) with invasive squamous
cell carcinoma of the vagina had a prior history of radiation
from 7 to 20 years prior to the development of their vaginal
cancer (4). However, Perez analyzed 1000 patients treated over
a 20 year period and found no increased incidence of pelvic
second neoplasia following radiation therapy (5).

Anatomical considerations

Vaginal cancers occur most commonly on the posterior wall of
the upper third of the vagina. Plentl and Friedman, in an extensive review of the literature, noted that 51.7% of primary
vaginal cancers occurred in the upper third of the vagina and
57.6% on the posterior wall (6). The next most common site
appears to be the anterior aspect of the lower third of the
vagina. It would appear that malignancies arising in the posterior aspect of the upper third of the vagina do not meta-
stasize as readily as those in other locations of the vagina
and are more successfully treated. Cancers of the lower third
of the vagina spread by way of the femoral nodes. Due to the
extensive lymphatic anastomosis around the vagina, malignancy
from the middle third may also spread to femoral nodes as
well as to pelvic nodes. The anterior vaginal tumors tend to
spread more frequently to the femoral regional nodes as compared to posterior lesions.

Pathology

Over 90% of vaginal tumors are squamous in origin. Adenocarcinoma accounts for approximately 5%. Tavassoli and Norris
reviewed the clinical and pathologic features of 60 smooth
muscle tumors of the vagina (7). The smooth muscle tumor is
the most common mesenchymal tumor of the vagina in the adult
woman. In their review of 60 smooth muscle tumors of the vagina, five neoplasms recurred. All five smooth muscle tumors

that later recurred were larger than 3 cm, with greater than
5 mitotic figures per ten high power fields (H.P.F.) and various degrees of atypia. Tavassoli and Norris conclude that
a neoplasm with moderate to marked atypia and greater than
5 mitotic figures per ten HPF merits the designation of leio-
myosarcoma.

Rare cases of malignant melanoma have been reported in the
vagina. Melanoma may arise from remnants of the urogenital
sinus containing pigment which may undergo malignant change.
These tumors have the characteristic deep pigmentation of
melanoma, forming an ulcerative lesion, involving bladder and
rectum, and spreading to vulva and cervix with infiltration
into the parametrium. Both hematogenous and lymphatic dissemination occurs and metastases have been noted to the brain
(8).

Sarcoma botryoides is generally found as a cancer of the vagina in childhood. It is a lesion of mixed mesodermal origin
with rhabdomyoblast elements but rarely, if ever, cartillage
and bone. The tumor rapidly fills the vagina and can be noted
protruding from the introitus with the characteristic grape-
like appearance. The tumor is locally invasive, but may involve femoral, parametrial, and aortic lymph nodes as well
as metastases to the lung.

Patterns of spread

Vaginal cancer may spread along the vaginal tube to involve
cervix or vulva. However, if the cervix is involved, it must
be considered a cervical lesion. The anterior vaginal cancers
penetrate into the vesico-vaginal septum early, giving the
characteristic bullous edema of the bladder mucosa. The posterior lesions tend to distend and displace the vaginal mucosa
and only after a considerable growth of tumor are the deep
layers invaded. Therefore, the posterior lesions tend to remain localized for longer periods than the anterior lesions
which can invade readily into the submucosa of the bladder
and eventually involve the bladder mucosa. The tumor spreads
by continuity, invading the parametrium and involving paracol-

pos tissue with extension into the obturator fossa, cardinal
ligaments, lateral pelvic sidewalls, and uterosacral ligaments.

The lymphatic drainage of the vagina consists of an extensive
intercommunicating network. The lymphatics in the upper portion of the vagina drain primarily via the lymphatics of the
cervix, while the lowest portion of the vagina drains either
cephalad to cervical lymphatics or following drainage patterns
of the vulva into femoral and inguinal nodes. The anterior
vaginal wall cancers drain most commonly into the deep pelvic
nodes, with the interiliac and parametrial nodes being the
first involved. However, due to the complex lymphatic system
of the vagina, drainage may occur to any of the many nodal
groups, regardless of the location of the lesion. The incidence
of lymph node metastasis is directly proportional to the stage
of the vaginal cancer. Plantl and Friedman, in their review
of the literature, reported 141 cases with positive nodes
(20.8%) in 679 cases. Metastases to the lungs or supraclavicular nodes in squamous cell carcinoma of the vagina tend to
occur in the more advanced stages.

Clinical presentation

Primary squamous cell carcinoma of the vagina is a disease of
the older woman. Herbst et al., noted that in their series,
one-half of the patients (47.1%) were 60 years of age or older,
with a peak incidence occurring in the 50 to 70 year age group
(2). Pride et al., in thier review noted that the mean age
for invasive squamous cell carcinoma was 62 years (4).

Symptoms

Most invasive squamous cell carcinomas of the vagina present
with vaginal bleeding. This may be in the form of postmeno-
pausal or intermenstrual bleeding or post-coital spotting.
Only in the advanced stages, with the disease spread to adjacent organs, are there symptoms of dysuria and pelvic pain.

Diagnosis and staging

The diagnosis of carcinoma of the vagina is best made by a
careful speculum examination and palpation of the vagina. Cytology is most helpful in detecting early squamous cell carcinoma of the vagina. Colposcopy is a particularly useful tool
for directing biopsies following abnormal cervical cytology.
Since many of the cancers originate from the posterior wall
of the vagina, a speculum must be carefullly rotated so as
not to obscure the lesion by the blades of the speculum. Once
the diagnosis of invasive carcinoma has been confirmed pathol-
ogically, the patient should undergo a staging evaluation
which should include cystoscopy and proctosigmoidoscopy. The
patient is best staged under anesthesia together with the
gynecologist and radiation therapist. Further biopsies of
the vagina are taken at various sites, down the vagina so as
to delineate the level of normal vaginal mucosa. The patients
are staged using the FIGO staging system (Table 1).

Table 1.   STAGING CLASSIFICATION FIGO nomenclature

Stage 0	Carcinoma in situ; intraepithelial carcinoma
Stage I	The carcinoma is limited to the vaginal wall
Stage II	The carcinoma has involved the subvaginal tissue but has not extended to the pelvic wall
Stage III	The carcinoma has extended to the pelvic wall
Stage IV	The carcinoma has extended beyond the true pelvis or has involved the mucosa of the bladder or rectum. Bullous edema as such does not permit a case to be allotted to Stage IV
Stage IVA	Spread of the growth to adjacent organs
Stage IVB	Spread to distant organs

Management of primary carcinoma of the vagina, except clear cell

In general, there has been poorer results in treating carcinoma of the vagina than the results obtained in the treatment
of cervical cancer. Some of the poor results in treatment is
due to the fact that the disease is often well advanced before proper diagnosis. The symptoms of vaginal bleeding or

pain often occur late and delay on the part of the physician
in establishing a diagnosis is not uncommon. Early spread of
vaginal cancer is due to the thin wall, loose areolar invest-
iture and rich lymphatic drainage system around the vagina.
Treatment for primary carcinoma of the vagina has generally
been radiation therapy only, radical surgery only and combined therapy. Plentl and Friedman reviewed large series of
five-year survival data by treatment regimen in vaginal cancer and found a 23.6% survival with radiation therapy only,
22.7% with radical surgery only, and 28.3% with combined therapy (6). Recently, Perez and Camel reported on the use of
radiation therapy of carcinoma of the vagina (5). Their results revealed a five-year survival of 90% for Stage I, 58%
for Stage IIA, 32% for Stage IIB, 40% for stage III and 0%
for Stage IV. It was of interest that in patients with Stage
I, the addition of external radiation did not significantly
increase survival or tumor control. In Stage II and Stage III
the combination of interstitial or intercavitary therapy plus
external irradiation was necessary for local control. Local
or parametrial metastases occurred more frequently in lower
stage recurrences while distal metastasis occurred more commonly in the more advanced stages. The incidence of distant
metastasis in Perez' series was slightly higher than observed
in invasive carcinoma of the cervix.
It does appear that the superiority of radiation therapy over
radical surgery for most carcinomas of the vagina has been
established. However, individualization is important which
considers the stage, grade, tumor size and location of the
lesion. In general our treatment plan is as follows:
Carcinoma in situ -and perhaps generally followed the recom-
mendations of Lee and Symmonds and performed either wide local
incisions or partial or total vaginectomy, depending upon
the location and whether there is multicentric origin of the
malignancy (9).
In treating patients with Stage I carcinoma of the vagina -
we have taken into account differences in prognosis according
to the location of the primary lesion. Radical hysterectomy

is considered only for small lesions of the upper third of the vagina. Vaginectomy is also necessary with pelvic lymph node dissection:

Other Stage I patients are treated with local irradiation providing the lesion is superficial. Patients that have a high propensity for lymph node metastasis (poorly differentiated tumors) are treated with an addition of external pelvic radiation.

All other stages, including Stage II and III are treated with either radium needles or intravaginal cylinders together with external radiation. Groin dissections are added if the lesions are in the lower third and anterior portion of the vagina. We have reserved the ultra-radical procedures for either surgery or radiation failures. However, some stage IV's, particularly with extension to bladder or rectum, are best treated by exenteration.

Clear cell carcinoma of the vagina

Diethylstilbestrol was introduced in the late 1940's in an
effort to decrease abortions in high risk mothers. In 1970,
Herbst and Scully reported on seven cases of adenocarcinoma
of the vagina in adolescence (3). Until that time, adenocarcinoma of the vagina and cervix in young women was recorded
only a few times in the medical literature. Careful epidemiologic evaluation of the mothers of these young women with
clear cell adenocarcinoma revealed an association with maternal
DES ingestion. In 1971, a special registry was established,
and as of June 1, 1980, 429 cases of both vaginal and cervical
clear cell adenocarcinoma have been accessioned into the registry (10). Of the 429 cases, 243 gave a positive history
for in utero exposure to Diethylstilbestrol. It also appeared
that the risk, both for clear cell carcinoma and vaginal adenosis, was related to the time of ingestion during pregnancy.
Eighty percent of the mothers of the cancer patients had begun treatment in the first twelve weeks of pregnancy, in comparison with only 50% of the mothers of a group of DES exposed
daughters who did not have cancer (11). The youngest DES exposed female to develop clear cell adenocarcinoma was seven
years old and the oldest,31 years of age with a peak incidence
at age 19. Ninety-five percent of the cases of clear cell developed in individuals 14 years of age or older. Whether women
over the age of 25 are at risk to develop clear cell carcinoma, is as yet, uncertain, as many of the exposed women have
not yet reached that age.

Office management of the DES exposed female

We do not perform a pelvic examination on the premenarchal
girl who has been known to be exposed to DES unless there is
a specific gynecological indication, e.g. bleeding or abnormal
leukorrhea. All the patients that we have managed with clear
cell adenocarcinoma have associated evidence of vaginal adenosis. Although clear cell adenocarcinoma of the vagina may
affect any region of the vagina, Robboy et al. reported that

three-fourths of the tumors are located in the anterior wall
usually in the upper third and have a surface area of less
than 12 cm² (12). These tumors often appear as a polypoid
or nodular reddened lesion, with the majority penetrating
less than 3 mms into the vaginal stroma. Often the tumor extends subepithelial so that the exact spread of the tumor is
difficult to ascertain by vaginal observation. Careful inspection and palpation of the vagina with cytology from both
the cervix and vagina, is essential. Most of the cancers that
we have managed have been diagnosed by observation and palpation. If the cytology is abnormal then colposcopy is essential to define specific areas for biopsy. The use of Schiller
stain has not been particularly helpful, due to the large
areas of adenosis that appear nonstained and therefore, make
biopsy of specific locations difficult. At the present time
there is no data to suggest that any contraceptive method
appears to be contraindicated in the DES exposed woman. However, the use of oral contraceptives must be carefully moni-
tored as exogenous estrogens for contraception may increase
the risk of estrogen related tumors by accumulating the life-
time estrogen dosage already received by this patient. Although there appears to be an abnormal intrauterine contour
in many patients with vaginal adenosis, the use of the intrauterine device (IUD) does not appear to be at greater risk
for the DES exposed woman. One of the perplexing questions
is the risk of squamous cell carcinoma of the vagina in DES
exposed women. This area is still a subject of some controversy, although at the present time there is no convincing
evidence for an increased occurrence of squamous cell malignant or pre-malignant lesions among the DES patients (13, 14).
However, there have been some reports which have shown an increased incidence of cervical intraepithelial neoplasia in
these women (15). As many of the exposed women have not yet
reached the age of maximum risk, controlled studies will be
needed to answer this important question.

Management and treatment of clear cell adenocarcinoma of the vagina

As part of the metastatic evaluation, we have recommended CAT
scan, or lymphangiography to determine possible aortic node
metastasis in all cases. Robboy et al., noted that in clear
cell carcinoma in young women, metastasis to the lungs or
supraclavicular nodes accounted for 1/3 of recurrence, a proportion much greater than for squamous cell carcinoma of the
cervix or vagina (16). Therefore, it is essential to properly
evaluate the aortic nodes before instituting any therapy. If
any of these nodes are suspected as positive, percutaneous
aspiration biopsies have been helpful. All patients are staged
under anesthesia, together with the radiation therapist.If
the patient is anticipated to have Stage I disease, preparation
is made for radical surgery at the time of the staging. Biopsies are taken down the vagina to determine areas of normal
vaginal mucosa and sent for frozen section. Fortunately, most
of the cancers are in the upper third of the vagina, but due
to the subepithelial spread of the malignancy, nearly the
entire vagina must be removed.

We have generally employed radical hysterectomy with partial
or complete vaginectomy, pelvic lymph node dissection and
aortic node sampling for Stage I clear cell adenocarcinoma
of the upper vagina. If the lower vagina is involved, we also
include a superficial and deep inguinal and femoral node dissection. We replace the vagina with a split thickness skin
graft which is inserted arount the 8th or 9th post-operative
day. Although some have recommended placement of the skin
graft at the time of radical hysterectomy, but due to serum
discharge from the operative site and possible infection, we
have found the graft takes more satisfactorily with the 8 or
9 day delay. One of the advantages of radical pelvic surgery
is ovarian conservation. Metastasis to the ovaries has been
rare and encountered only in patients with spread to other
organs as well. Recently, two of our patients who have had
ovarian conservation developed benign serous cysts of the
left ovary. Whether this is a coincidence or results from a
compromised blood supply with encasement of the ovary by the

rectal-sigmoid mesentary is not celar. If pelvic nodes are
positive, we have added external radiation giving 4,000-4,500
rads to the whole pelvis postoperatively. The morbidity has
not been high, however, these patients must be maintained on
exogenous estrogen. Our indication for postoperative radiation
is the high incidence of recurrence and poor survival in patients with positive nodes. Of 122 patients with vaginal carcinomas and negative nodes, only 14% died in contrast to 52%
of the 25 patients with positive nodes (10). Among the 239
patients with Stage I clear cell carcinomas, the overall survival rate was 90%.

Patients with Stages II and III are usually treated with radiation therapy, utilizing both external radiation, intracavitary radiation and/or needle implants to the tumor. As in
cervical carcinoma, survival becomes progressively worse with
higher stages. Stage II survival is 80%, decreasing to 37%
for patients with Stage II vaginal carcinoma. In Stages II
and III, we perform an extraperitoneal node dissection prior
to primary radiation therapy to determine if there is aortic
metastasis.

The use of pelvic exenteration, either total, anterior or
posterior, has been the primary therapy in 20 cases (10). Some
of these cases had received preoperative radiation therapy
and 12 of the 20 are free of disease one to 10 years postoperatively. Twenty-six patients received postoperative radiation
therapy because of pelvic lymph node involvement. Seven of
these patients have died and 19 are currently living and well
without recurrences. After primary treatment, the patient must
be closely evaluated, particularly with chest x-rays, pelvic
and cytologic examinations. The possibility that serum cathepsin B-1 may be helpful as a marker is currently being investigated (17).

Recurrences

Most recurrences of clear cell carcinoma occur within three
years after initial treatment. However, in two patients the
interval was as long as seven years. Pulmonary and supracla-

vicular nodal metastases are more frequent as compared to squamous cell carcinoma of either the cervix or vagina. If local recurrences occur without side wall involvement pelvic exenteration may be considered. If either aortic or pelvic nodes are involved, exenteration is not indicated. A variety of chemotherapeutic agents have been used with poor response. At the present time our plan would be to use cisplatinum adriamycin and cytoxan, alternating on a three week interval for six months.

References

1. Rutledge, F. 1967. Cancer of the vagina. Am. J. Obstet. Gynecol. 97:635.
2. Herbst, A.L., Green, T.H. Jr., Ulfelder, H. 1970. Primary carcinoma of the vagina. Am. J. Obstet. Gynecol. 106:210.
3. Herbst, A.L. and Scully, R.E. 1970. Adenocarcinoma of the vagina in adolescence: A report of 7 cases including 6 clear cell adenocarcinomas (so-called mesonephromas). Cancer 27:745.
4. Pride, G.L., Schultz, A.E., Chuprevich, T.W. et al. 1979. Primary invasive squamous carcinoma of the vagina. Obstet. Gynecol. 53:218.
5. Perez, C.A. and Camel, H.M. 1982. Long-term follow-up in radiation therapy of carcinoma of the vagina. Cancer 49: 1309.
6. Plentl, A.A., Friedman, E.A. 1971. Lymphatic System of the Female Genitalia: The Morphologic Basis of Oncologic Diagnosis and Therapy, pp 51-74, Philadelphia, W.B. Saunders.
7. Tavassoli, F.A., Norris, H.J. 1979. Smooth muscle tumors of the vulva. Obstet. Gynecol. 53:213.
8. Chung, A.F., Woodruff, J.M., Lewis, J.L. 1975. Malignant melanoma of the vulva. Obstet. Gynecol. 45:638.
9. Lee, R.A., Symmonds, R.E. 1976. Recurrent carcinoma in situ of the vagina in patients previously treated for in situ carcinoma of the cervix. Obstet. Gynecol. 48:61.
10. Herbst, A.L. and Bern, H.A. 1981. Developmental effect of Diethylstilbestrol (DES) in Pregnancy. New York, N.Y., Thieme Stratton, Inc.
11. O'Brien, P.C., Noller, K.L., Robboy, S.J., et al. 1979. Vaginal epithelial changes in young women enrolled in the National Cooperative Diethylstilbestrol Adenosis (DESAD) Project. Obstet. Gynecol. 53:300.
12. Robboy, S.J., Scully, R.E., Herbst, A.L. 1975. Pathology of the vaginal and cervical abnormalities associated with prenatal exposure to Diethylstilbestrol. J. Reprod. Med. 15-13.
13. Burke, J., Antonioli, D., Rosen, S. 1978. Vaginal and cervical squamous cell dysplasia in women exposed to Diethylstilbestrol in utero. Am. J. Obstet. Gynecol. 132:537.

14. Robboy, S.J., Keh, P.C., Nickerson, R.J., et al. 1978. Squamous cell dysplasia and carcinoma in situ of the cervix and vagina after prenatal exposure to diethylstilbestrol. Obstet. Gynecol. 51:528.
15. Fowler, W.C., Schmidt, G., Edelman, D.A., et al. 1981. Risks of cervical intraepithelial neoplasia among DES-exposed women. Obstet. Gynecol. 58:720.
16. Robboy, S.J., Herbst, A.L., Scully, R.E. 1974. Clear cell adenocarcinoma of the vagina and cervix in young females: Analyses of 37 tumors that persisted or recurred after primary therapy. Cancer 34-606.
17. Pietros, R.J., Szego, C.M., Mangon, C.E., et al. 1978. Elevated serum Cathepsin B-1 and vaginal pathology after prenatal DES exposure. Obstet. Gynecol. 52:321.

5. CIN - DEFINITION, EPIDEMIOLOGY AND DIAGNOSIS

J.A. Jordan

Definition

Most pathologists still use the terminology described in the
World Health Organisation classification (1975), but many now
use the new classification of cervical intraepithelial neoplasia grades I to III (CIN I-III). The W.H.O. (1975) classification is as follows:

Dysplasia: A lesion in which part of the thickness of the
epithelium is replaced by cells showing varying degrees
of atypia.

The epithelial abnormalities designated as dysplasia occur
in either the squamous epithelium of the portio or in metaplastic epithelium of the endocervical mucosa. The changes
may be observed in the cervical glands. The lesion may also
accompany carcinoma in situ or invasive cervical carcinoma.
Dysplasia may be separated into three grades - mild, moderate and severe - according to the degree of cellular a-
typia and epithelial architecture:

(a) *Mild dysplasia* - loss of polarity and of regular stratification are minimal. The nuclei are always enlarged,
often irregular, and are darkly stained. Mitoses are
often found and occasionally are abnormal; they are
confined to the lower third of the epithelium. The cytoplasm is generally well preserved and keratinisation
of single cells or of the epithelial surface is a common feature.

(b) *Moderate dysplasia* - the degree of epithelial abnormality
is intermediate between mild and severe dysplasia.

(c) *Severe dysplasia* – atypia is very pronounced. There is
   loss of polarity and the crowded cells have large,
   darkly stained nuclei. Mitoses, occasionally including
   atypical forms, are seen. The abnormal cells tend to
   be present in the upper third, as well as the middle
   and lower thirds of the epithelium. The superficial
   cells show a degree of maturation. A layer of flattened cells may form the surface.

Carcinoma in situ: A lesion in which all or most of the
epithelium shows the cellular features of carcinoma.
There is no invasion of the underlying stroma.

In the classical form small hyperchromatic nuclei are
surrounded by scanty cytoplasm with little, if any,
squamous differentiation. Orderly stratification is lacking and cellular polarity is often vertical or diagonal
rather than horizontal. Mitoses, normal and abnormal, are
found scattered throughout the epithelium. Flattened
parakeratotic cells may be present on the surface. The
lesion often involves the cervical glands.

Variants of the classical form occur. These include a
keratinising form found characteristically in the portio,
and a large-cell, non-keratinising form around the squamo-
columnar junction or in the endocervix. These variants
may be difficult, if not impossible, to distinguish from
dysplasia.

However a new terminology has been introduced, namely
cervical intraepithelial neoplasia (CIN). There are two
reasons why this term has been introduced. First, it does
not use the word carcinoma as in carcinoma in situ.
Second, and most important is that the premalignant disease currently referred to as dysplasia or carcinoma in
situ is really a continuum of epithelial abnormality
ranging from the mildest form of dysplasia to carcinoma
in situ (Richart, 1967).

The CIN terminology corresponds with the W.H.O. classification
as follows:

CIN I - mild to moderate dysplasia

CIN II - moderate dysplasia

CIN III - severe dysplasia and carcinoma in situ

An accurate histological diagnosis is not easy, and reference to Table I shows the many criteria which have to be assessed when deciding whether an epithelial lesion is CIN, and if so, what degree it is.

TABLE I

The histological diagnosis of Cervical Intraepithelial Neoplasia
From Anderson (1982)

1. Differentiation (Maturation, Stratification)
   a. Present or absent
   b. Proportion of epithelium showing differentiation
2. Nuclear abnormalities
   a. Nucleus: cytoplasm ratio
   b. Hyperchromasia
   c. Nuclear pleomorphism and anisokaryosis
3. Mitotic Activity
   a. Number of mitotic figures
   b. Abnormal configuration
   c. Height in epithelium

Epidemiology

The association between carcinoma of the cervix and sexual activity is well established. Women with cervical carcinoma report more sexual and marital partners; earlier age at first intercourse, marriage and first pregnancy; and a higher prevalence of venereal disease and marital breakdown than do comparable women without the disease (Boyd and Doll, 1964, Wynder et al, 1954, Rotkin, 1967, and Kessler, 1976). The strongest associations are with the number of sexual partners, age at first intercourse and venereal disease and other associations are probably secondary to an association with one or other of these factors. Observed correlations with low social economic class (Thomas, 1973, Wright et al, 1978, and Harris et al, 1980) and cigarette smoking could also be indirect, re-

flecting the inference of associated sexual characteristics.
Similar associations have also been found for CIN.

A likely explanation for these observations is that the man
contributes a carcinogenic agent during intercourse. Several
infectious agents have been suggested including chlamydia,
mycoplasma, cytomegalovirus, herpes simplex type II virus
(Nahmias and Sawanabori, 1978). Alternatively, reactions to
components of the semen of some men might themselves initiate
or promote carcinogenises (Coppleson, 1970, Singer, 1979,
Singer et al, 1976, and Reid et al, 1978). It is difficult on
the basis of the sexual history of women with cervical cancer
to distinguish between an infectious and a non infectious
agent. Sexual histories of husbands of patients and controls
have therefore been studied recently to differentiate between
hypotheses, because sexual promiscuity will increase the
cancer risk only if the husband is capable of acquiring a
carcinogenic agent through sexual contact and passing the
agent to his wife.

A recent study by Buckley et al (1981) has confirmed that if
the husband is "promiscuous" then the wife is much more likely to develop cervical cancer than the husband and wife who
have never had any other partner!

A further infectious agent which is receiving much attention
now is the human papilloma virus and it is now generally believed that some patients with genital warts will develop
CIN because of this virus (Syrjanen, 1980).

Diagnosis

It is believed that if CIN can be detected and treated then
this will reduce significantly the mortality rate from cervical cancer. Since CIN is asymptomatic and unrecognisable to
the naked eye, then special investigation is necessary for
its detection. The only practical way in which its presence
can be suspected is by the use of cervical cytology. Description of the technique of cytology is beyond the scope of this
chapter. However, it is worth pointing out that cytology
screening programmes in Canada (Miller et al, 1976), United

States (Cramer, 1974), Finland (Hakama and Rasanen-Virtanen, 1976); Iceland (Johannesson et al, 1980) and Scotland (MacGregor and Teper, 1978) have shown significant reductions in the incidence and death rate from cervical cancer if properly planned cytology screening programmes are introduced. There are some who advocate the use of routine colposcopy but most Gynaecologists feel that this it totally unnecessary and time consuming if a proper cytology service is available.

References
1. Anderson, M.C. 1982. The Patholgy of CIN - errors in diagnosis in "Pre-clinical neoplasia of the cervix". Ed. Jordan, J.A.,
2. Sharp, F., and Singer, A. Pub. The Royal College of Obstetricians and Gynaecologists, London, 133 - 140.
3. Boyd, J.T., Doll, R. 1964. A study of the aetiology of carcinoma of the cervix uteri. Brit. J. Cancer, 18: 419-34.
4. Buckley, J.D., Harris, R.W.C., Doll, R., Vessey, M.P. and Williams, P.T. 1981. Case-control study of the husbands of women with dysplasia or carcinoma of the cervix uteri. Lancet, 8254, 1010-1015.
5. Coppleson, M. 1970. The origin and nature of premalignant lesions of the cervix uteri. Int. J. Gynaecol Obstet. 8: 539-50.
6. Cramer, D.W. 1974. The role of cervical cytology in the declining morbidity and mortality of cervical cancer. Cancer, 34: 2018-2027.
7. Hakama, M. and Rasanen-Virtanen, U. 1976. Effect of a mass screening programme on the risk of cervical cancer. Am. J. Epid, 103(5): 512-517.
8. Harris, R.W.C., Brinton, L.A., Cowdell, R.H., et al 1980. Characteristics of women with dysplasia or carcinoma in situ of the cervix uteri. Br. J. Cancer, 42: 359-68.
9. Johannesson, G., Geirsson, G., Day, N. and Tulinius, M. 1980. Screening for cancer of the uterine cervix in Iceland 1965-1978. To appear in Acta Path Scand.
10. Kessler, H. 1976. Human cervical cancer as a venereal disease. Cancer Res, 36: 783-91.
11. MacGregor, J.E., and Teper, S. 1978. Mortality from carcinoma of cervix uteri in Britain. Lancet, October 7: 774.
12. Miller, A.B., Lindsay, J. and Hill, G.B. 1976. Mortality from cancer of the uterus in Canada and its relationship to screenning for cancer of the cervix. Int. J. Cancer, 17: 602-612.
13. Nahmias, A.J. and Sawanabori, S. 1978. The genital herpes-cervical cancer hypothesis - 10 years later. Prog Exp Tumour 2: 117-39.
14. Reid, B.L., French, P.W., Singer, A., Heigen, B.E. and Coppleson, M. 1976. The role of a high-risk male in the etiology of cervical carcinoma. Am. J. Obstet Gynaecol, 126: 110-15.
15. Richart, R.M. 1967. Natural history of cervical intraepithelial neoplasia. Clin. Obstet. Gynecol, 10: 748-784.

16. Rotkin, I.D. 1967. Adolescent coitus and cervical cancer: Associations of related events with increased risk. Cancer Res, 27: 603-17.
17. Singer, A. 1979. Further evidence for high risk male and female groups in the development of cervical carcinoma. Obstet Gynecol. Surv., 34: 867-68.
18. Singer, A., Bevan, I.R. and Coppleson, M. 1976. A hypothesis: The role of a high-risk male in the etiology of cervical carcinoma. Am J. Obstet Gynecol., 126: 110-15.
19. Syrjanen, K.J. 1980. Current views on the condylomatous lesions in uterine cervix and their possible relationship to cervical squamous cell carcinoma. Obstet. Gynecol Surv. 35: 11, 685-694.
20. Thomas, D.B. 1973. An epidemiologic study of carcinoma in situ and squamous dysplasia of the uterine cervix. Am J. Epidemiol., 10: 19-28.
21. World Health Organisation 1975. International Histological classification of tumours 13. Poulson, H.E., Taylor, C.W. in collaboration with Sobin L.H. and other pathologists from nine countries. W.H.O., Geneva.
22. Wright, N.H., Vessey, M.P., Kenward, B. et al 1978. Neoplasia and dysplasia of the cervix uteri and contraception: a possible protective effect of the diaphragm. Br. J. Cancer 38: 273-79.
23. Wynder, E.L., Cornfield, J. Schroff, P.D. et al 1954. A study of environmental factors in carcinoma of the cervix. Am J. Obstet Gynecol. 63: 1016-52.

6. THE TREATMENT OF CERVICAL INTRA-EPITHELIAL NEOPLASIA BY SURGICAL CONE BIOPSY

J.A. Wijnen

Introduction

The treatment of cervical intra-epithelial neoplasia (CIN) today, falls into two categories: excision and destruction. Excisional methods, hysterectomy with or without vaginal cuff
or cone biopsy have given excellent results (1) and in most
parts of the world form the mainstay of therapy. The terminology generally used for this procedure is a bit confusing: is
it a conization, a cone, an exconization or a cone biopsy? Probably cone biopsy and exconization are the preferred terms;
they stress the diagnostic, the therapeutic character of this
procedure respectively.
Reservations about the reproductive performance following cone
biopsy and a decline in the age of CIN-patients, stimulated
consideration of a more conservative approach. The initial results of local treatment by destruction are relatively encouraging and may justify a long-term evaluation.
This paper will be restricted to the excisional methods, especially the surgical cone biopsy.
The important first step in deciding the therapeutic approach
to CIN, is to establish the diagnosis clearly and to eliminate
the possibility of invasive cancer. So, in what kind of patient
should we consider a surgical cone biopsy to be indicated?

Criteria for selection of patients

As we use cytologic smears of the uterine cervix as a screening tool, we will have to evaluate patients with abnormal
smears to exclude invasive cancer.
PAP-smears of the uterine cervix can be false-negative and

false-positive; they can overestimate or underestimate the
grade of the lesion (2, 3).
Verschoof (4) recently presented some results of the cervical
screening program in The Netherlands. In a further evaluation
of cases with cytologically PAP IIIA (mild to moderate dysplasia) more severe lesions were found in 5-20% and in 0.1-0.4%
invasive cervical cancer was found. Thus histologic evaluation
of patients with abnormal PAP-smears seems to be indicated.
Whether or not the lesions require treatment is another subject.
If expert colposcopy is not available and no suspicious lesion
is present, the only reliable diagnostic method to exclude more
severe dysplastic lesions and invasive cancer in persistant
abnormal cervical smears, is a diagnostic cone biopsy. All other
sampling methods have been reported to be unreliable without
colposcopy: they will miss some cancers (1)*. Diagnostic cone
biopsy is preferably done using Schiller's iodine staining test
to include the entire abnormal area in the excision. The value
of this Schiller's test is debatable, but in the absence of
colposcopy it is better than nothing.
Cone biopsy should aim to be diagnostic as well as therapeutic
and remove the entire lesion.
A thorough histopathologic evaluation is then indicated. The
resection margins and clockwise sections of the cone specimen
should be carefully studied and reported.
When expert colposcopy is available, it has been possible to
exclude invasive cancer in 80-90% of women with abnormal cervical cytology in an outpatient evaluation. With expert colposcopy the number of diagnostic cone biopsies could be reduced
to about one tenth.
Heinzl and Szalmay (5) found a histopathologic correlation in
82.1% of cases, when comparing colposcopically directed punch
biopsies and specimens obtained through following exconization
or hysterctomy.

* Ed. note: See also chapters 1, 3, 4, 5.
  Sometimes a blind biopsy can prevent conisation in cases of
  invasive carcinoma (eds).

If colposcopy is available cone biopsy can be limited to the
following indications:

1. Lesions colposcopically suspect for invasive cancer: when
   the histopathology of the biopsies is not correlating, or
   where cytology indicates a greater likelihood of invasive
   disease than is indicated by the colposcopically directed
   punch biopsy.
2. When the entire squamo-columnar junction or the entire lesion
   cannot be seen (unsatisfactory colposcopy). Cone biopsy has
   to be performed especially when the endocervical curettings
   show serious anomalies.
3. If there is supicion of micro-invasion or invasion on colposcopically directed biopsy.
4. A therapeutic indication for exconization can be the unreliable patient who is not likely to return for follow-up
   visits after conservative management.

Techniques

Generally, al techniques which produce a cone, small enough to
prevent surgical and reproductive complications and large
enough to encompass the entire lesion, will do. The cone has
to be well oriented for the laboratory and damage of the surface epithelium must be avoided.
Another advantage of colposcopy before taking a cone biopsy
is that colposcopy will allow the size and shape of the cone
to be tailored to the needs of the individual patient.
Hospitalization and general or regional anesthesia are required in most patients.
We use the following technique:
The patient under general or regional anesthesia is placed in
the dorsal lithotomy position. The position and the extent of
the lesion is located first by colposcopy and then by Schiller's
iodine solution to determine the shape and the size of the
cone biopsy. Small marking incisions made under colposcopic
vision can be used also.
The normal equipment for vaginal gynaecologic surgery is used.
Primary hemostasis is attempted by ligating descending cervical

branches of the uterine artery. Care is taken to prevent
abrasion of the cervical epithelium by rough vaginal examination or by any surgical instrument. Sometimes intracervical
injection of a hemostatic agent to the cervical stroma is used.
After reproduction is completed, the endo-cervical canal can
be completely removed. However, in women desirous of further
childbearing, the excision should be no more radical than
necessary. Correspondingly, the uncommon downward extension
of the lesion to the vagina should be encompassed in the excision.

When the epithelium of the endocervical canal is not entirely
removed in the cone biopsy, endocervical curettage (ECC) up to
the internal os is done after the cone specimen has been excised
Electro-surgical cutting devices should not be used to excise
the cone specimen. They will interfere with subsequent histological interpretation of the margins. Repair and hemostasis is
achieved with hemostatic whip sutures, which take the edges of
the remaining upper and lower cervical lip several times.
Currently Vicryl [R] or Dexon [R] sutures are used. Other authors
recommend no suturing at all in order to leave the surface free
for epithelialization without the fear of occluding neoplastic
tissue rests (6,7). They use cautery or hemostatic pressure
gauze.
Accessability of the uterine cavity has to be maintained.

Complications

The overall incidence of complications of cone biopsy is reporte
to vary from 3-11 percent and even as high as 25 percent (6,8).
The percentage of complications seems to be related to the size
of the cone removed.
Intra-operative complications:
- excessive bleeding
- uterine perforation with damage to adjacent organs
Pre-operative hemostatic precautions, i.e. well-placed hemostatic sutures, care in assessing the direction of the endocervical canal and the use of smaller or specially designed
scalpel blades will diminish these risks.

Post-operative complications:
- secondary hemorrhage, especially following deeper incisions
- post-operative pelvic infection is rarely seen.

Late complications:
- cervical stenosis, causing menstrual disorders and dysme-
  norrhea. This can probably be prevented by accurate hemostasis and suturing.
- reproductive problems
     . infertility because of removal of most of the glandular
       epithelium of the endocervix with subsequent dry cervix
       or stenosis.
     . pregnancy and labour problems, especially immature or
       premature labour may occur because of cervical incom-
       petency after a large cone biopsy, taking much of the
       cervical subepithelial tissues. Fibrosis may cause
       cervical dystocia during labour.
       Moinian and Andersch (1982) (9) analysed 923 pregnancies
       in 414 patients before and after cone biopsy with the
       use of hemostatic sutures and intracervical injection
       of a hemostatic agent and cold-knife technique. They
       reported post-operative bleeding in 22 percent of cases,
       cervical stenosis in 4.8 percent of cases and severe
       dysmenorrhea in 5.5 percent. They found a complicating
       cervical factor in pregnancies after cone biopsy in 20.5
       percent. This resulted in subsequent cervical cerclages
       during pregnancy and caesarean sections during labour.
       The late spontaneous abortion rate in this study was
       reported to be seven times higher after cone biopsy than
       before.

In pregnancy the advance of colposcopy has enhanced the safety
of a conservative diagnostic approach of patients with abnormal
PAP-smears. In Stafl and Mattingly's series (10), cone biopsy
was found unnecessary in all pregnant patients with CIN.
There was no histological evidence of progress of the lesion
when the definitive cone biopsy after delivery was compared
with colposcopically directed punch biopties made during pregnancy.

Follow-up

If therapeutic exconization or hysterectomy was used, 80% of recurrences, which in fact are residual lesions, will appear in the first year of follow up (11). We take separate endocervical and ectocervical cytology smears, 4 and 10 months after surgical intervention and when these are negative, yearly smears are taken for the following 4 years and once every 3 years up to the age of 65.

Results

In the absence of colposcopy, a Schiller directed cone biopsy aiming for cure and to remove all of the endocervical canal, can expect to cure up to 98% of patients witn CIN I and II and 93% with CIN III (table 1).

The historical dictum: 'Conization is too much for diagnosis and too little for therapy', seems not to be true.

Colposcopically directed cone biopsy will give similar cure rates, but will allow the average cone biopsy to be much smaller than the non-colposcopically directed one and this might lower the complication rate.

Hysterectomy for CIN gives cure rates of 96-97% (table 2) (1). Addition of a vaginal cuff in patients with colposcopic extension of the lesion to the vaginal vault (estimated to be near 4%) (1) can expect to cure almost all.

Most reports indicate that recurrences of invasive cancer after cone biopsy or hysterectomy in the cervix or elsewhere are rare and that recurrence of persistance of CIN is uncommon (1). Recurrences of CIN or invasive cancer, even in cases where the cervical margins were reported to be free on histopathologic exam, showed no significant difference after cone biopsy and hysterectomy (13, 14).

The literature on hysterectomy studies performed within weeks of cone biopsy shows residual CIN lesions in 12-60% (15, 16). Many authorities have recommended hysterectomy for cases of non-radical conization. However, one might expect that residual lesions must also exist in some women who have been treated by cone biopsy only. Yet paradoxically these residual lesions

Table 1   Results of treatment of carcinoma in situ by cone
           biopsy or amputation of cervix

Author	Year	No. of cases	Time of follow-up	Subsequent overt in- vasive cancer
Mussey and Soule	1959	53	Over 5 yrs (9), less than 5 yrs (44)	0
Friedell, Hertig and Younge	1960	36	To 16 yrs (24), less than 5 yrs (12)	0
Parker et al	1960	124	1 month - 10 yrs	0
Schuller	1962	166	Over 5 yrs (41), less than 5 yrs (125)	0
Jordan, Bader and Day	1964	54	1 - 12 yrs	0
Anderson	1965	51	All over 5 yrs	0
Lewis	1966	30	All over 5 yrs	0
Devereux and Edwards	1967	77	2 - 6 yrs	0
McLaren	1967	113	1 - 14 yrs	0
Hulme and Eisenberg	1968	111	Over 5 yrs (57), 2 - 5 yrs (54)	
Way, Hennigan and Wright	1968	140	Over 5 yrs (108)	1
Krieger and McCormack	1968	314	Over 5 yrs (157)	3
Boyes, Worth and Fidler	1970	808	6-16 yrs (165), 1-5 yrs (643)	2
Green	1970	325	15 months - 22 yrs	1
Creasman and Rutledge	1972	65		1
Davidson and Taylor	1973	54	All over 5 yrs	0
Brudenell, Cox and Taylor	1973	103	5 - 15 yrs	1

Table 1 (continued)

Coppleson	1976	593	Over 5 yrs (132)	0
Kolstad and Klem	1976	795	5 - 25 yrs	7
Bjerre, Eliasson, Linel et al	1976	1430	not stated	2

Source: M. Coppleson. 1981, Gynecologic Oncology

almost never seem to progress to invasive cancer.

Long term follow-up of conization cases still shows a very low incidence of recurrent CIN or invasive disease. Recurrences of CIN after therapeutic conization are reported less often than one would anticipate from the residual lesion rates in the cone-hysterectomy studies discussed before. Coppleson (17), Kolstad (14) and Boyes (18) found recurrence rates of CIN in 1.6-3.2%, which are very low compared with the 12-60% residual lesions in the hysterectomy studies (15, 16).

Some of the residual lesions reported in these hysterectomy studies may be immature metaplastic squamous epithelium, associated with repair after cone biopsy and histologically indistinguishable from carcinoma in situ. Hysterectomy performed within a few weeks of cone biopsy, would be likely to expose these changes and so produce a high incidence of so-called 'residual lesions'.

The use of cone biopsy as therapy places a burden on the histopathologist in determining from the cone margins whether excision is complete or incomplete. Free margins are considered to be prognostically favourable. However, Kolstad and Klem, (1976) (14) and Schulmann and Caveneck, (1961) (13) report recurrences of CIN where the biopsy margins were free of CIN. Nevertheless, even when the margins are involved in the cone specimen and no further treatment is undertaken, only a minority of patients will show evidence of persistent disease.

Conclusions

- Most centres now believe that hysterectomy is over-treatment for the majority of patients with CIN.
- Hysterectomy for CIN only is indicated particularly in those women in whom the cone biopsy cannot be carried out for technical reasons.
- CIN in the margins of the cone biopsy is not necessarily an indication for hysterectomy: follow-up is necessary after both cone biopsy and hysterectomy.
- If other gynaecological disorders requiring hysterectomy are present with CIN, hysterectomy seems to be warranted.
- The results of adequate surgical cone biopsy in the treatment of CIN are excellent. But long term cytological follow-up needs to be pursued.
- Cone biopsy is not a minor surgical procedure. The complication rate, late sequelae, costs and impact on the histopathologist are relatively high, as is the psychological burden for the patient. Considering that colposcopy affords an improved accuracy of pre-operative diagnosis and the present results of a more conservative management of CIN in selected patients, it can be stated that even cone biopsy is over-treatment of many cases of CIN.
- Treatment results of CIN will continue to depend on the quality of primary diagnosis.
- Indications for cone biopsy should be defined precisely, cone biopsy should be used primarily as a diagnostic tool and secondarily as treatment. The operation should be restricted only to those patients in whom it is mandatory.

58

References

1. Coppleson, M.: Cervical intra-epithelial neoplasia: clinical features and management. In: Gynaecologic Oncology. Ed. M. Coppleson, Churchill Livingstone, p. 408-433, 1981.
2. Stafl,A., Friedrich, E.G.Jr. & Mattingly, R.F.: Detection of cervical neoplasia-reducing the risk of error. Clin. Obstet. Gynecol. 16, 238, 1973.
3. Shingleton, J.M., Partridge, E.E. & Austin, J.M.Jr.: The significance of patients with atypical Papanicolaou smears, Obstet. Gynecol. 49, 61, 1977.
4. Verschoof, K.J.H.: Meeting Dutch Society for Colposcopy and cervical pathology, 1982.
5. Heinzl, S. & Szalmay, G. (1981): Importance of colposcopic specimen-biopsy to the diagnosis of CIN. Zentralbl. Gynäkol. 103, 997, 1981.
6. Bjerre, B., Eliasson, G., Linell, F., Soderberg, H. & Sjoberg, N.: Conization as only treatment of carcinoma in situ of the uterine cervix. Am. J. Obstet. Gynecol. 125, 143, 1976.
7. Sekiba, K., Nawachi, K. & Endo, S.: A conization technique to prevent complications associated with conventional method Fourth World Congress Int. Fed. for Cervical Pathology and Colposcopy, London (1981).
8. Claman, A.D. & Lee, N.: Factors that relate to complications of cone biopsy. Am. J. Obstet. Gynecol. 120, 124, 1974.
9. Monian, M. & Andersch, B.: Does cervix conization increase the risk of complications in subsequent pregnancies? Acta Obstet. Gynecol. Scand. 61, 101, 1982.
10. Stafl, A. & Mattingly, R.F.: Colposcopic diagnosis of cervical neoplasia. Obstet. Gynecol. 41, 168, 1973.
11. Bevan, J.R. Attwood, M.E., Jordan, J.A. et al: Treatment of pre-invasive disease of the cervix by cone biopsy. Br. J. Obstet. Gynaecol. 88, 1140, 1981.
12. Noumoff, J., Kohan, S., Strider, W. & Douglas, G.W.: Surgical (cold knife) conization in the management of cervical intra-epithelial neoplasia. Fourth World Congress Int. Fed. for Cervical Pathology and Colposcopy, London, 1981.
13. Schulmann, H. & Cavanagh, D.: Intra-eptihelial carcinoma of the cervix. The predictability of residual carcinoma in the uterus from microscope study of the margins of the cone biopsy specimen. Cancer, 14, 795, 1961.
14. Kolstad, P. & Klem, V.: Long term follow-up of 1121 cases of carcinoma in situ. Obstet. Gynecol. 48, 125, 1976.
15. Creasman, W.T. & Rutledge, F.: Carcinoma in situ of the cervix. An analysis of 861 patients. Obstet. Gynecol. 41, 501, 1972.
16. Nagell, J.R. van, Parker, J.C.Jr., Hicks, L.P., Conrad, R. & England, G.: Diagnostic and therapeutic efficacy of cervical conization. Am. J. Obstet. Gynecol. 124, 134, 1976.
17. Coppleson, M.: Treatment of preclinical carcinoma of the cervix. In: The Cervix Uteri. Jordan, J.A. and Singer, A. Eds. London, Saunders, 1974.
18. Boyes, D.A., Worth, J.A. & Fidler, H.K.: The results of treatment of 4389 cases of preclinical cervical squamous carcinoma. J. Obstet. Gynaecol. Br. Commonw. 77, 769, 1970.

7. TREATMENT OF CIN BY DESTRUCTION - LASER

J.A. Jordan and J. Mylotte

Introduction

The word laser is an acronym derived from the first letters of
the words Light Amplification by Stimulated Emission of Radiation. The laser is a device which converts some form of energy
such as heat, light or electricity into radiant energy of a
special kind at one or more discrete wavelengths. When the
wavelength and radiant energy lies within the visible portion
of the electro-magnetic spectrum it is called light with which
we are all familiar. Not all lasers emit their radiant energy
as light but the radiation emitted by all lasers has three special qualities. It is coherent (all the waves are exactly in
phase with each other in both space and time); it is collimated
(the rays are parallel to each other); and it is monochromatic
(all the waves are exactly the same wavelength).
The early lasers, such as the Ruby Lasers, were first manufac-
tured in the 1950s (1) and were very inefficient, converting
only a small proportion of their energy into coherent radiant
energy. Now we have the gas lasers, the most efficient of which
is the carbon dioxide (CO_2) laser which is more efficient than
the Ruby lasers but still relatively inefficient because it
converts no more than 15% of its energy into coherent output
radiation. The laser produces its light at a wavelength of
10.6 microns which is in the infra-red portion of the spectrum
where it is invisible to the naked eye. When used for the treatment of CIN, the laser is attached to a colposcope and by a
system of mirrors the laser beam is directed to the tissue
which is to be destroyed. Unmodified laser light is parallel,
in theory can travel to infinity, and contains no energy which
is of practical use unless it is focused by a simple lens. Comparison can be made with the rays of the sun which in themselves are relatively harmless but when focused with a lens can

produce intense heat at the focal point of the lens. So it is
with the laser, and tissue at the focal point of the laser is
destroyed by vaporising the intra-cellular fluid at the speed
of light. The diameter of the laser beam at its focal point is
approximately 1.8 mm and the beam is easily controlled by a
micromanipulator attached to the colposcope, with the result
that it is totally under the control of the surgeon, thereby
allowing him to destroy tissue with great precision.

The treatment of CIN

As with any destructive technique the following criteria must
be met before treatment by destruction can be considered.

1. The patient is seen and assessed by an expert colposcopist.
2. The expert colposcopist can see the entire lesion, i.e.
   can see the squamo-columnar junction.
3. The expert colposcopist must exclude invasive carcinoma
   by biopsy or biopsies.
4. The expert colposcopist must perform the laser vaporisation himself.
5. There must be a good cytological and colposcopical follow-
   up.

In most cases the CIN can be removed as an out-patient procedure without any form of anaesthesia (97% of cases) but occasionally a paracervical block may be helpful, or, less commonly, general anaesthesia. For laser vaporisation the patient
is placed in the routine colposcopy position i.e. a modified
lithotomy position. No pre-operative preparation of the vagina
is needed, nor is it necessary to use antibiotics of antiseptic
creams of pessaries post-operatively.

Technique of laser vaporisation

The key to eradication of CIN by laser vaporisation is depth
of destruction, and this is a function of two parameters, namely power density (watts per cm^2) and time. The power density
is a physical term which signifies the amount of energy released at the focal point of the laser beam, i.e. on the cervix

and is controlled by a simple watt regulator on the laser con-
sul; the usual wattage recorded is 20-30 watts and this will
give a power density at the point of impact of 400-600 watts
per cm^2. The time for which the beam is released is controlled
by the operator by a simple foot switch; the surgeon can
pre-set the machine to release the laser beam for a fixed
period of time such as 0.1 second, or 0.5 seconds, or alternatively the beam can be released in a continuous fashion
and be controlled only by the foot switch. When the laser
surgeon is using laser microsurgery for the first time he
will use the simple and safe intermittent therapy, i.e. each
time he presses the foot pedal the beam will be released for
a set time of less than one second. However, very quickly the
operator finds that the continuous beam is equally safe, is
quicker and is more effective.

The laser was first used for the treatment of CIN as recently
as 1974 (2-5) and the first laser used outside the United
States was introduced to the Birmingham and Midlands Hospital
for Women in August 1977. Preliminary results from the original users of laser vaporisation were extremely poor (Table 1)
with a very high proportion of patients having residual abnormality following a single laser vaporisation. It was quickly apparent however, that the failures could be explained
quite simply. The operator had not destroyed tissue to e great
enough depth! By trial and error the Birmingham group arrived
at the figure 5-7 mm depth of destruction as being the ideal (6)
and later results from the same centre (Table 1) show that
laser vaporisation to a depth of 5-7 mm will give an apparent
cure rate of 91.4% with a single laser vaporisation.

In 1979 Anderson and Hartley (7) concluded that destructive
methods of treatment should reach a minimum depth of 4 mm and
this was based on the study of cervical crypt or cleft or gland
involvement by CIN as studied in cone biopsy specimens. They
concluded that in 99.8% of patients with CIN the lesion did
not extend in the clefts more than 4 mm below the surface.
It is obviously impossible to measure 4 mm with any degree of
accuracy and therefore the figure of 5-7 mm is a good guide
for the clinician.

Table 1   Depth of vaporisation of CIN and a apparent cure with single laser application
(Birmingham and Midlands Hospital for Women 1977-1980)

Depth of Vaporisation	CIN I		CIN II		CIN III		CIN I-III	
	Successes	Cure Rate	Successes	Cure Rate	Successes	Cure Rate	Successes	Cure Rate
1-2 mm	3/6	50%	1/7	14.3%	4/26	15.4%	8/39	20.5%
2-4 mm	17/27	63%	11/18	61%	20/60	33.3%	48/105	45.7%
4-5 mm	4/5	80%	5/5	100%	14/20	70%	23/30	77%
5-7 mm	33/36	91.7%	45/45	100%	114/129	88.4%	18/210	91.4%

The depth of destruction is not difficult to measure and with experience the clinician will have no problem in determining his depth of destruction.

Complications of laser vaporisation

Most patients are aware of some discomfort but this is usually minimal and described as a warm feeling, a cramp-like feeling or tiny needles sticking into the cervix. Some patients feel no discomfort whatsoever but occasionally some form of anaesthesia is necessary. A study of 91 consecutive patients attending the laser clinic at the Birmingham and Midlands Hospital for Women shows the reaction of patients to the treatment (Table 2). Some of the early reports relating to laser vaporisation gave the impression that patients felt nothing and that the treatment could be carried out with impunity! This of course is not so but nevertheless, in the majority of cases, treatment can be carried out easily without analgesia. If there is a problem then the operator can of course revert to the use of paracervical block or even general anaesthesia.

Bleeding during treatment is not a problem because one of the characteristics of the laser beam is to seal off the small capillaries during the vaporisation process. The 91 patients already mentioned were assessed for bleeding and reference to Table 2 will show that no bleeding occurred in over 80% of patients subjected to laser vaporisation. Troublesome bleeding does occur from time to time, particularly in the presence of inflammatory changes, but is not usually a problem. Secondary haemorrhage occurs infrequently with 1.5% of patients seeking advice within a few days of treatment.

Regeneration following laser destruction

Re-epithelialisation of the cervix occurs very rapidly and within eight to ten days new immature metaplastic cells cover the entire surface of the lesion no matter how extensive the vaporisation has been: in all cases the treated area will be covered by relatively mature squamous epithelium within four weeks.

Table 2   Laser vaporization 5-7 mm deep Discomfort and bleeding during treatment in 91 consecutive patients (Birmingham and Midlands Hospital for Women)

Discomfort

Degree:	None/minimal	Easily tolerable	Tolerable	Painful	Para Cx. block	Anaesthesia
Patient No.	10	45	27	3	2	4

Bleeding

Type:	None	Slight	Moderate	Troublesome
Patient No.	78	7	3	3

Because the epithelium subjected to vaporisation disappears
"in a puff of smoke" there is no necrotic tissue such as that
which is left following diathermy or cryocautery and for this
reason there is minimal discharge, and to all intents and
purposes no post-operative fibrosis or stenosis. Furthermore
the squamo-columnar junction is almost always visible follow-
wing laser vaporisation, a factor which is thought to be important when relying on colposcopy and cytology for follow-up.
The healing process has been studied by electron-microscopy (8)
and it was this study which formed the basis of the conclusions
mentioned above, namely that new squamous cells appear on the
surface of the vaporised tissue within eight to ten days. The
electron-microscopy healing study has revealed one other important factor. A constant criticism of destructive methods
has been the problem of inadequate destruction of tissue with
the possibility of residual CIN being covered by new squamous
epithelium and remaining undetected until it suddenly appears
as invasive carcinoma. Following laser vaporisation any abnormal
epithelium which has been undestroyed, either because surface
epithelium has not been destroyed deeply enough or because the
abnormal epithelium extends into the depths of the crypt or
gland beyond the depth of destruction, will remain on the
surface during the healing process and be recognisable when the
patient is followed-up by colposcopy or cytology. Such residual
abnormality can be readily destroyed by further laser vaporisation and reference to Table 3 will show the average number of
treatments for each patient based on the histological diagnosis.
For example patients with CIN I require on average 1.21 treatments while patients with CIN III required on average 1.35
treatments. Overall, the 358 patients followed-up received an
average of 1.27 treatments. These figures of course include the
patients in the early part of the study where destruction was
too superficial and if the initial treatment is designed to
destroy tissue to a depth of 5-7 mm then the overall treatment
sessions will be less than that described in Table 3.

Table 3

Details of Laser tratment for CIN (Birmingham and Midlands
Hospital for Women 1977-80)

	Patient No.	No. of treatments	Treatment rate
CIN I	75	91	1.21
CIN II	80	97	1.21
CIN III	203	274	1.35
CIN I-III	358	462	1.27

Laser failures

Reference to Table 4 shows how 11 patients deemed "laser failures" were subsequently treated and it is quite clear that the majority of so-called failures were due to inadequate laser vaporisation or poor patient selection. All of them occurred in the early days of the study and we would now conclude that if a patient is properly selected for treatment and treatment is carried out by an expert colposcopist to a depth of 5-7 mm, then the number of patients who cannot be "cured" by one or more laser treatments is minimal.

We can be criticised particularly for cases 10 and 11, patients who had CIN III extending into the endo-cervical canal. Although the squamo-columnar junction could be seen in both of these patients, it was obviously a mistake to try to eradicate the disease in this way and both patients should have had cone biopsy as the primary treatment. Extension of the disease into the lower part of the canal is not necessarily a contraindication to laser vaporisation because if it extends a very short distance then a properly planned vaporisation may indeed remove the entire lesion.

Cone biopsy via laser

Laser vaporisation as described above destroys and thereby removes the same amount of tissue as a ring biopsy or small cone biopsy and of course we accept the comment that there is a possibility that unsuspected invasive carcinoma may be destroyed in this way. We believe however, that with careful patient selection by expert colposcopists this is more of a theoretical than a pratical risk. However, to overcome this problem a cone biopsy performed by the laser beam can be performed (9) The advantage of this being that the laser allows a proper cone biopsy to be taken for adequate histological assessment and by virtue of the capillary co-agulation property of the laser beam, bleeding is minimal. This particular technique is worthy of further investigation.

Table 4   Laser Failures (Birmingham and Midlands Hospital for Women 1977-80)

	Histology	Depth of vaporisaton	Final treatment	Final diagnosis	Reason for failure
1	CIN III	2 mm	Cone Biopsy	CIN III	Bleeding during 2 laser treatments.
2	CIN I	1-2 mm	Cryosurgery	CIN I	Inadequate depth.
3	CIN III	2-3 mm	Diathermy	CIN III	Inadequate depth.
4	CIN III	3 mm	Cone Biopsy	CIN III	Inadequate depth.
5	CIN I	2-3 mm	Cryosurgery	CIN I	Inadequate depth.
6	CIN III	2-3 mm	Hysterectomy	CIN III	Endocervical lesion.
7	CIN III	5 mm	Cone Biopsy	CIN I	Not clear.
8	CIN III	5 mm	Cone Biopsy	CIN III	Bleeding during laser treatments.
9	CIN III	3 mm	Cone Biopsy	CIN III	Inadequate depth.
10	CIN III	5 mm	Cone Biopsy	CIN III	Endocervical lesion.
11	CIN III	4 mm	Cone Biopsy	CIN III	Endocervical lesion.

Vaginal extension of CIN

In three to four per cent of patients the CIN will be so extensive
that it involves part of the upper vagina. Using traditional
methods this is a very difficult situation to treat but laser
vaporisation of vaginal intra-epithelial neoplasia has given
excellent results. In the majority of cases it can be treated
in the out-patient clinic although extensive areas are probably
treated most thoroughly under general anaesthesia. It is important
to note that the depth of vaporisation when treating vaginal
lesions should not be as deep as for cervical lesions and depths
of vaporisation of 3-4 mm will give excellent results. As with
the cervix healing is extremely rapid with minimal or no fibrosis.

Conclusion

Long term follow-up of patients treated by laser vaporisation
is not yet available because the method was not used to any
great extent until 1976-1977 and in many of the early cases
treatment was unsatisfacory because of inadequate depth of
destruction. However, sufficient cases have now been followed
for three to four years to allow us to predict with the same
confidence as those of our colleagues who have used cryocautery
or deep radical diathermy, that we can expect cure rates in the
region of 96-97%. The key of course to this is careful patient
selection, and laser vaporisation, like other methods of
destruction, should never be used unless the five criteria
mentioned at the beginning of this chapter can be adhered to.
If these five points cannot be guaranteed, then the surgeon
should resort to the well tried and trusted methods of treatment such as cone biopsy or even hysterectomy, or better still
refer the patient to someone who can consider the possibility
of destruction.

Finally, let us not forget that there are many ways in which
CIN can be t?   and the method selected will vary from place
to place depend g on the views of the person undertaking
treatment, but although the same problem may be treated differently by different gynaecologists, I am sure that we are all agreed
that treatment should never be undertaken unless the patient has
been seen and assessed by a skilled colposcopist.

REFERENCES

1. Patel, C.K.N. 1968. High power carbon dioxide laser. Sci Am 219:22
2. Bellina, J.H. 1977. Laser in gynecology. Ann Obstet and Gynec 6:371
3. Stafl, A., Wilkinson, E.J. and Mattingly, R.F. 1977. Laser treatment of cervical and vaginal neoplasia. Am J Obstet Gynecol 128:128
4. Baggish, M.S. 1980. High-power density carbon dioxide laser therapy for early cervical neoplasia. Am J Obstet Gunecol 138:1, 117
5. Carter, R., Krants, K.E., Hara G.S., Lin, F. Masterson, B.J. and Smith, S. 1978. Treatment of cervical intraepithelial neoplasia with the carbon dioxide laser beam. Am J Obstet Gynecol 131:8, 831
6. Mylotte, M.J. and Jordan, J.A. 1981. Rev. Fr. Gynecol Obstet 76:5, 353
7. Anderson, M.C. and Hartley, R.B. 1979. Cervical crypt involvement by intraepithelial neoplasia. Obstet Gynecol Survey 34:852
8. Mylotte, M.J. and Jordan, J.A. Unpublished results 1981
9. Dorsey, J.M. and Diggs, E.S. 1979. Microsurgical conization of the cervix by carbon-dioxide laser. Obstet Gynecol 54:565

8. DESTRUCTION OF CERVICAL INTRAEPITHELIAL NEOPLASIA AT 100°C WITH THE SEMM COAGULATOR

I. Duncan

Ten years ago the traditional treatment for squamous carcinoma in situ (CIS) of the uterine cervix in most centres in the Western World was either cone biopsy or hysterectomy (1). The latter course of action deprived the patient of future childbearing while cone biopsy, although in theory permitting continued fertility, did so at the cost of increased rates of spontaneous abortion, premature labour and instrumental delivery (2). Since then there has been an increase in the number of patients diagnosed as having CIS and simultaneously the mean age of these patients has fallen (Fig. 1).
Thus, there has been greater need for conservative management. Fortunately, the last ten years have also seen a marked re-kindling of interest in colposcopy and where this has been available locally destructive methods of treating the whole spectrum of cervical intraepithelial neoplasia (CIN) using heat and cold have been tried.
High temperature electrocautery is well established (3). Cryo-surgery has found many advocates and was reviewed recently by Charles and Savage (4). The most sophisticated approach employs laser which so far has proved to be as effective as older methods (5, 6). Each modality has its advantages and disadvantages. The ideal method of local tissue destruction should be effective and safe, economical in capital outlay, maintenance and time, simple to use and highly acceptable to the ambulant patient, preserving her fertility where desired. As the need for cone biopsy and hysterectomy has fallen in the author's institution (Fig. 2), various ablative techniques have been used (Fig. 3). The most recent technique "Cold Co-agulation" has been in regular use since April 1978, a pilot

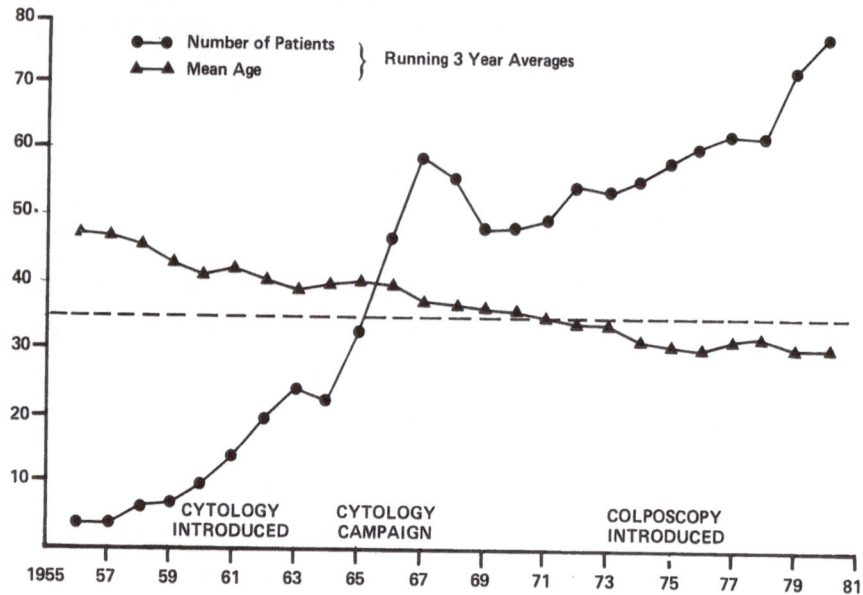

CA-IN-SITU – DUNDEE LABORATORIES CATCHMENT AREA

Fig. 1

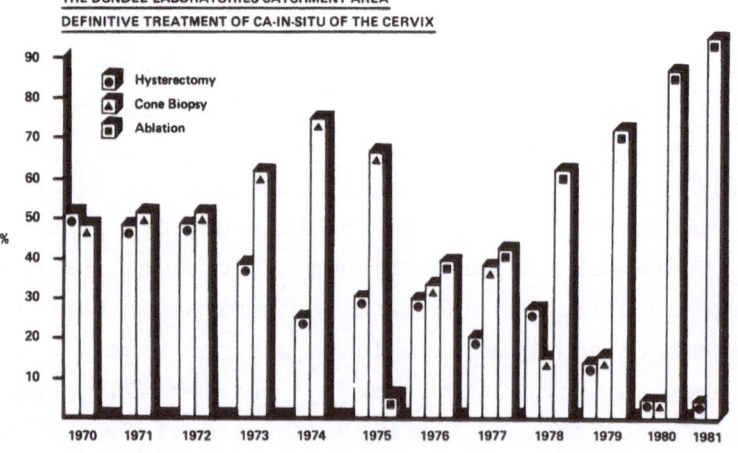

THE DUNDEE LABORATORIES CATCHMENT AREA
DEFINITIVE TREATMENT OF CA-IN-SITU OF THE CERVIX

Fig. 2

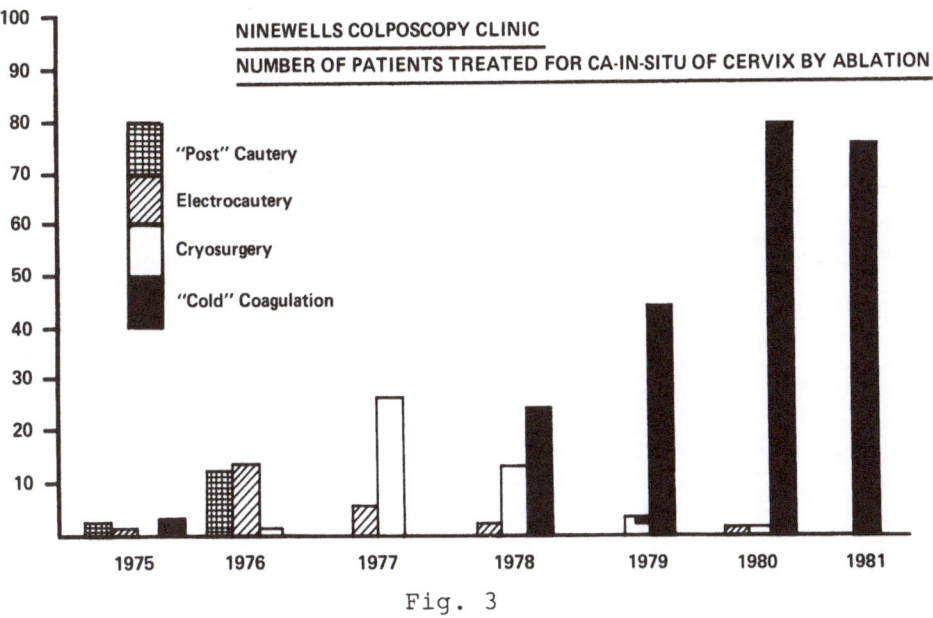

Fig. 3

study with three patients having been performed in 1975.
The term "Cold Coagulation" was coined by Semm, the inventor
of the instrument, in 1966 (7), but is an unfortunate one and
confusion arises with the terms "cryosurgery" and "cryocautery". "Thermocoagulation" is an alternative since the instrument employs heat not cold but this term has been used synonymously with high temperature electrocoagulation and electro-
diathermy. "Caloric Coagulation" may be a more acceptable and
accurate description, the latin noun "calor" meaning moderate
heat in distinction to "ardor".

The Apparatus

The instrument consists of a small portable electronic monitor powered by mains electricity. A range of temperatures between 50°C and 120°C is available with the latest model. A
working temperature is pre-selected and is maintained by a
thermocouple. The heat is conveyed to the tissues via a choice
of thermosounds two of which can be connected to the monitor
simultaneously. These Teflon-coated thermosounds are easily
cleaned and can be sterilised at 140°C at the press of a but-
ton. Treatment areas are overlapped (Fig. 4).
In this study thermosounds were applied to the tissue for 20
seconds at 100°C at each of the overlapping areas until the
whole of the transformation zone was destroyed.

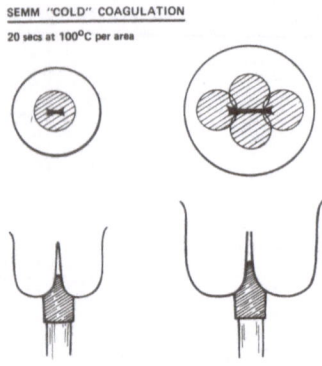

SEMM "COLD" COAGULATION
20 secs at 100ºC per area

Fig. 4

Patients

CIN is screened for by cervical cytology. Patients with abnormal smears are referred to the Ninewells Colposcopy Clinic which serves Tayside Region and adjacent parts of Scotland. Cervical smears are repeated and colposcopic examination is carried out by or under the direct supervision of an experienced operator. Directed punch biopsies are taken from areas of most significantly abnormal appearance and the histology reported.

If the squamo columnar junction cannot be seen in the endocervix or when, even with the aid of an endocervical speculum the lesion extends out of sight cranially or there is any suggestion of micro invasive carcinoma then cone biopsy is indicated. This approach is preferred to blind endocervical curettage (ECC) which is not performed routinely. When the lesion can be seen in its entirety and has been accessible to punch biopsy even although it extends into the endocervix, then coagulation is carried out.

Following treatment triple sulphonamide cream is given to the patient for nightly application per vaginam for one week but no restriction is made on sexual intercourse or the use of menstrual tampons. Repeat cervical cytology is obtained in the Ninewells Colposcopy Clinic at four monthly intervals for one year, and six monthly intervals for a second year. Further

smears are taken in the community annually when the initial
lesion was CIN. III (Carcinoma in situ or severe dysplasia) and
biennially when it was CIN I (mild dysplasia) or CIN II (moderate dysplasia). The Ayre's spatula used has been modified
in an attempt to obtain cells both distal and proximal to the
original lesion (8). Cervical cytology is thus used again for
rescreening treated patients. Persistent or recurrent abnormal
smears demand re-evaluation with the colposcope exactly as
for a new referral.

By 1st January 1982 there were 403 patients treated for histologically proven CIN with the Semm Coagulator and who had
been seen for follow-up on at least one occasion (Table I).
These patients form the subject of this report.

NINEWELLS COLPOSCOPY CLINIC
"COLD" COAGULATION STUDY 1.1.82

			Mean Age
CIN 3	C.I.S.	224	29.6 ± 5.9
70%	SD	59	29.9 ± 5.7
	CIN 2	73	29.3 ± 6.8
	CIN 1	47	31.1 ± 7.7
ALL CIN		403	29.8 ± 6.3

Table I

The mean age of the patients was 29.8 $\pm$ 6.3 with a range of
18-52 years. Table I reveals no significant difference in the
mean ages with varying degrees of CIN and 79 per cent were
under the age of 25 years (Fig. 5). Figure 6 reveals that 60
per cent of the patients had had two or fewer pregnancies
prior to treatment.

76

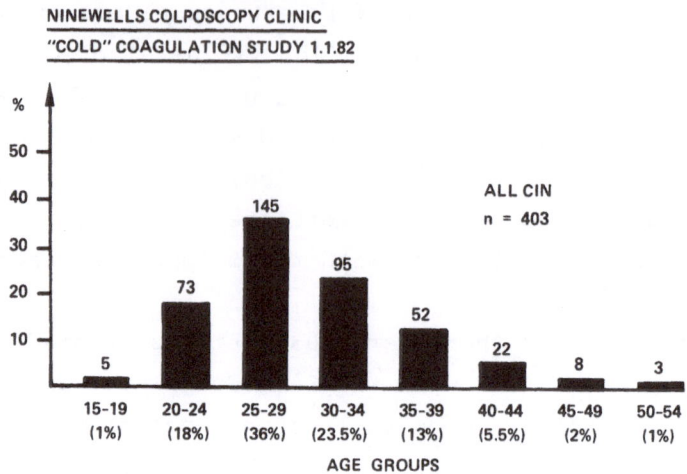

NINEWELLS COLPOSCOPY CLINIC
"COLD" COAGULATION STUDY 1.1.82

ALL CIN
n = 403

AGE GROUPS

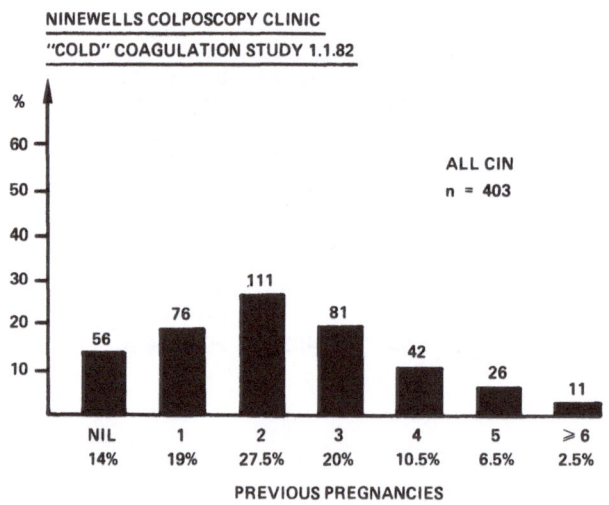

NINEWELLS COLPOSCOPY CLINIC
"COLD" COAGULATION STUDY 1.1.82

ALL CIN
n = 403

PREVIOUS PREGNANCIES

Figs. 5 and 6

Results

The failure rates are shown in Table II - 2.5 per cent in the first six months of follow-up, 2 per cent in the second six months and 1 per cent in the third. To date there have been no recurrences after 18 months of negative follow-up but the long term results remain to be determined. There was no significant difference between the degrees of CIN 1, 2 and 3 al-

NINEWELLS COLPOSCOPY CLINIC – "COLD" COAGULATION STUDY 1.1.82

FAILURE RATES

	1st six months	2nd	3rd	4th	3rd Year	4th Year	5th Year
C.I.S.	7/224 = 3%	4/153 = 2.5%	2/103 = 2%	0/61 = NIL	0/25 = NIL	0/2 = NIL	0/2 = NIL
S.D.	0/59 = NIL	0/45 = NIL	0/25 = NIL	0/14 = NIL	0/6 = NIL		
CIN 2	2/73 = 2.5%	1/39 = 2.5%	0/24 = NIL	0/10 = NIL	0/1 = NIL		
CIN 1	1/47 = 2%	1/30 = 3.5%	0/22 = NIL	0/14 = NIL	0/1 = NIL		
ALL CIN	10/403 = 2.5%	6/267 = 2%	2/174 = 1%	0/99 = NIL	0/33 = NIL	0/2 = NIL	0/2 = NIL

Table II

Table II

NINEWELLS COLPOSCOPY CLINIC – "COLD" COAGULATION STUDY 1.1.82

TREATMENT FAILURES

Patient	Age	Original Lesion	Recurrence Persistence	Further Treatment	Current Cytology	
J.A.	25	CIS	CIS	"Cold" Coag	Neg	
J.C.	28	CIS	CIS	"Cold" Coag	Neg	
I.C.	43	CIS	CIS	"Cold" Coag	Neg	Also VIN → Laser
K.McL.	36	CIS	CIS	"Cold" Coag	?	
M.B.	30	CIS	CIS	Cone Biopsy/Hyst	Neg	
L.D.	28	CIS	CIS	Hyst	Neg	
P.N.	34	CIS	CIS	Hyst	Neg	
J.C.	27	CIS	SD	"Cold" Coag	Neg	
M.S.	40	CIS	SD	Hyst	Neg	
C.McR.	25	CIS	CIN 2	Hyst	Neg	
C.C.	32	CIS	CIN 1	Hyst	Neg	
M.R.	30	CIS	CIN 1	"Cold" Coag	Neg	
W.W.	23	CIS	CIN 1	"Cold" Coag	?	
M.C.	28	CIN 2	? CIS	Hyst	Neg	
P.McD.	30	CIN 2	CIN 2	"Cold" Coag	?	
M.H.	39	CIN 2	CIN 1	"Cold" Coag	?	
M.M.	27	CIN 1	CIS	Cone Biopsy	Neg	Previous Cryo for CIS
G.B.	28	CIN 1	CIN 1	"Cold" Coag	?	

Mean Age 30.7 ± 5.4

Table III

though, probably by chance, there have been no failures so far with severe dysplasia as opposed to CIS. The 18 individuals where a single treatment was not effective are described in Table III. Treatment with the Semm Coagulator was repeated in 10 of these patients with apparent succes in 5. The outcome is not yet known in the other 5. Only in two patients was the recurrent or persistent lesion greater in degree than the initial one. The histology in the first of these patients is in doubt, the reporting pathologists split between CIS and an atypical warty lesion. The second patient had previously been treated for CIS with cryosurgery and perhaps this degree of CIN had persisted undetected.

There have been no cases of micro invasive or frankly invasive carcinoma developing after coagulation.

The mean age of patients with treatment failure was no different from the study group.

Integrity of Follow-Up

Lost to follow-up are 29 patients, 8 of whom have not returned at all after treatment and are otherwise excluded from the series (Table IV). Of the remaining 21 patients, 2 had had 5 follow-up smears, 2 had had 4 smears, 4 had had 3 smears, 4 had had 2 smears and 9 had had 1 smear. All of these patients had normal cervical cytology when last seen.

NINEWELLS COLPOSCOPY CLINIC

"COLD" COAGULATION STUDY 1.1.82

DEFAULTERS OR LEFT AREA WITHOUT TRACE

C.I.S.	10	NO PATIENT HAD ABNORMAL CYTOLOGY
S.D.	5	WHEN LAST SEEN
CIN 2	6	8 patients have had no
CIN 1	8	follow up smear
	29	

Table IV

Fourteen of the 29 patients are known to have left the area
while the remainder, despite enthusiastic recall, are presumed to have defaulted. The resulting integrity of the follow-up is shown in Table V.

NINEWELLS COLPOSCOPY CLINIC
"COLD" COAGULATION STUDY 1.1.82
INTEGRITY OF FOLLOW UP

		%
at 6 months	403/411	98
1 year	267/282	94.5
18 months	174/189	92
2 years	99/112	88.5
3 years	33/41	80.5
4 years	2/3	

Table V

Side Effects and Complications

Menstrual-like pelvic cramp was experienced by most patients
while coagulation was proceeding but resolution of pain occurred almost immediately the thermosound was removed. In many
patients no discomfort was appreciated. Anaesthesia was restricted to use in one patient where treatment was only tole-
rated after paracervical block.
There were no complaints of excessive vaginal discharge. No
patient required hospitalisation or treatment for secondary
haemorrhage, although approximately 2 to 3 per cent of patients experienced slight bleeding persisting for up to one
month. Superficial dyspareunia and slight adnexal tenderness
recorded in one patient, four and eight months after coagulation, resolved with metronidazole. Coagulation was carried
out inadvertently at 5 weeks gestation in a patient with irregular menses and she aborted one week later.
In the longer term 2 patients required cervical dilatation to
break down adhesions formed between the anterior and posterior
cervical lips.

Subsequent Pregnancy

Of 74 patients exposed to pregnancy since treatment, 9 had established pre-existing infertility. Sixty of the remaining 65 patients have conceived, twice in two instances. Four of the remaining 5 patients have been exposed to pregnancy for less than six months. The outcome of pregnancy is presented in Table VI where it can be seen that there were no complications related to the previous coagulation.

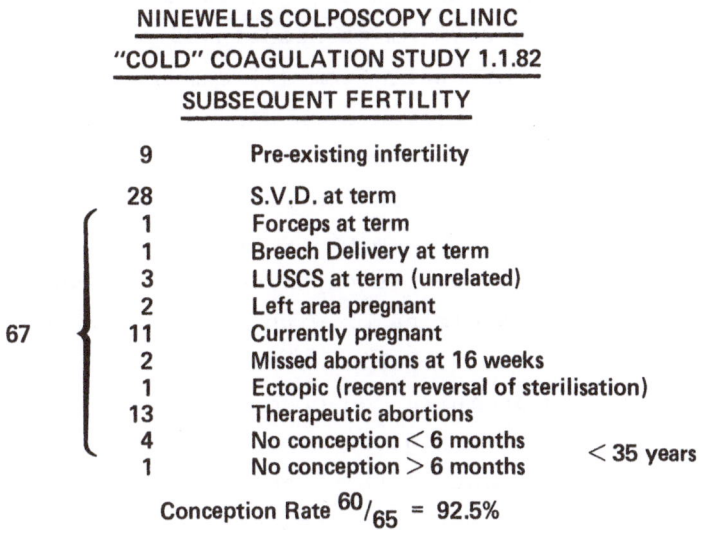

NINEWELLS COLPOSCOPY CLINIC

"COLD" COAGULATION STUDY 1.1.82

SUBSEQUENT FERTILITY

9	Pre-existing infertility	
28	S.V.D. at term	
1	Forceps at term	
1	Breech Delivery at term	
3	LUSCS at term (unrelated)	
2	Left area pregnant	
11	Currently pregnant	
2	Missed abortions at 16 weeks	
1	Ectopic (recent reversal of sterilisation)	
13	Therapeutic abortions	
4	No conception < 6 months	< 35 years
1	No conception > 6 months	

(67 braces the rows from 28 through 1)

Conception Rate $^{60}/_{65}$ = 92.5%

Table VI

Thirteen patients (20 per cent) wishing to avoid pregnancy failed to do so and therapeutic abortion was carried out in each case. This figure is only marginally higher than the history of therapeutic abortion before treatment in 17.5 per cent of the 403 patients. Cervical cerclage was avoided except in one patient treated for CIN 3 persisting after cone biopsy.

Discussion

The rationale for local destruction of CIN depends upon expert colposcopic evaluation so that areas of epithelial abnormality may be selected for histological confirmation and

the presence of invasive disease excluded. Provided then that
the destructive process, albeit by burning, freezing, vaporisation or whatever, is capable of destroying all the abnormal epithelium, then similarly good results are to be expected.
The abnormal epithelium is present not only on the surface but
also in the cervical crypts. Przubora and Plutowa (9) found
in 52 of 56 cases of CIS that the depth of crypt involvement
was less than 3 mm and in no patient was it more than 4 mm.
More recently, Anderson and Hartley (10) found the mean depth
of crypt involvement with CIN 3 was 1.24 mm in 343 therapeutic
cone biopsies, being 2.92 mm or less in 95 per cent and 3.8
mm or less in 99.7 per cent. Semm (7) demonstrated that the
depth of destruction achieved with his coagulator was a function of the temperature and duration of application and in
theory the parameters used in the present series were adequate
to achieve at least 3 to 4 mm of destruction. This may well
be an underestimate as Semm's experiments were performed on
fresh hysterectomy specimens or with coagulation carried out
4 hours pre-hysterectomy. Kubista, Grunberger and Ulm, from
Vienna (11), using an infra-red coagulator at approximately
100°C reported that for a given exposure time there was an
increase in the apparent depth of necrosis when the cervix was
treated 24 to 48 hours prior to hysterectomy, compared to 30
minutes before or after hysterectomy, i.e. the zone of destruction takes time to develop.
Theoretically then the Semm coagulator is capable of destroying CIN and to date in practice, it is as successful as any
of the alternatives. Encouraging results reported earlier in
the series from the same centre (12, 13 and 14) continue to
be borne out. The long term results of the present study are
awaited with interest. In 1978, Staland (15) reported treating
CIN with the Semm coagulator. Thirty-nine of his 71 patients
had been followed for more than 3 years. Abnormal cytology
was encountered in only 2 patients after treatment, one where
suspicious smears persisted but neither colposcopy nor cone
biopsy revealed any pre-malignancy and the cytology subsequently reverted to normal. In the other patient abnormal cytology

recurred at 6 months but returned to normal after cryosurgery. Javaheri, Balin and Meltzer (16) describe treating 25 patients with CIN 1 and 18 patients with CIN 2 using a "modest heat apparatus with a working temperature of 70 to 90°C". Their failure rate was 4 per cent for CIN 1 and 5.5 per cent for CIN 2.

No significant complications have occurred in the present series nor did Staland report any in his. Fergusson and Craft (17) reported a comparison of patients with benign cervical erosion randomised to treatment by cryosurgery or coagulation with the Semm coagulator. They concluded that the latter "has the advantage of reducing the post-operative watery discharge associated with cryosurgery but suffers the disadvantage of being painful in a small number of patients". The use of anaesthetic is not mentioned by these authors but by implication none was used. Staland used local anaesthetic combining injection with local spray. Javaheri et al used spray only. Anaesthetic was used in only one of the 403 patients reported above.

The short treatment time and lack of noise, smoke and smell all contribute to high acceptability by patients and doctor alike.

As patients become younger the preservation of reproductive ability assumes greater importance and is amply demonstrated in this series. The few failures of conception are more likely to be related to the brevity of exposure than a complication of coagulation and are likely to be self limiting. Indeed the performance of the treated cervices in subsequent pregnancy would indicate normality of the tissues with minimal scarring. Staland likewise reports no complication in subsequent pregnancy.

The apparatus itself is light and portable and costs approximately the same as portable cryosurgical equipment. In so many respects therefore "cold coagulation" or as suggested "caloric coagulation" approaches the ideal locally destructive method as defined above and is certainly an option when high temperature electrocautery, cryosurgery or laser therapy are appro-

priate. In the management of CIN, like any other method of
local destruction, it will fall into disrepute unless prece-
ded by expert colposcopic assessment and the rules adhered
to of treating only non-invasive lesions which can be entirely visualised with the colposcope. Figure II must not be in-
terpreted as indicating that therapeutic cone biopsy has no
place in modern treatment. Indeed, a few cone biopsies following colposcopy were performed in Ninewells Hospital in 1981
but in no case did the histology show squamous carcinoma in
situ. Cone biopsy still has an important role in the modern
management of CIN but in centres using colposcopy and local
destruction, it is no longer the mainstay of treatment.

REFERENCES

1. Kottmeier, H. Ed. Annual Report on the Results of treatment in Gunaecological Cancer. Vol. 17, 112-113, FIGO,
   Stockholm.
2. Jones, J.M., Sweetham, P. The hazards of cone biopsy of
   the cervix. International Federation for Cervical Pathology and Colposcopy. Fourth World Congress, London, 13-17th
   October 1981 (in press).
3. Chanen, W. 1982. Treatment of CIN by Destruction - Electrocoagulation Diathermy in Pre-clinical Neoplasia of the
   Cervix - Proceedings of the Ninth Study Group. Ed. Jordan
   J.A., Sharp, F., Singer, A. 191-196, RCOG, London.
4. Charles, E.H., Savage E.W. 1980. Cryosurgical treatment
   of cervical intra epithelial neoplasia. Obstet. Gynecol.
   Surv. 35 : 539-548.
5. Bellina, J.H., Wright, V.C., Voros, J.I., Riopelli, M.A.
   and Hohenschutz, V. Carbon dioxide laser management of cervical neoplasia[2]. (In Press).
6. Jordan, J.A., Mylotte, J. 1982. Treatment of CIN by Destruction - Laser[3], 205-211.
7. Semm, K. 1966. New apparatus for the "Cold Coagulation" of
   benign cervical lesions. Am. J. Obstet. Gynecol. 95, 963-
   966.
8. Duguid, H.L.D., Parrat, D., Traynor, R. 1980. Actinomyces-
   like organisms in cervical smears from women using intrauterine contraceptive devices. Br. Med. J. 281, 534-537.
9. Przybora, L.A., Plutowa, A. 1959. Histological topography
   of carcinoma in situ of the cervix uteri. Cancer 12, 263-
   277.

10. Anderson, M.C., Hartley, R.B. 1980. Cervical crypt in-
    volvement of intra epithelial neoplasia. Obstet. Gynecol.
    55, 546-550.
11. Kubista, E., Grunberger, W. and Ulm, R. Histological
    findings after infra-red coagulations of the portio ute-
    ri[2]. (In Press).
12. Duncan, I.D., 1981, at the 17th Bi-annual meeting of the
    Scottish Association for Clinical Cytology, in The Medi-
    cal Technologist and Scientist, 11, 20-21.
13. Duncan, I.D. Cryosurgery and "cold" coagulation in the
    treatment of cervical intra epithelial neoplasia.
    International Conference on Gynaecological Oncology, Dublin,
    1st-3rd September 1981. Raven Press, New York. (In Press).
14. Duncan, I.D. 1982. Treatment of CIN by Destruction - "Cold"
    Coagulator[3], 197-204.
15. Staland, B. 1978. Treatment of premalignant lesions of
    the uterine cervix by means of moderate heat thermo-sur-
    gery using the Semm Coagulator. Ann. Chir. Gynecol. 67,
    112-116.
16. Javaheri, G., Balin, N., Meltzer, R.M. 1981. Role of cryo-
    surgery in the treatment of intra epithelial neoplasia
    of the uterine cervix. Obstet. Gynecol. 58, 83-87.
17. Fergusson, I.L.C., Craft, J.L. 1974. A new "Cold Coagula-
    tor" for use in the outpatient treatment of cervical ero-
    sion. J. Obstet. Gynecol. Br. Commw. 81, 324-327.

9. THE TREATMENT OF CIN BY CRYOTHERAPY

M. van Lent

Introduction

The use of local cold application in the treatment of gynaecologic cancer was first reported by Openchowski in 1883 (1),
but only after the pioneering efforts of Cooper (2), a neuro-
surgeon, and after the development of economical and safe
equipment, which began two decades ago, could cryosurgery
gain a place in the therapeutic options of the gynaecologist
in his treatment of cervical intraepithelial neoplasia. The
acceptance of this method was also stimulated by the increasing number of young patients with CIN, which was identified
by large scale screening programs. The understandable desire
of these women to preserve a normal chance of pregnancy with
a favourable outcome justified the search for less radical
treatments than hysterectomy.
Although, conisation is an effective treatment for CIN (3),
the socio-medical drawbacks and high rate of "irradicality"
of the procedure are serious limitations in its use as a
diagnostic procedure.
In a large literature survey dealing with over 6,500 patients
mentioned in 19 different reports we found an average irradicality of over 30 per cent. Certainly there is a bias in these figures to be found with those authors who prefer hysterectomy as definitive treatment.
Nevertheless in the gynaecologic department of the Leyden
University Hospital, the number of cones without free margins
was about 18 per cent in the years 1972 till 1977.
During those years the existing tradition of colposcopy in
our institution was further developed without a change in

our therapeutic regimen.

As shown in figure 1 only minimal stromal invasion was over-
looked by colposcopic evaluation. The efficacy of colposcopically directed biopsies was recently confirmed by Kirkup et al
(1980) (4).

Figure 1:

COMPARISON COLPOSCOPICALLY DIRECTED BIOPSY - FINAL HISTOLOGY.
(S.C.J. VISIBLE).

BIOPSY	FINAL HISTOLOGY			TOTAL
	CIN I/II	CIN III	INVASION	
CIN I/II	2	1	-	3
CIN III	1	46	3*	50
INVASION	-	1	2	3
TOTAL	3	48	5	56

* Only minimal stromal invasion.

In view of these favourable results and supported by some encouraging reports in the literature (5, 6) we started in January 1977 an experimental program to treat CIN III by means
of cryosurgery.

The program was ended in January 1979. The results of 75 patients treated during these years are presented with a follow-
up of 3-5 years.

Material and methods

Between January 1st, 1977 and January 1st, 1979 CIN III was
found in 85 patients with persistently abnormal cervical
smears in our department. The diagnosis was confirmed histologically in all patients by colposcopically guided punch
biopsies of the cervix.

The conditions for admitting patients in ths tudy were as follows:

   I : Full visualization of the entire transformation zone at colposcopy.

  II : No suspicion of invasion in either cytological reports or biopsies.

 III : Sufficient guarantees for later follow-up.

  IV : Diameter of the transformation zone less than approximately 2 cm.

The first criterion is the most important of all for any conservative treatment.

In my opinion the value of endocervical curettage in the selection of patients is exaggerated in most reports. For those who do not trust their own eyes an ECC is invaluable. Another reason for our hesitation to accept ECC as the most decisive factor to the exclusion of local therapy lies in the fact that the number of patients with a positive ECC is twice as big as the number with a hidden squamocolumnar junction. The simple explanation is that you can look into the cervical canal at colposcopy, especially with the aid of the Kogan endocervical speculum.

The prediction of invasive disease by the cytologist is based on additional findings in the smear. In our preliminary study we checked the accuracy of the cytological department. As demonstrated in figure 2, our cytologist predicted invasion correctly in 9 of our 13 patients; on the other hand in 27 patients invasive disease was present. This observation sufficiently explains the exclusion of all patients with a Pap. V cytological report. In our study only two patients were lost for follow-up due to immigration to another country.

The importance of the extent of the lesion, as a limiting criterion we learned through one of our failures that we will discuss later.

Figure 2

COMPARISON CYTOLOGY - HISTOLOGY (1972 - 1977)

CYTOLOGY	HISTOLOGY					TOTAL
	NEG.	M.D.	S.D.	CIS.	INV.	
S.D.	1	2	2	15	1	21
CIS		2	6	70	17	95
INV.				4	9	13
TOTAL	1	4	8	89	27	129

M.D. = mild to moderate dysplasia

S.D. = severe dysplasia

CIS. = carcinoma in situ

INV. = invasive disease

The above mentioned conditions were satisfied by 63 of the 85 patients. This means that in about 75 per cent of our patients a conisation was spared. The reasons for exclusion from cryotherapy were as follows:

- 14   Unsatisfactory colposcopic findings
- 4*   Pap. V smear
- 1*   Discrepancy cytology-histology
- 1   Adenocarcinoma in situ
- 1   Lesion too extensive
- 2   Reliable follow-up impossible
- 5(1*)Microinvasion in biopsies

* S.C.J. Not visible.

There fore, with 20 patients colposcopy was unsatisfactory.

The median age of the treated patients was 34 years (range
20-52 years) and that of the excluded patienis was 43,5 years
(range 30-63 years). The relationship between unsatisfactory
colposcopic findings and increasing age has long been noticed
and explains the significantly higher age of the excluded
patients. In one patient an adenocarcinoma in situ was found
and in five patients microinvasion was present in the biopsies.

Apart from the 63 patients in the study group, 12 patients
from affiliated clinics that were participating in the trial
were treated by cryotherapy in our department. The characteristics of these patients are shown in Table I.

Table I

TREATED PATIENTS (N = 75)

	S.D.	CIS	CIN III
"OWN PATIENTS"	36	27	63
REFERRED PATIENTS	3	9	12
TOTAL	39	36	75

S.D. = severe dysplasia
CIN = carcinoma in situ

The same treatment criteria as mentioned before were applied
to them before therapy.

Hypothermia can be achieved by the evaporation of a liquid
gas, a change of phase or by the expansion of a compressed
gas through a small orifice. In our trial we used a Krymed[R]
equipment which is based on the last mentioned principle.
Crisp had determined that using a freeze-thaw-freeze cycle
tissue destruction to a depth of 5-6 millemeters can be a-
chieved (7). As Anderson and Hartley have demonstrated in

their survey about the depth of crypt involvement by CIN this
depth is sufficient to destroy all pathological tissue in
virtually all patients with CIN (8).

Because of the fact that the boiling point of the type of gas
determines the lowest possible temperature of the cryoprobe,
we preferred to use nitrous oxide as a refrigerant. This gas
is generally available in every hospital.

In all instances a Creasman probe was used with a long endocervical protrusion.

The cervix was cleaned of mucus with 3% acetic acid. To improve the contact with the tissue to be frozen, K-Jelly[R] was
applied on the cryoprobe. Cryosurgery was performed using a
3-minute freeze, 3-minute thaw, 3-minute refreeze technique.
Follow-up consisted of cytologic and colposcopic examination
at fixed intervals: 6 weeks, 12 weeks, 6 months, 9 months,
12 months, 18 months and once a year therafter.

Endocervical curettage was performed once a year. Although
it has little value in the selection of patients, this procedure should not be omitted in the follow-up of patients
treated by cryosurgery.

All patients had a copious watery discharge lasting till
their next menstrual period. No one needed analgetics. One
patient developed signs of pelvic inflammatory disease and
was treated accordingly. She had a history of salpingitis.

Results

Cure rates after cryosurgery vary considerably as reported
in the literature (9). This is partly explained by a lack of
uniformity in the assessment of failures and the fact that
results are presented after more than one treatment. Charles
and Savage (9) (1980) recommended in a recent review the following characteristics of failure at 4 months or more after
a single treatment.

Table II

CHARACTERISTICS OF FAILURES

PRETREATMENT		POSTTREATMENT	
CYT.	HIST.	CYT.	HIST.
IIIB	S.D.	6 wks IIIB	TISSUE REPAIR
IV	S.D.	6,12 wks IIIB	CIN III
IV	CIS	6 wks IIIB	CIN I
IV	CIS	6,12 wks IIIB	CIN I

S.D. = severe dysplasia
CIS   = carcinoma in situ
IIIB = suggestive for severe dysplasia
IV   = suggestive for carcinoma in situ

Tissue healing after cryotherapy takes a prolonged time and
the histological differentiation between regenerative processes and CIN is difficult even for experienced pathologists
(12).
The discrepancy between cytology and histology after treatment in 3 or 4 patients occurred only in the beginning of
this study and as our cytologist gained experience in the
judgment of postcryosurgery smears, overreading became less
frequent. Within 4-6 months after cryosurgery a reluctance to
consider further treatments seems justified unless there is
convincing proof of failure. So, in a follow-up of 3-5 years
only one patient with a histological confirmed failure was
encountered. This patient had a very extensive lesion and
needed 5 applications of the probe. Mistakes will come home
to roost. According to the earlier mentioned criteria she
should not have been treated at all.
In our opinion these results, that are in accordance with
other recent reports (13, 14), confirm the statement that
cryosurgery is the treatment of choice for patients with
CIN III, provided that a meticulous preoperative screening

by colposcopy is performed and a careful selection is made of
the patients suitable for this treatment.

References

1. Openchowski, P.H. 1881. On the local effects of cold C.R.
   Soc. Biol. 5, p. 38.
2. Cooper, I.S. and Lee, A.S.J. 1961. Cryothalamectomy-hypo-
   thermic congelation: a technical advance in basal glanglia
   surgery. Preliminary report J. Am. Geriatr. Soc. 9, p. 714.
3. Larsson, G. 1981. Conisation for cervical dysplasia and
   carcinoma in situ. A long-term follow-up of 1013 women.
   An. Chir. Gynaecol., 70, p. 79.
4. Kirkup, W. et al. 1980. The accuracy of colposcopically
   directed biopsy in patientw with suspected intraepithelial
   neoplasia of the cervix. Br. J. Obstet. Gynaecol. 87, p. 1.
5. Crisp, W.E. 1972. Cryosurgical treatment of neoplasia of
   the uterine cervix. Obstet. Gynecol. 39, p. 495.
6. Creasman, W.T. et al. 1973. Efficacy of cryosurgical treatment of severe cervical intraepithelial neoplasia. Obstet.
   Gynecol. 41, p. 501.
7. Crisp, W.E. 1971. In: Cryosurgery in the treatment of
   abnormal cervical lesions: An invitational symposium.
   J. Reprod. Med. 7, p. 147.
8. Anderson, M.C. and Hartley, R.B. 1980. Cervical crypt
   involvement by intraepithelial neoplasia. Obstet. Gynecol.
   55, p. 546.
9. Charles, H.E. and Savage, E.W. 1980. Cryosurgical treatment
   of cervical intraepithelial neoplasia. Obstet. Gynecol.
   Surv. 35, p. 539.
10. Townsend, D.E., Ostergard, D.R. 1971. Cryocauterisation
    for preinvasive cervical neoplasia. J. Reprod. Med. 6,
    p. 171.
11. Elmfors, B., and Stormby, N. 1979. A study of cryosurgery
    for dysplasia and carcinoma in situ of the uterine cervix.
    Br. J. Obstet. Gynaecol. 86, p. 917.
12. Norum, M.L. et al 1969. Ultrastructural changes in normal
    ectocervical epithelium immediately following cryosurgery.
    Lab. Invest. 21, p. 11.
13. Einerth, Y. 1978. Cryosurgical treatment of dysplasia and
    carcinoma in situ of the cervix uteri. Acta Obstet. Gy-
    necol. Scand. 57, p. 361.
14. Popkin, D.R. et al. 1978. Cryosurgery for the treatment
    of CIN. Am. U. Obstet. Gynecol. 130, p. 551.

10. DIAGNOSIS AND TREATMENT OF MICROINVASIVE CERVICAL CANCER

K.J. Lohe

Still today the opinions as to the diagnosis and most appropriate treatment of microinvasive cervical cancer may be called a confusing dilemma. The problems arise because there is no standardized nomenclature, no standardized histologic definition, no standardized size delimitation, no standardized assessment of microscopic vascular invasion, and, finally, no uniform concept about type and extent of the treatment for these lesions.

As to nomenclature, the terms "Mikrokarzinom" in German and "microinvasive carcinoma" in English are most frequently and, in the majority of cases, synonymously used for "carcinoma Stage IA". Other commonly used synonyms are summarized in table I.

Table I
_____

Mikrokarzinom-microinvasive carcinoma-
carcinoma Stage IA
_____

carcinoma in situ with early invasion or minimal stromal invasion, with microscopic or microinvasive foci, with extension on microinvasion, with early invasive changes, or with an invasive focus: intraepithelial carcinoma with microinvasive foci: early cancer: early and very early invasive invasive carcinoma: minimally or microscopic invasive carcinoma: carcinoma with early stromal invasion: cipient or early syperficial carcinoma: superficially invasive or superficial infiltrating carcinoma: early Stage I or IM (micro): small, preclinical, or occult carcinoma: and hidden covert, or possibly clinically latent cancer.
_____

Histologic definition is confusing. The same term is applied
to variably advanced stages of early cancer. Some authors use
the term "microinvasive carcinoma" and mean the morphologic
equivalent of the classical early stromal invasion and include at least some cases with merely suspicious invasive
changes. Others apply the name to a genuine cancer of microscopic dimension but imply that it is no more than stromal
invasion.

The size of the early cervical cancer is given differently
by the authors (Table II). The dimensions of stromal invasion
established by microscopic examination refer to the visual
field, to the tumor diameter, the tumor depth, length, and
width, and, finally, to objects of known size as a pea or a
coffee bean.

Table II
_____

Different parameters used for the definition
of the size of cervical microcarcinoma.
_____

A. Visual field by microscopic examination
    1. Up to one visual field with 40x magnification
    2. Up to two and one-half visual fields with a 10x objective
    3. Up to one visual field with 200 and 400x magnification
    4. Up to one visual field with medium magnification

B. Tumor Diameter
    1. Up to 5 mm
    2. Up to 10 mm

C. Tumor depth
    1. Up to 3 mm
    2. Up to 3-4 mm
    3. Up to 3-5 mm
    4. Up to 5 mm

D. Superficial tumor extent (length, width)
    1. Up to 0.5 cm
    2. Up to 1 cm

E. Objects of known size
    1. Up to a grain of rice, a lentil, a pea, or a coffee bean
_____

Likewise, tumor invasion into blood or lymph vessels proven
by microscopic examination is assessed differently. Especially in view of a possible therapy, some authors attach great
importance to this event, while others do not.

A uniform opinion about the type and scope of treatment for
microinvasive cervical cancer does not exist. Some favour
conservative management and others favour radical methods of
treatment.

In order to find a solution to the problems of beginning cervical cancer, it is necessary to give an exact morphologic
definition of it. From a prognostic and therapeutic point of
view we distinguish today two different forms of beginning
cervical carcinoma: the early stromal invasion and the microcarcinoma (MC).

In early stromal invasion (ESI) variably shaped projections
growing down from the epithelium of the portio, the cervical
canal, or the cervical glands, penetrate the subepithelial
connective tissue. Confluent neoplastic formations have not
yet developed.

In MC a network of infiltrating formations of atypical cells
can be seen. What is true of extended stromal invasion by
carcinoma is also true of microcarcinoma: from the first moment a carcinoma invades the stroma, tumor cells may be found
in lymph- or blood vessels. Qualitatively, MC corresponds in
every respect to the pathologic diagnosis of cancer. The diagnosis of MC implies not only a qualitative evaluation of a
carcinomatous lesion, but also a quantitative assessment of
it. We were the first to introduce a three-dimensional tumor
definition in microinvasive cervical cancer (Fig. 1). Since
1972 we define MC as a carcinoma with a maximum length and
width of 10 mm and a maximum depth of 5 mm. Thus, its maximum
volume measures 500 mm^3. These dimensions are based on the
results of our histologic examination of radically operated
patients suffering from cervical cancer. In small carcinomas
lymph node metastases were detected only in a few cases. In
minute tumors of the above dimensions metastases were never
found. The question whether the size delimitation of MC to

the above-stated magnitude is justified, will be answered
only by an evaluation of an adequately long disease-free survival time after treatment of such patients.

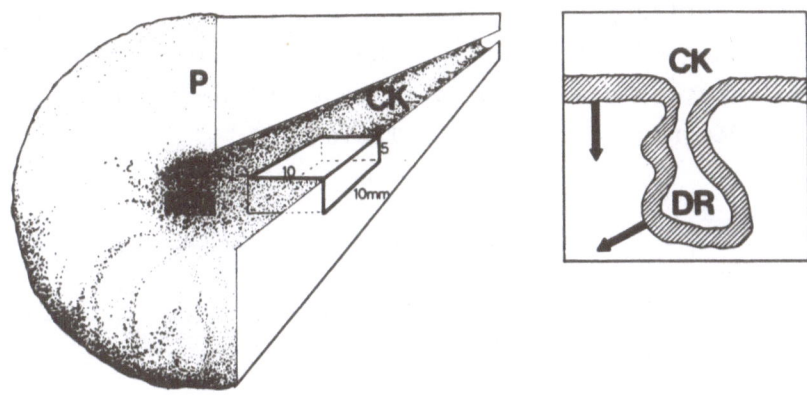

Fig. 1. Half of a conization specimen contains a schematical-
ly represented microcarcinoma with a maximum volume of 500 mm³.
The invasion depth has to be measured vertically to the direction of the atypical epithelium at the surface of the cervical
canal or gland. P. portio vaginalis; MM, external cervical
os; CK. cervical canal; DR, cervical gland.

If the diagnosis of early cervical cancer is to include the
consideration of dimensional parameters, it is essential that
the total abnormal area be available for histologic examination. Strictly speaking, only conization or hysterectomy
will, with a high degree of certainty, guarantee a correct
histologic diagnosis of this beginning cancer. To us, ESI and

MC are not clinical, but histological diagnoses which are closely linked to strict morphological criteria and quantitative assessment.

As a contribution to the controversal problem concerning the proper treatment of early cervical cancer, I collected from six University hospital departments of gynecology the therapeutic results in 285 patients with ESI and 134 patients with MC according to the criteria I have just mentioned. In all six departments, clinical investigation and histologic studies are carried out in a comparable manner. A diagnosis of ESI or MC was made for each of the 419 patients with early cervical cancer on a tissue speciment which guaranteed a reliable diagnostic statement (Table III).

Table III

Clinic	ESI	MC	Total	%
Erlangen	25	17	42	10
Freiburg	60	22	82	20
Graz	99	33	132	32
Heidelberg	10	8	18	4
Cologne	88	52	140	33
Munich	3	2	5	1
TOTAL	285	134	419	100

The different therapeutic modalities applied to the 419 patients with beginning cervical cancer are summarized in Figure 2. The therapy ranges from conization to radical operation with subsequent radiation treatment. Cases with postoperative radiation therapy are indicated by white columns. Vaginal hysterectomy was the preferred therapy in 42% of the 285 patients with ESI and 28% of the 134 patients with MC. With the conization of 23% of the patients with ESI and 12% of the patients with MC, a very restricted method of treatment was chosen. In table IV the patients with conization and

vaginal or abdominal hysterectomy, 72% of all patients with
ESI and 41% of all patients with MC were given minimal or
restricted cancer treatment. A treatment more in line with
the usual cancer therapy was given to 28% of the patients
with ESI and to 59% of the patients with MC, if we add together the radical operations according to the methods of
Schauta-Amreich, Te Linde and Wertheim-Meigs, and all cases
with postoperative radiation treatment.

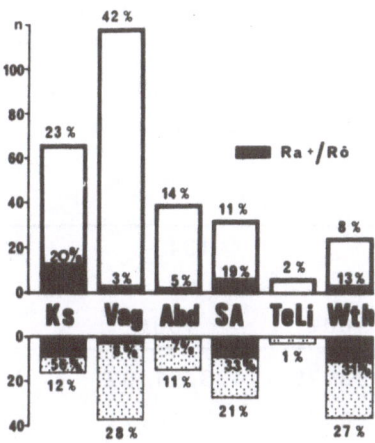

Fig. 2. The different treatments applied at the six clinics
in 285 patients with early stromal invasion (top) and 134 patients with microcarcinoma (bottom); cases with postoperative
radiation therapy are indicated by black columns. Ks,conization
Vag., vaginal hysterectomy; Ab, abdominal hysterctomy; SA,
vaginal radical operation according to the method of Schauta-
Amreich; TeLi, radical operation according to the method of Te
Linde; Wth, radical operation according to the method of Wertheim-Meigs.

Table IV

		TREATMENT	
		restricted (Ks - Vag - Abd)	radical (SA - TeLi - Wth)
285	ESI	72%	28%
134	MC	41%	59%

As I know from looking into the outcome of the 419 patients with early cervical cancer (Table V), none of our patients with ESI, but three of our patients with MC died of cancer, even if a causal association between MC and death was not definitively proven. Table VI gives the so-called survival rates of the 419 treated patients with early squamous cancer of the cervix including all patients lost to follow-up or deceased. The survival rate for our patients with early cervical cancer is on the average 10% higher than that for our patients with stage IB cervical cancer.

Table V

	285 ESI 100%	134 MC 100%	419 EARLY CA. 100%
Alive and well	267/93.7%	123/91.8%	390/93.1%
"Further growth"	2/ 0.7%	1/ 0.7%	3/ 0.7%
Recurrence	4/ 1.4%	3/ 2.2%	7/ 1.7%
Lost to follow-up	6/ 2.1%	4/ 3.0%	10/ 2.4%
Dead			
By early ca.	---	3/ 2.2%	3/ 0.7%
By other causes	12/ 4.2%	4/ 3.0%	16/ 3.8%

Table VI

Survival-rates	ESI	MC	Early ca.
Total	267 of 285 93.7%	123 of 134 91.8%	390 of 419 93.1%
5-years	167 of 176 94.9%	92 of 98 93.9%	259 of 274 94.5%
10-years	63 of 73 86.3%	35 of 41 85.4%	98 of 114 85.9%

For the purpose of discussing and comparing the therapeutic
results presented here, with those reported in the literature,
I tried to apply our definition and classification of cases
of ESI and MC to the published cases. According to our histologic tumor definition, three fairly comparable groups could
be set up:

1) 1203 observations reported in the literature largely
   corresponding to our definition of ESI (Table VII),
2) 435 observations reported in the literature largely
   corresponding to our definition of MC (Table VIII),
3) 1623 observations reported in the literature which, by
   our definition, do not allow a clear separation into
   ESI and MC (Table IX).

The therapeutic results in the three groups of patients are
summarized in Table X. In each group the ratio between radical and restricted treatment of cancer patients is similar.
If I examine the prognosis of all therapeutic procedures taken
together, I come to the conclusion that the risk of dying of
ESI is rather ... Out of our 285 patients none and out of
the 1203 cases ... ported in the literature at the most 4 patients died from their cancer. On the other hand, the risk
of dying of MC seems to be higher. This statement is support-

Table VII

1203 observations reported in the literature, largely corresponding to our definition of ESI

Latour 1957, Dilworth 1962, Christopherson 1964, Ullery 1965,
Green 1966, Margulis 1967, Thompson 1968, Kottmeier 1969, NG
1969, Kolstadt 1969, Boyed 1970, Marcuse 1971, Boutselis 1971,
Averette 1976, Duncan 1977, Wilkinson 1978.

Table VIII

---

435 observations reported in the literature, largely corresponding to our definition of MC

Kottmeier 1969, Boyes 1970, Mestwerdt 1973

Table IX

1623 observations reported in the literature which, by our
definition, do not allow a clear separation into ESI and MC

Held 1961, Holtorff 1962, Way 1964, Przybora 1965, Uhlmann
1966, Coppleson 1967, Roman 1967, Myssey 1969, Foushee 1969,
Mosler 1970, Brandl 1970, Artner 1971, Tscharf 1972, Christopherson 1976, Ruch 1976, Leman 1976, Seski 1977, Sedlis
1979

---

ed by the fact that 14 of 435 patients with MC reported in
the literature died of cancer as well as three of our 134 patients, even if a causal association between MC and death
was not definitely proven.

Table X

	ESI		MC		ESI/MC	
	285	1203	134	435	419	1263
	own	published	own	published	own	published
	cases	cases	cases	cases	cases	cases
Radical treatment	28%	30%	59%	50%	38%	49%
Restricted treatment	72%	70%	41%	50%	62%	51%
Cancer death	--	0.3% (4)	2% (3)	3% (14)	0.7% (3)	0.5% (7)

Table XI

Early cervical carcinoma: Lymph node metastases

Up to 1%: Braitenberg 1962, Kauffmann 1965, Fettig 1969, Hil-
          lemanns 1969, Ruch 1970, Mosler 1970, Stark 1972,
          Friedberg 1972, Benson 1977, Fennell Jr. 1978

Up to 2%: Zinser 1963, Ober 1969, Castano-Almendral 1969,
          Käser, 1969, Seski 1977

Up to 3%: Younge 1959, Bajardi 1976, Kolstadt 1969

Up to 4%: Belliveau 1966, Averette 1976

Up to 6%: Boutselis 1971

Up to 10%: Levitt 1965

The large number of patients cured of early cervical cancer after restricted treatment indicates that in most cases the decisive criterion for a successful treatment is the total elimination of the tumor from the cervix. Morphologic tumor characteristics may be of importance for prognosis. The tissue specimens of the three MC's from our deceased patients show in each case an intensely dissociating tumor growth with marked lymphatic invasion. The importance of lymphatic invasion in MC is well demonstrated by the one fatal case within the series of Burghardt and Holzer. They report a very carefully investigated MC with a maximum tumor volume of 315 mm³ and striking lymphatic vascular invasion. The patient died three years after hysterectomy of fulminant metastatic spread to lymph nodes and distant organs. Therefore, for the moment, one should take these morphologic characteristics into consideration when choosing therapy.

Metastases in lymph nodes of the pelvic wall play an important part within the whole set of problems regarding early cervical cancer. Reported frequencies range from 0.1 to 10% (Table XI). Examining the frequency of histologically proven lymph node metastases in the published cases of early cervical cancer as defined by us, in which surgical treatment included lymphadenectomy. I found metastatic tumor invasion of the pelvic lymph nodes in only 3 of 1050 patients (0.3%). Follow-up examination of these 3 patients did not reveal any recurrence (Table XII).

Table XII

Early cervical cancer: 1050 lymphonodectomies and 3 cases with nodal involvement

Held 1961, Christopherson 1964, Way 1964, Ullery 1965, Margulis 1967, Coppleson 1967, Thompson 1968, NG 1969, Kolstadt 1969, Myssey 1969, Foushee 1969, Brandl 1970, Boutselis 1971, Artner 1971, Tscharf 1972, Mestwerdt 1973, Roche 1975, Christopherson 1976. Ruch 1976, Leman 1976, Averette 1976, Seski 1977, Boronow 1977, Duncan 1977, Deslis 1979

On the other hand, under critical assessment and in the light of our criteria, out of 35 cases of so-called MC with lymph node metastases published in the literature, only 5 cases, at best, may actually be regarded as such. The fact that none of these 5 patients died of her disease is of particular significance (Table XIII).

Table XIII
_____

So-called Microcarcinomas with lymph node metastases

Lax 1953, Decker 1956, Schüller 1958, Friedell 1959, Fanger 1960, Lange 1960, Lock 1961, Walz 1962, Braitenberg 1962, Zinser 1963, Christopherson 1964, Enterline 1965, Mussey 1969, Foushee 1969, Kolstadt 1969, Sidhu 1970, Brandl 1970, Froewis 1971, Ruch 1976

_____

Therefore, metastatic involvement of the regional lymph nodes in early cervical cancer as defined by us, is the exception, indeed, and it is observed in less than 1% of the patients. In all these cases only lymph nodes of the pelvic wall were involved. The literature discloses not a single case in which early cervical cancer was accompanied by metastatic invasion of parametrial lymph nodes.

These statements explain the fact that the so-called extended cancer management applied to early cervical cancer, does not guarantee a 100% cure. In few fatal cases reported in the literature, tumor spread seems to have taken place before therapy was instituted.

From my investigations I conclude that

1) to cure ESI as well as carcinoma in situ a total elimination of the lesion by conization or simple hysterectomy is sufficient;

2) MC, due to the higher risk involved as compared with ESI, calls for a more extensive therapy according to the morphologic criteria of the primary tumor. In the majority of cases a simple hysterectomy is sufficient.

If vascular tumor invasion is diagnosed before operation, additional lymphadenectomy is advisable. However,
radical removal of the parametrial tissues is unneccess-
ary and, thus, the most severe postoperative complications, such as ureteric lesions, can be avoided;

3) it would be desirable if such definite microscopic
   criteria for early cervical cancer were accepted inter-
   nationally. Worldwide standardized diagnostic procedure
   is the prerequisite for determining the minimal, effective and safe treatment of this lesion.

References

1. Artner, J., and Holzner, H. 1971. Zur Frage der beginnenden Stromainvasion des Zervixkarzinoms, Zschr. Geburtsh.
   Gynäkol. 175, 209-217.
2. Antoine, T. 1962. Symposium on cervical lesions: May one
   treat the "early invasive carcinoma (microcarcinoma)"
   less radically than the more extensive invasive carcinoma; Acta Cytol. 6, 173.
3. Artner, J. and Holzner, H. 1972. Zur Definition und Behandlung des histologischen Stadiums IA des Cervixcarcinoms,
   Arch. Gynäkol 212, 195-216.
4. Bajardi, F. 1966. Das frühinvasive Kollumkarzinom, Krebs-
   arzt 22, 110-111.
5. Belliveau, R.R. and Grayson, J.W. 1966. Current concepts
   in microinvasive carcinoma of the uterine cervix, Rocky
   Mt. Med. J. 63, 40-42.
6. Boutselis, J.G., Ullery, J.C. and Charme, L. 1971. Diagnosis and management of stage IA (microinvasive) carcinoma of the cervix, Amer. J. Obstet. Gynecol. 110, 984-
   989.
7. Boyes, D.A., Worth, A.J. and Fidler, H.K. 1970. The results of treatment of 4389 cases of pre-clinical cervical
   squamous carcinoma. J. Obstet. Gynaecol. Brit. Commonw.
   77, 769-780.
8. Braitenberg, H., and Schüller, E. 1962. 700 Konisationen
   der Portio vaginalis uteri zur histologischen Abklärung
   bei Krebsverdacht, Geburtsh. Frauenheilk. 22, 701-731.
9. Brandl, K., Georgiades, E. and Kraus, U. 1970. Die Bedeu-
   tung der Portioamputation und Konisation als diagnostische
   und therapeutische Massnahme nach suspekter oder positiver
   Routineuntersuchung der Portio vaginalis uteri. Zschr.
   Geburtsh. Gynäkol. 172, 113-130.
10. Castano-Almendral, A. and Käser, O. 1969. Probleme der
    Behandlung des Collumcarcinoms, Gynäkologe 1, 187-197.
11. Christopherson, W.M. and Parker, J.E. 1964. Microinvasive
    carcinoma of the uterine cervix, Cancer 17, 1123-1131.

12. Coppleson, M. and Reid, B. 1967. Preclinical carcinoma of the cervix uteri. Its nature, origin and management, Pergamon press. Oxford.
13. Decker, W.M. 1956. Minimal invasive carcinoma of the cervix with lymph node metastases, Amer. J. Obstet. Gynecol. 72, 1116-1119.
14. Dilworth, E.E. and Maxwell, G.E. 1962. Superficially invasive carcinoma and carcinoma in situ of the uterine cervix, Amer. J. Obstet. Gynecol. 84, 83-88.
15. Enterline, H.T. 1965. Management of microinvasive carcinoma, J. Amer. Med. Assoc. 193, 220-222.
16. Fanger, H. and Murphy, T.H. 1960. Carcinoma in situ of the uterine cervix. Surg. Gynecol. Obstet. 111, 177-182.
17. Fettig, O. 1969. Zur Klinik des Mikrokarzinoms (Collum-Ca. Stad. Ia), Mitt. Ges. Bekämpf, Krebskrankh. Nordrhein-Westfalen e.V. 5, 561-562.
18. Fidler, H.K. and Boyd, J.R. 1960. Occult invasive squamous carcinoma of the cervix. Cancer 12, 764-771.
19. Foushee, J.H.S., Greiss, F.C. and Lock, F.R. 1969. Stage IA squamous cell carcinoma of the uterine cervix. Amer. J. Obstet. Gynecol. 105, 46-58.
20. Frick, H.C., Janovski, N.A., Gusberg, S.B. and Taylor, H.C. 1963. Early invasive cancer of the cervix, Amer. J. Obstet. Gynecol. 85, 926-937.
21. Friedberg, V., Käser, O., Ober, K.G., Thomasen, K. and Zander J. 1972. Behandlung der Uteruskarzinome, in Gynäkologie und Geburtshilfe (O. Käser, V. Friedberg, K.G. Ober, K. Thomsen, and J. Zander, Eds.), Thieme, Stuttgart, Bd. III.
22. Friedell, G.H. and Graham, J.B. 1959. Regional lymph node involvement in small carcinoma of the cervix, Surg. Gynecol. Obstet. 108, 513-517.
23. Froewis, J. 1962. Zur Frage der karzinomatösen Lymphknotenbesiedlung beim Collumkarzinom (kasuistischer Beitrag), Wien, Klin. Wochenschr. 74, 357-358.
24. Froewis, J., Zischka-Konorsa, W., and Kremer, H. 1969. Der tatsächliche Krebsbefall von Parametrien und Lymphknoten bei örtlich anatomischem Stadium I des Kollumkrebses, Wien. Klin. Wochenschr. 81, 667-672.
25. Froewis, J. and Ulm, R. 1971. Untersuchungen über den Karzinomsbefall der Lymphknoten bei 1358 operierten Karzinomen des Collum uteri, Wien. Klin. Wochenschr. 83, 153-156.
26. Green, G.H. 1966. The significance of cervical carcinoma in situ, Amer. J. Obstet. Gynecol. 94, 1009-1022.
27. Held, E. 1961. Wann und wie operieren wir Collumcarcinome? Gynaecologia 151, 89-94.
28. Hillemanns, H.G. 1969. Das Cervixcarcinom, Gynäkologe 1, 150-166.
29. Hillemanns, H.G. and Limburg, H. Dysplasie-Carcinoma in situ-Mikrokarzinom, in Handbuch der speziellen pathologische Anatomie und Histologie (O. Lubarsch, F. Henke, R. Rössle, and E. Uehlinger, Eds.), Springer, Berlin, Bd.VII/4.

108

30. Hochuli, E. 1970. Die vaginale Hysterektomie, Geburtsh.
    Frauenheilk. 30, 589-601.
31. Holtorff, J. 1962. Zur Therapie des Mikrokarzinoms am
    Collum uteri. Geburtsh. Frauenheilk. 22, 1097-1101.
32. Huhn, F.O. 1964. Die Lymphknotenveränderungen beim Zer-
    vixkarzinom und die Beziehungen Tumorgrösse und lympho-
    gene Tumorausbreitung, Habilitationsschrift, Köln.
33. Käser, O. 1969. Die formale und klinische Problematik des
    beginnenden Cervixcarcinoms, in Rundtischgespräch zum
    IV. Hauptthema, Arch. Gynäkol. 207, 353.
34. Kaufmann, C., Ober, K.G. and Huhn, F.O. 1965. Das begin-
    nende Karzinom der Cervix uteri (sog. Microkarzinom). Ein
    Erfahrungsbericht zur Prognose und Therapie an Hand von
    130 Beobachtungen, Geburtsh. Frauenheilk. 25, 112-131.
35. Kern, G. 1964. Carcinoma in situ. Vorstadium des Gebär-
    mutterhalskrebses, Springer, Berlin.
36. Kirkland, J.A. 1966. The cytological and histological
    diagnosis of dysplasia, carcinoma in situ and early in-
    vasive carcinoma of the cervix, Aust. N.Z. J. Obstet. Gy-
    naecol. 6, 15-19.
37. Kolstadt, P. 1969. Carcinoma of the cervix stage IA. Diag-
    nosis and treatment, Amer. J. Obstet. Gynecol. 104, 1015-
    1022.
38. Kottmeier, J.L. 1969. Erfahrungen des Radiumhemmet. Stock-
    holm, mit der Behandlung des Oberflächencarcinoms und des
    frühinvasiven Carcinoms der Cervix, Arch. Gynäkol. 207,
    332-342.
39. Lange, P. 1960. Part II. Pelvic node metastasis in early
    cancer of the cervix, in Clinical and histological studies
    on cervical carcinoma: Precancerosis, early metastases
    and tubular structures in the lymph nodes, Acta Pathol.
    Microbiol. Scand. Suppl. 143 50, 52-119.
40. Latour, J.P.A., Brown, L.B. and Turnbull, L.A. 1957. Pre-
    clinical carcinoma of the cervix, Amer. J. Obstet. Gyne-
    col. 74, 354-360.
41. Lax, H. 1953. Das Oberflächencarcinom, Zschr. Geburtsh.
    Gynäkol. 138, 105-153.
42. Levitt, S.H. and Rubin, P. 1965. Early invasive carcinoma
    of the cervix. A problem of definition and treatment. Ra-
    diology 85, 711-715.
43. Lock, F.R. 1961. Discussion to: J.P.A. Latour: Results
    in the management of preclinical carcinoma of the cervix,
    Amer. J. Obstet. Gynecol. 81, 511-520.
44. Lohe, K.J. 1978. Early squamous cell carcinoma of the
    uterine cervix. I. Definition and histology, Gynecol. On-
    col. 6, 10-30.
45. Marcuse, P.M. 1971. Incipient microinvasive carcinoma of
    the uterine cervix. Morphology and clinical data of 22
    cases, Obstet. Gynecol. 37, 360-367.
46. Margulis, R.R., Ely, C.W. and Ladd, J.E. 1967. Diagnosis
    and management of stage IA (microinvasive) carcinoma of
    the cervix, Obstet. Gynecol. 29, 529-538.
47. Mestwerdt, G. and Wespi, H.J. 1973. Atals der Kolposlopie,
    Fischer, Stuttgart, 4th ed.
48. Mosler, W., Kaiser, P. and Randow, H. Die abgestufte Be-

handlung der Vor- und Frühstadien des Zervixkarzinoms,
Deut. Gesundheitsw. 25, 2222-2225.

49. Mussey, E., Soule, E.H. and Welch, J.S. 1969. Microinvasive carcinoma of the cervix. Late results of operative
treatment in 91 cases, Amer. J. Obstet. Gynecol. 104,
738-744.

50. Ng, A.B.P. and Reagan, J.W. 1969. Microinvasive carcinoma
of the uterine cervix, Amer. J. Clin. Pathol. 52, 511-529.

51. Ng, A.B.P., Reagan, J.W. and Lindner, E.A. 1972. The cellular manifestations of microinvasive squamous cell carcinoma of the uterine cervix, Acta Cytol. 16, 5-13.

52. Ober, K.G. and Huhn, F.O. 1962. Arch. Gynäkol. 197, 262-
290.

53. Ober, K.G., Kaufmann, C., and Hamperl, H. 1961. Carcinoma
in situ, beginnendes Karzinom und klinischer Krebs der
Cervix uteri. - Ihre Diagnose und Therapie sowie ihr Ein-
fluss auf Ergebnisse der Kregsbehandlung, Geburtsh. Frauenheilk. 21, 259-297.

54. Ober, K.G. 1969. Die formale und klinische Problematik
des beginnenden Cervixcarcinoms, in Rundtischgespräch zum
IV. Hauptthema, Arch. Gynäkol. 207, 354.

55. Przybora, L.A. 1965. Incipient invasion of cervical cancer: Morphological aspects of carcinogenesis in 74 cases,
Gynaecologia (Basel) 160, 69-86.

56. Roman, T.N. and Latour, J.P.A. 1967. The effect of early
diagnosis on survival statistics in carcinoma of the uterine cervix, Amer. J. Obstet. Gynecol. 97, 739-749.

57. Ruch, R.M. 1970. Microinvasive carcinoma of the cervix -
a confusing dilemma, South. Med. J. 63, 1123-1126.

58. Schüller, E. 1958. Carcinoma colli uteri incipiens, Arch.
Gynäkol. 190, 520-548.

59. Sidhu, G.S., Koss, L.G. and Barber, H.R.K. 1970. Relation
of histologic factors to the response of stage I epidermoid
carcinoma of the cervix to surgical treatment, analysis
of 115 patients, Obstet, Gynecol. 35, 329-338.

60. Silverberg, S.G., Frable, W.J. and Dunn, L.L. 1971. Dysplasia and early carcinoma of the uterine cervix - Detection, diagnostic evaluation and management, Virginia Med.
Monthly 98, 444-448.

61. Stark, G. 1972. Die klinische Früherkennung von Karzinomen in der Gynaekologie, in Schnelldiagnostik und Sofort-
therapie - Krebsfrüherkennung, Schriftenreihe der Bayeri-
schen Landesärztekammer, Bd. 28, München.

62. Thompson, W.R. 1968. Microinvasive carcinoma of the uterine cervix, J. Arkansas Med. Soc. 65, 139-144.

63. Tscharf, H. 1972. Zur Behandlung der Frühstadien des Zervixkarzinoms, Ärztl. Prax. 24, 4608.

64. Uhlmann, G. 1966. Therapie und Heilungsergebnisse bei
Frühkarzinomen des Collum uteri, Geburtsh. Frauenheilk.
26, 775-780.

65. Ullery, J.C., Boutselis, J.G. and Botschner, A.C. 1965.
Microinvasive carcinoma of the cervix, Obstet. Gynecol.
26, 866-875.

66. Ulm, R. 1972. Kollum-Ca: Lymphknoten mitentfernen, Med.
Tribune Kongressber. 7, 1.

110

67. Walz, W. 1962. Symposium on cervical lesions: May one treat the "early invasive carcinoma (microcarcinoma)" less radically than the more extensive invasive carcinoma? Acta Cytol. 6, 176.
68. Way, S. 1964. Microinvasive carcinoma of the cervix, Acta Cytol. 8, 14-15.
69. Younge, P.A. and Kevorkian, A.Y. 1959. Carcinoma in situ of the cervix. The problems of detection and evaluation in regard to therapy, in CIBA Foundation Study Group No 3, Cancer of the cervix. DIAGNOSIS of early forms, London, 83-96.
70. Zinser, H.K., Meissner, H. and Bötzelen, H.P. 1963. Diagnostische und therapeutische Betrachtungen an 403 Frühfällen, Geburtsh. Frauenheilk. 23, 321-342.

11.SURGICAL TREATMENT OF CERVICAL CANCER BY THE WERTHEIM-OKABAYASHI PROCEDURE

F.B. Lammes, K. Sekiba

Okabayashi published as early as 1921 his technique of radical abdominal hysterectomy. It was not proposed by him as a new technique but more as a modification of the operation performed by his teacher Prof. Takayama, who perfected the original Wertheim procedure by operating on 200 cases each year. Okabayashi places emphasis on the extended radicality of extirpation of the parametrium and perfecting the technique in detail. Later on, in 1955, Yagi wrote again from Okayama about the Okabayashi modification.

The principles of the Okabayashi procedure can be found in three points:
1. the usage of avascular spaces
2. cleavage of recto-uterine ligaments before managing the vascular web
3. dissecting the ureter at the end of the procedure because of the increased mobility of the uterus.

Okabayashi himself rarely removed lymphglands; in the modification of Sekiba it is an indispensable part of the operation. It is very important to use the anatomical possibilities of the avascular spaces in the pelvis. Knowledge of these opportunities gives the operation the combination of great radicality and low morbidity.

There are different modifications of the Okabayashi procedure in Japan. Sakamoto in Tokyo developed a method to separate the pelvic nerves and parasymphatic plexus hopefully trying to prevent the difficulties of the neurogenic bladder[*]. Not every

* See also chapter 9 (Eds).

one in Japan is convinced that this problem can be prevented
by this method. Sekiba in Okayama thinks that the risks of
undertreatment by less radicality cannot be neglected, while
the advantages of this modification are not statistically
proved.

The experience in Rotterdam with the Okabayashi operation has
shown that the pure anatomical dissection gives the possibility
of an extensive dissection of the pelvis with very little morbidity. The brilliance of the operation is however also dependant of the possibility to repeat the operation frequently.
The different steps of Sekiba's modification of Okabayashi
procedure are:

1. no cauterisation of the tumour or other vaginal surgical
   procedure
2. median laparotomy
3. inspection and palpation
4. ligation of lig. rotunda not far from uterus for leaving
   peritoneum for closure
5. opening of retroperitoneum as high as the bifurcation
6. lymphadenectomy from bifurcation until internal inguinal
   nodes
7. sliding behind ramus pubis the paravesical fossa is
   opened and the fossa is widened with blunt dissection
   and retractors
8. separation of the iliac vessels from psoas muscle and
   complete clearing of the obturator fossa. The dissection
   is done partly laterally and partly under the iliac
   vessels
9. careful opening of the pararectal fossa and widening with
   retractors
10. separating umbilical artery by placing retractor between
    vesical artery and uterine artery
11. ligation of uterine artery at origin
12. isolation of ureter from posterior leaf of peritoneum
    and following dissection along medial side of ureter
    wall until crossing with uterine artery
13. ligation and cleavage of infundibudal pelvic ligament,

or displacement of ovaries

14. incision of peritoneum of Douglas extending over the
    sacral uterine ligaments
15. dissecting space between vagina and rectum and wide ex-
    posing sacro-uterine ligaments
16. placing the wide retractors in the fossa pararectalis
17. stepwise cleavage of sacro-uterine ligaments on safe
    but short distance of rectum until the approachment with
    cardinal ligament
18. clamping of cardinal ligaments closely to the lateral
    pelvic wall in one or two steps with strong curved for-
    ceps
19. same procedure left side
20. the uterus is pulled anterior out of the pelvic towards
    the ceiling by holding the cervix
21. the uterine artery is hold with forceps and gauze; by
    squeezing at the crossing, the uretercanal is visualized
22. the ureteric tunnel is bluntly dissected with the point
    of special scissors on the medial side of the ureter
23. the anterior part of the vesico uterine ligament is
    stepwised ligated with slender curved forceps, clamped
    and incised after ligation
24. the posterior vesico uterine ligament is stretched and
    bluntly pierced in the avascular triangle. Two straight
    forceps are placed. Incision and ligation of this liga-
    ment
25. suturing the paravaginal tissue with non-absorble suture
    and clamping and cleavage thereafter
26. incision of the vagina wall with diathermy
27. drainage of bilateral dead pelvic space in the corners
    of the vagina. The rest of the vagina is closed by con-
    tinuous dexon sutures
28. peritonisation with interrupted sutures
29. Sekiba dilates the urethra with Hegar 16 afterwards for
    preventing urineretention.

The results of the operation performed in Okayama University
Hospital are presented in Table I, II, III and IV.

Table I

Relation between Postoperative   Histological Extension
and 5 Year Survival Rate (1970-1975, Okayama Univ.)

Postoperative histological extension		Cases	5 year surv. rate
Extrauterine extension	−	358	98.0% (351/358)
	+	250	80.4% (201/250)
Lymph node metastasis	−	526	94.5% (497/526)
	+	82	67.1% (55/ 82)
Parametrial extension	−	503	94.8% (477/503)
	+	105	71.4% (75/105)
Vaginal extension	−	457	93.2% (426/457)
	+	150	84.0% (126/150)
Total		608	90.8% (552/608)

Table II   Duration of operation

Cases	Minutes	
53	60- 90	
141	90-120	
108	120-150	Total : 387 cases
59	150-180	Minimum: 65 min.
16	180-210	Maximum: 310 min.
7	210-240	Average: 133 min.
1	240-270	
2	270-300	

1975-1979 Okayama University

Table III   Amount of Blood Loss.

Cases	ml		
4	0- 250		
32	250- 500		
73	500- 750		
92	750-1000		
99	1000-1250		
31	1250-1500	Total	: 387 cases
32	1500-1750	Minimum:	200 ml
11	1750-2000	Maximum:	2713 ml
4	2000-2250	Average:	1037 ml
4	2250-2500		
5	2500-2750		

1975-1979 Okayama University

Table IV

Complication of Radical Hysterectomy	%
Death during operation	0 %
Pyelitis	9.0%
Urinary fistula	0 %
Retroperitoneal inflammation	7.5%

1970-1975, 608 cases in Okayama University

References

Okabayashi, H. 1921. Surg. Gyn. Obst. 33, 335-341
Yagi, H. 1955. Am. J. Obst. Gyn. 69, 33-47
Sakomoto, S. 1982. Gyn. Oncology, vol. 2 ed Churchill

12. SURGICAL TREATMENT OF CERVICAL CANCER BY THE A.V.R.U.E.L.
PROCEDURE

B.W. Ketting, O.P. Bleker

Introduction

The first attempts to surgically remove cancerous lesions of
the uterine cervix, date from the second half of the 19th century. Radical hysterectomy war performed vaginally by Schauta,
abdominally by Wertheim.
Between 1920 and 1940 surgical treatment was generally replaced
by radiotherapy. After that period operation again became more
the method of choice in stage I and IIA cases.

Description of the A.V.R.U.E.L. procedure

This operation is a combination of an abdominal transperitoneal
lymphadenectomy and a vaginal radical hysterectomy. (Abdominal
and Vaginal Radical Uterus Extirpation and Lymphadenectomy).
Sindram developed this procedure in 1957 and published a description in 1959 and 1960 (11, 12). Aartsen (1) published an
atlas of the operation. The operative procedure combines the
advantages of parts of the Wertheim operation, the abdominal
lymphadenectomy after Taustig (13) and the Schauta operation.
The first phase is an abdominal examination to determine the
local extent of the tumour process and of metastatic growth.
A transperitoneal pelvic lymphadenectomu is performed and the
operative specimen is freed from the infundibulopelvic and
round ligaments and the large vessels.
In the second or vaginal phase, a vaginal cuff is prepared,
followed by completion of the radical hysterectomy per vaginam.
_The performance of the transperitoneal lymphadenectomy as
opposed to the extraperitoneal method, advocated by Mitra, enables examination of the lymph nodes, by inspection and pal-

pation in the pelvis as well as along the aorta. The Schauta
hysterectomy, following the lymphadenectomy, is considered
superior because it allows the removal of more parametrial
tissue than can be removed when using the abdominal Wertheim
procedure.

A. The abdominal phase of the operation:
Before the operation, the bladder is emptied by a urethral
catheter and a rectal cannula is introduced to prevent distention of the rectosigmoid. After preparation of the skin, the
abdomen is draped. A median or paramedian incision is made.
The peritoneum is opened and a Semm's retractor is inserted.
The internal genitalia, parametria and lymph nodes along the
large vessels are palpated. Palpable lymph nodes above the bifurcation of the aorta or above the sacral promontory, are dissected and submitted for frozen section examination by the
pathologist. The planned operation is performed if the parametria seem non-invaded, no tumour is detectable outside the
cervix or in the pelvic or extrapelvic lymph nodes. In the remaining cases, primary radiotherapy is preferred and the operation is discontinued. After inspection and palpation of the
ureter, the infundibulopelvic ligament is doubly ligated and
cut as high as possible, with an aneurysm needle. The round
ligament is also doubly ligated and cut, but care must be taken
to leave the pelvic portion long enough to allow fixation to
the apex of the vagina at the end of the operation. The uterus
is pulled aside by traction, the ovary and tube with an ovary
clamp (fig. 1). Using both sharp and blunt dissection, the
layers of the broad ligament are opened. Lymph node dissection
with polyp forceps begins along the external iliac artery (fig.
2). Afterwards, the lymph nodes along the common iliac artery
are dissected. This procedure often causes small haemorrhage.
During slight traction on the round ligament, the internal
inguinal lymph nodes are grasped by polyp forceps and dissected.
The obturator fossa is opened by bluntly dissecting the external iliac vessels, from the psoas muscle. The external iliac
artery and vein are pushed medially, while the psoas muscle is

118

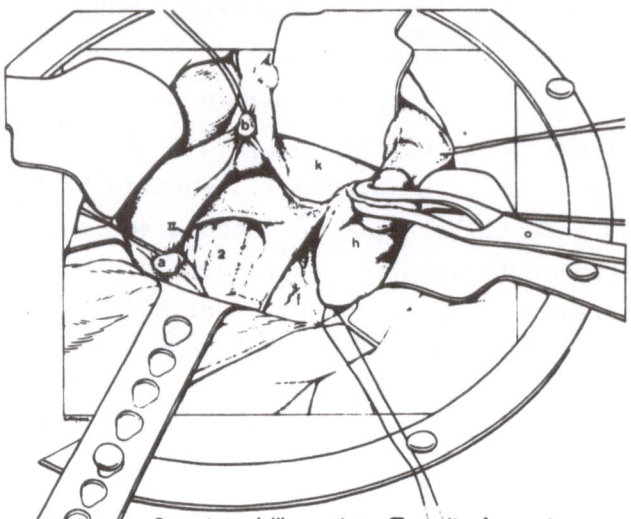

2. external iliac artery; II genito-femoral nerve;

Fig.1   a. infundibulo pelvic ligament

b. round ligament; f. sigmoid; h.uterus; k. bladder

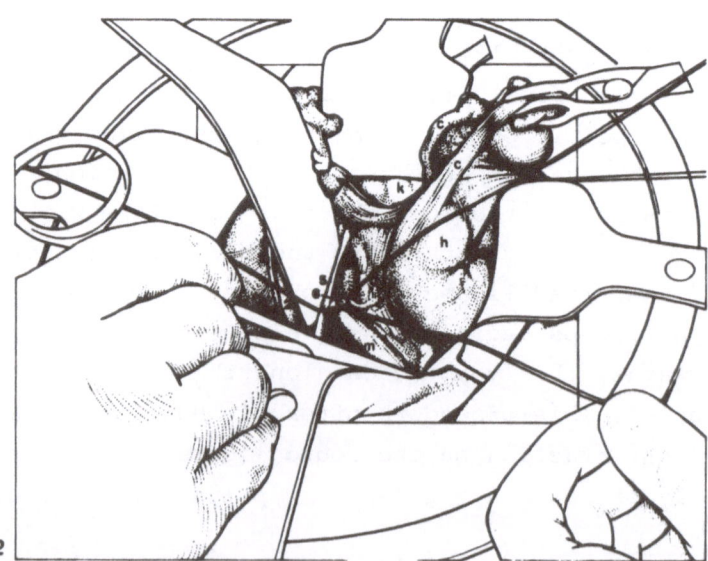

Figure 2

2. external iliac artery; 5. lateral umbilical ligament; 6.uterine artery; c. Fallopian
tube; h. uterus; k. bladder, m. ureter.

held laterally by a retractor. The obturator nerve is located
and fat and lymph nodes along that nerve are mobilized distally
with the polyp forceps (fig. 3).
Special care is taken not to damage the veins at the bottom of
the obturator fossa. The external iliac vessels are kept behind the retractor and the tissue around the obturator nerve
is dessected "en-bloc" along the obturator nerve towards the
pelvic side-wall guided by the index finger (fig. 3).

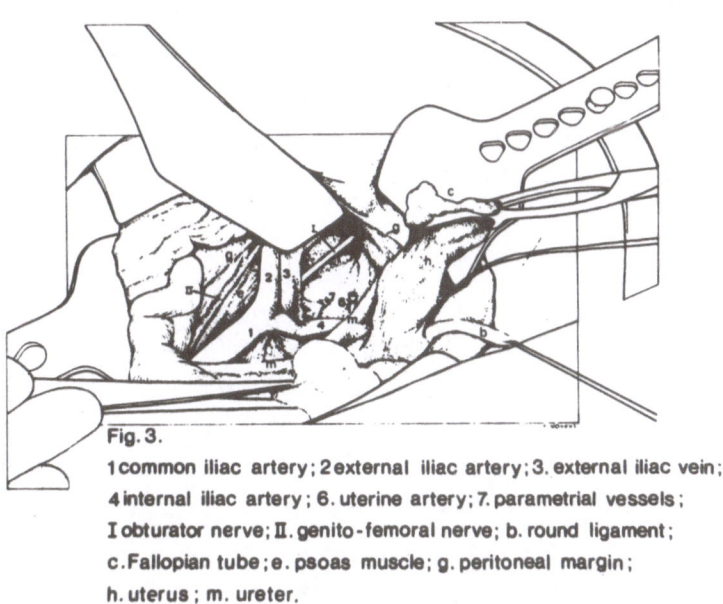

Fig. 3.

1 common iliac artery; 2 external iliac artery; 3. external iliac vein;
4 internal iliac artery; 6. uterine artery; 7. parametrial vessels;
I obturator nerve; II. genito-femoral nerve; b. round ligament;
c. Fallopian tube; e. psoas muscle; g. peritoneal margin;
h. uterus; m. ureter.

The paravesical space is opened bluntly to the pelvic floor.
With polyp forceps, all adipose tissue and pelvic nodes are
dissected from the paravesical space and from the parametrium.
Care must be taken to grasp only tissue to be removed and not
the blood vessels in the polyp forceps. The tension applied to the
forceps in order to prevent serious haemorrhage is a matter of
experience.
Dissected vessels should be ligated and cut.

By blunt dissection, the ureter is mobilized from the large
vessels. The uterine artery and vein and the lateral umbilical
ligament (= obliterated hypogastric ligament) are now identified. The uterine vessels are ligated and cut near the internal
iliac artery and vein. The lateral umbilical ligament is freed
from the bladder and may be removed or left on the specimen
to be removed later. Lymph node dissection along the internal
iliac vessels is now performed. After careful inspection of
the haemostasis, the same procedure is performed on the opposite side.

After lymphadenectomy and ligation of the uterine vessels on
both sides, the bladder is dessected from the uterus in the
conventional way, until it is reflected below the cervical
tumour. The bladder peritoneum is partly dissected from the
bladder itself, in order to obtain a greater peritoneal flap
to cover the pelvis (fig. 4).

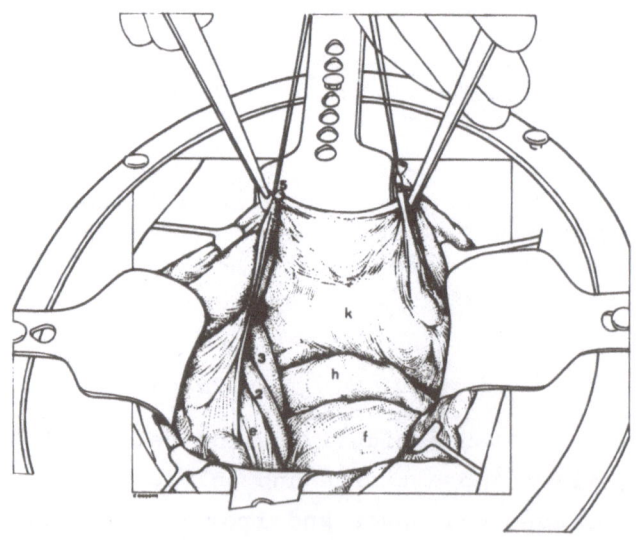

Figure 4

2. external iliac artery; 3. external iliac vein; 5. lateral umbilical ligament; e. psoas
muscle; f. sigmoid; h. uterus; k. bladder.

The round ligament sutures are kept long, lossely tied together and left underneath the peritoneum to be picked up at
the end of the operation and fixed at the transected vagina.
On both sides the peritoneal margins of the broad ligament
are sutured together in order to leave the cut ovarian vessels
underneath the peritoneum. Care must be taken not to touch
the ureter. The bladder peritoneum is sutured to the sigmoid
and in this way the true pelvis is closed from above and the
specimen to be removed later is left underneath that peritoneal abdominal floor (fig. 5). The abdominal wall is closed as
usual.

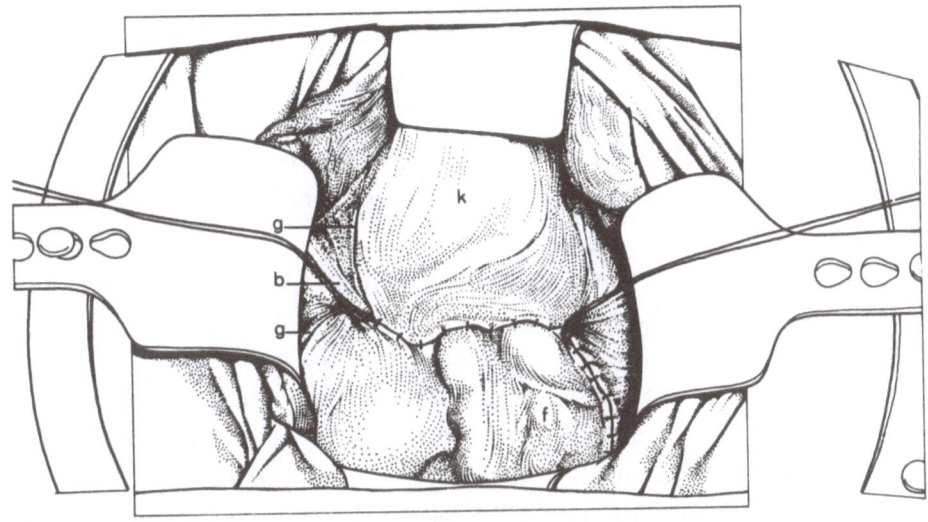

Figure 5
  b. round ligament f. sigmoid; g. peritoneal margin; k. bladder.

B. The vaginal phase of the operation.
The patient is now placed into an extended lithotomy position,
using special leg-holding-stockings. The bladder is again emptied with a urethral catheter and the vulvar area is prepared
and draped. The vagina is desinfected by the surgeon. In the
case of large exophytic tumours, reduction with electrocoagulation may be safely performed, since all important nourish-

ing vessels have already been ligated during the abdominal
stage of the operation. A gauze,drenched in 96% alcohol, is
placed against the surface of the tumour. Infiltration with
a 1:200.000 nor-adrenalin solution (about 30 ml. on each side)
is now performed in the areas of the Schuchardt incision which
will be made later.

The area of the intended vaginal cuff is then infiltrated to
reduce subsequent haemorrhage. The vaginal cuff is now dissected. The anterior and posterior vaginal walls are grasped
by tenaculae at a tumour-free distance from the cervical tumour,
and the vaginal wall is incised in a circular fashion. After
further dissection of the vaginal cuff with scissors, the cuff
is closed over the alcohol gauze with nylon sutures and tied
together with two adjacent sutures in order to obtain more
space (fig. 6). The vagina is thoroughly washed with alcohol
96% to prevent any spill of tumour cells. After renewed preparation and draping of the vulvar area and change of instru-
ments, draping sheets, gowns and gloves the operation is continued.

Two mediolateral perineal Schuchardt incisions are made and
haemostasis is carefully obtained. While the vaginal cuff is
pulled upward, the rectum is dissected up to the peritoneum
of the posterior cul-de-sac (fig. 7). The rectum is covered
with a surgical pad and a retractor holds it downwards.

The vaginal cuff is pulled downwards. The bladder is dissected
from the vagina and uterus with scissors. In this way the anterior fold of the peritoneum, already opened during the abdominal
stage, is reached (fig. 8). A large bladder retractor is now
introduced. Care should be taken to perforate neither the
bladder nor the vaginal cuff.

The dissection of the ureter from the vesico-uterine pillar
and the ureteral tunnel is now started (fig. 9). The specimen
is pulled in the opposite direction and by blunt dissection
an entrance is achieved towards the united paravesical and
pararectal space, demonstrated by the appearance of a certain
amount of old blood (fig. 10). The vesico-uterine pillar is
stretched by the bladder retractor and a lateral retractor is

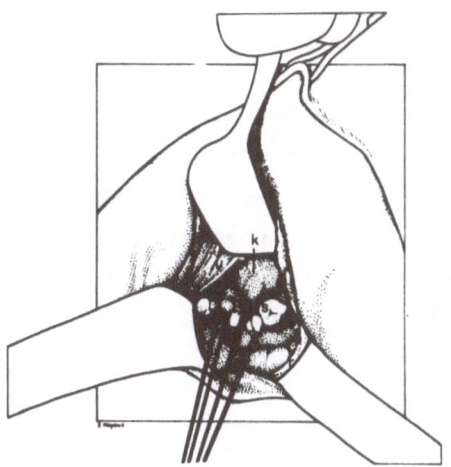

Figure 6

k. bladder; s. vaginal cuff.

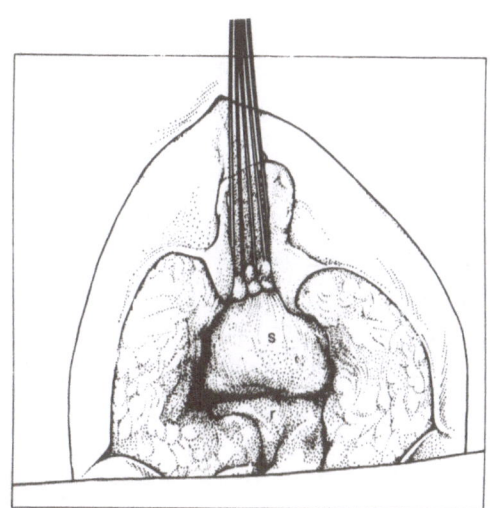

Fig. 7.

r. posterior vaginal wall; s. vaginal cuff.

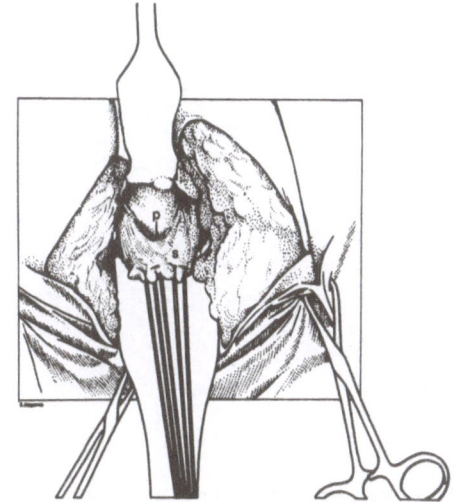

Figure 8

s. vaginal cuff; p. anterio plica

introduced. In most cases the ureter can now be palpated between thumb and index-finger in the vesico-uterine pillar.
From lateral onwards and in small steps, the overlying layers
of connective tissue and vessels are dissected by means of
the aneurysm needle until the lateral aspect of the so-called
ureteral "knee" is reached. More laterally the ureteral tunnel, or "van Bouwdijk Bastiaanse canal", is now opened and
widened by slightly opened scissors or clamp. After introduction of the index-finger into that tunnel, thus protecting
the ureter, the lateral wall is step by step ligated and cut,
using the aneurysm needle (fig. 11).

Figure 9

The retinaculum uteri, consisting of the vesico-uterine, cardinal
and sacro-uterine ligaments, is shown in its relation to the ureter
and the uterine artery For technical reasons the
upper part of the vesico-uterine ligament is not shown in the
subsequent drawings.

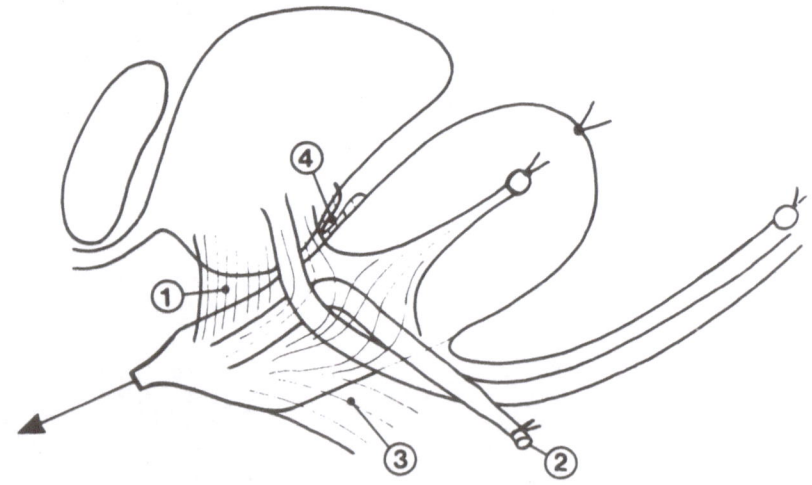

1: vesico-uterine pillar

2: uterine artery

3: sacro-uterine ligament

4: anterior fold of the peritoneum

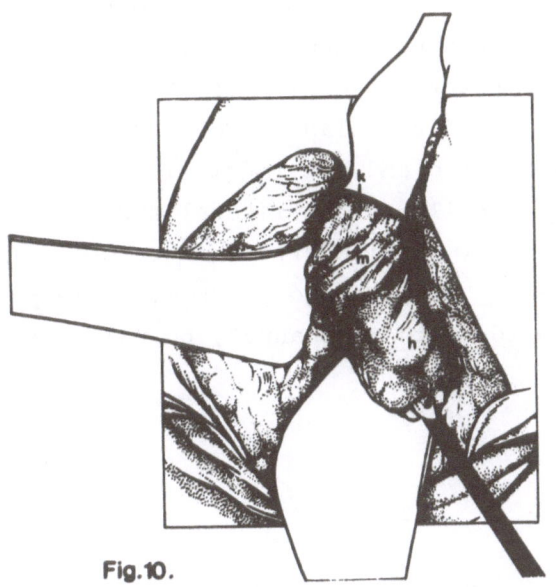

Fig. 10.

h. uterus; k. bladder; m. ureter; s. vaginal cuff.

Figure 11

Dilation of the ureteral tunnel in the lateral view, with the ureter localized medial to the index finger.

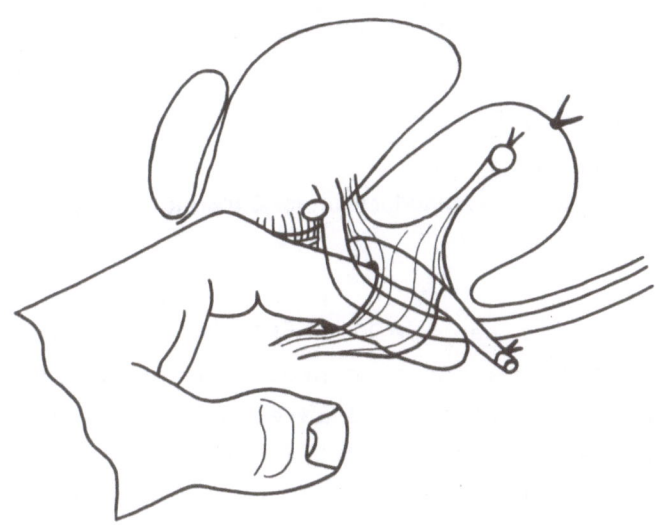

After the ureter is freed laterally, it is mobilized from the
(medial) underlying parametrium by some sharp dissection with
scissors but mostly by pushing it upwards with small tampons
(so-called "peanuts"). After dissection of the ureter and after careful localisation of the bladder boundaries, the vesico-uterine pillar is ligated and cut in small stept by means
of the aneurysm needle until, at the lateral side of the specimen, the ligated and cut uterine artery is reached. The uterine artery is grasped by a clamp and can now, while pushing
the ureter gently upwards with a "peanut", be pulled from
underneath the ureter (fig. 12).

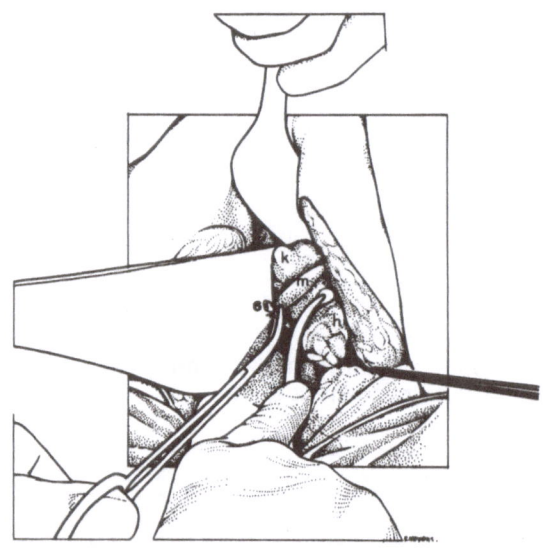

Figure 12

h. uterus; k. bladder, m. ureter; 6. uterine artery

The bladder and ureter can now be gently pushed upward and
freed from the specimen. The same procedure is carried out
on the other side. The peritoneal layer of the cul-de-sac is
now opened and a wide posterior retractor is introduced. The
rectum is separated stepwise from the posterior part of the
parametrium as far from the uterus as possible, using the

aneurysm needle (fig. 13). The uterosacral ligament is ligated
and cut laterally and extraperitoneally. Finally the posterior
layer of the peritoneum is cut with scissors after visualisa-
tion of the ureter. Having applied the same procedure to the
opposite side, the radical hysterectomy specimen can be re-
moved(fig. 16). After careful examination for haemostasis, the
round ligaments are picked up and stiched to the upper margins
of the anterior and posterior, transsected, vaginal walls (fig.
14).

Before the stitch is tied, the possibility that the ureter has
become involved must be excluded by palpation. On both sides
suction catheters are introduced into the extraperitoneal pelvic space, according to Symmonds and Pratt (12), brought through
the Schuchardt incisions and fixed to the skin with individual
nylon sutures. The top of the vagina is closed to minimize
air leak. The Schuchardt incisions are now closed (fig. 15).

Patient Material

From 1957 through 1979, 517 patients were treated in our department by the A.V.R.U.E.L. procedure (6).

In table 1 the number and mean age of 513 stage I and II patients are demonstrated. Two of these patients belonged to
stage IA, 9 to stage IIB. Four patients, who were operated
on in the period 1957-1960 with a stage III disease, are not
included.

After 1960 no stage III patient was treated surgically.

The majority of A.V.R.U.E.L. procedures were performed between
1970 and 1980. Within that decade nearly all stage I cases
were stage IB and all stage II cases were IIA. Stage IA cases
underwent a hysterectomy with vaginal cuff and stage IIB cases
received radiotherapy.

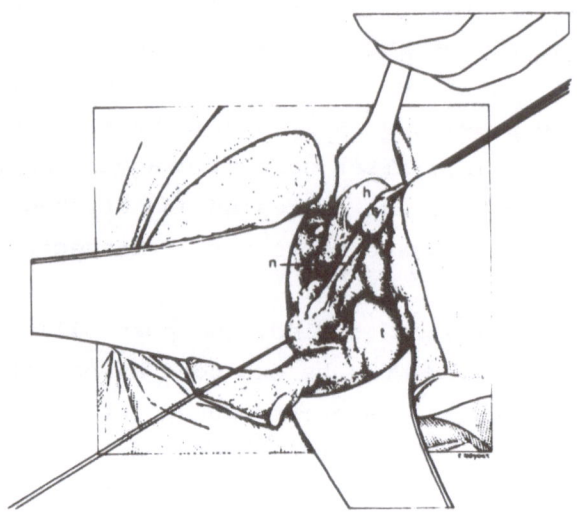

Fig.13.

h.uterus; n.posterior part of parametrium;

s.vaginal cuff; t.rectum

Figure 14

The round ligaments are fixed to the apex of the vagina, making sure that the ureter is not included in the ligature.

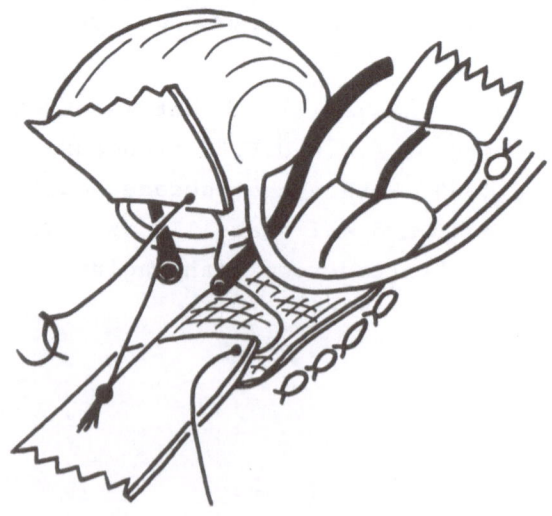

Figure 15

The Schuchardt incisions have been closed over the Redon drains. A balloon catheter has been inserted.

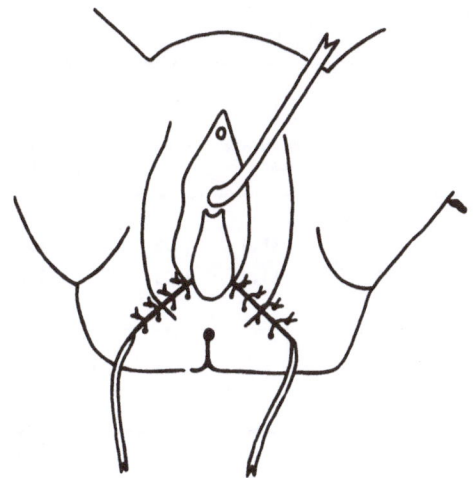

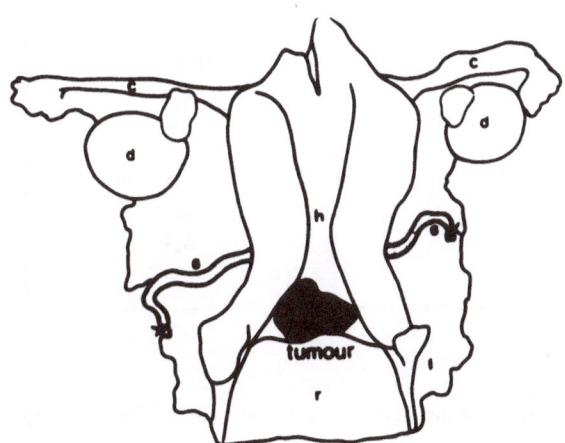

Figure 16

6. uterine artery ; c. Fallopian tube ;

d. ovary ; h. uterus ; r. posterior vaginal wall.

TABLE I

Number and mean age of 513 patients with invasive carcinoma
of the cervix, stages I and II, treated with the A.V.R.U.E.L.-
procedure from 1957 through 1979.

	1957-1960			1961-1969			1970-1979			1957-1979	
	No	mean age years	S.D.	No	mean age year	S.D.	No	mean age year	S.D.	No	mean age year
Stage I	65	44,1	10,0	43	48,0	11,2	212	46,8	10,8	320	46,4
Stage II	74	47,1	9,2	43	51,0	10,9	76	51,3	11,2	193	49,6

TABLE II

Short-term complications of treatment with the A.V.R.U.E.L.
procedure in 517 patients (1957-1979 incl.)

	No	Percent
Primary operative mortality.	7	1,3
Post-operative fistulae: Bladder	14	2,7
Ureter	19	3,7
Bowel	10	1,9
Post-operative ileus	14	2,7
Thrombosis and/or embolism.	23	4,4

Complications of the A.V.R.U.E.L. procedure

In table II the short-term complications of the operation are
demonstrated. We consider "primary operative mortality" to
have occurred when there is a direct connection between the
operation and the cause of death, including blood transfusion
complications, anaesthesia accidents, embolism etc. In accordance with Morris and Meigs (8) we maintain that the time between operation and death is irrelevant. The post-operative
mortality rate (total 1.3) decreased from 2.2 in the period

1957-1969 to 0.7 in the period 1970-1979.

Two patients died from massive pulmonary embolism, two from excessive blood loss, two from anaesthetic complications and one patient died as a result of a surgical incident. Postoperative fistulae occurred in 8.3% of patients, but the incidence was only 5% during the period 1970-1979. Thrombosis and embolism occurred in 4.4% over the whole period under survey, but this percentage decreased steadily in time, due to more widespread use of anti-coagulant therapy.

In table III the long-term complications of the operation are demonstrated. As can be seen in this table, urinary tract complaints make up the majority of the long-term complications. The removal of as much of the lower parametrium as possible may be responsable for the high incidence (nearly 26%) of urinary tract complaints*. Intestinal complications were comparatively rare and of no practical consequence. The fact that the incidence of sexual complaints, is also relatively low, can be explained by the fact that our data are derived from a retrospective study and can therefore only give an impression of the frequency of these complaints. Future prospective studies may reveal a higher incidence of sexual malfunction after extended surgery.

TABLE III

Long-term complications of treatment with the A.V.R.U.E.L. procedure in 517 patients (1957-1979 incl.)		
	No	**Percent**
Urinary incontinence	92	17,8
Urinary retention	18	3,5
Urinary incontinence and retention	23	4,4
	133	25,7
Intestinal complications	16	3,1
Sexual complications	34	6,6

* See also chapter 9 (eds)

Histology of 517 A.V.R.U.E.L. operation specimens

Histological examination of the tumours revealed a squamous cell carcinoma in 433 cases (83.7%), adenocarcinoma in 52 cases (10.1%) and other forms of carcinoma (totally undifferentiated, clear-cell carcinomas etc.) in 32 cases (6.2%).

Involvement of lymphnodes

In table IV metastatic lymph node involvement is shown in relation to the histological type of tumour and stage of disease. An increase in the incidence of lymph node involvement in relation to increasing the stage of disease is demonstrated. Although not shown in table IV, lymph node involvement, in relation to substages, was found by us to be as follows: 0% in stage IA (only 2 cases), 19.0% in stage IB, 22.7% in stage IIA and 5 out of 9 in stage IIB.

TABLE IV

Metastatic involvement of lymph nodes in 517 A.V.R.U.E.L. operation specimens in relation to the histological type of tumour and the stage of disease.

	Squamous cell	Adenocarcinomas	Others	Total
Stage I	40/263	7/38	4/19	51/320= 15,9%
Stage II	41/166	4/14	3/13	48/193= 24,9%
Stage III	1/4	----	----	1/4
All stages	82/433 = 18,9%	11/52 = 21,1%	7/32 = 21,9%	100/517 = 19,3%

The differences between squamous cell carcinomas and adenocarcinomas are statistically not significant, the difference between stage I and II is. (P < 0,05)

Involvement of parametrium

From 1961 through 1979 the surgically removed parametrial tissue was thoroughly microscopically examined in the Department of Pathology (Head Prof. dr. C.A. Wagenvoort). From 1957-1961 microscopic examination of removed parametrium was inconsistent. For this reason table V demonstrates the metastatic involvement in 376 A.V.R.U.E.L. operation specimens in relation to the stage of disease from 1961 through 1979. Microscopic tumour involvement of removed parametrial tissue was found in 14.6% of stage IB and 21,8% of stage IIA cases. We also found that in 25 out of 37 stage I cases with metastatic involvement of the parametrium lymph node involvement was also present. In stage II these numbers were 15 out of 28 cases. As is shown in Table V in about half of the cases the parametrial involvement was bilateral.

In agreement with Christensen and Folgmann (4), Averette et al (2) and Baltzer et al (3), we found that the clinical estimation of the stage of disease in carcinoma of the uterine cervix, has its limitations. As described above, under-staging may occur in stage IB and IIA. The relatively high involvement of the parametria in these stages clearly justifies the extensive removal of parametrial tissue in the surgical treatment of these stages of the disease.

Involvement of the ovaries

The incidence of metastatic involvement of the ovaries in cases of cervical carcinoma could be studies because, util recently, the performance of a radical hysterectomy nearly always included a bilateral oöphorectomy in our department. Metastatic involvement of the ovaries occurred in 0.5% of stage I cases and in 0.4% of stage II cases. This finding has changed our attitude towards the removal of the ovaries in our Department in patients under the age of 40 years. In these cases, if the laparotomy does not reveal macroscopic changes of the ovaries, they are preserved.

Survival of patients with invasive carcinoma of the uterine
cervix after treatment with the A.V.R.U.E.L. procedure (1957
through 1974)

Patient survival is generally accepted as the principal criterion for measuring the effectiveness of cancer treatment.
Although the survival rate, i.e. the proportion of patients
surviving a specified interval of time, is a simple concept,
there has been a considerable lack of uniformity in computing
it. Many physicians exclude death from other causes, apparently because they consider it unfair to charge non-cancer death
to the therapy being evaluated; some exclude only operative
death; others exclude death in which the cancer in question
was not known to be present at the time of death (5). Our calculation of survival rate is made on the assumption that patients who are "lost-sight-of" should be included with those
who died from cancer. The operative deaths are also included
in this category. Patients who died from intercurrent disease
however, are excluded from the calculated material.
(Death is only considered as intercurrent, if it has resulted
from some condition which could safely be regarded as uncon-
nected with the treated carcinoma or the treatment.)
From 1957 through 1974, 345 patients were treated with an
A.V.R.U.E.L. operation. We are therefore able to calculate
the five year survival rates and, in 225 cases the ten year
survival rates. From the 345 patients treated from 1957 through
1974, 185 were in stage I and 156 in stage II. Only four patients (two treated in period 1957-1960 and two in 1961-1969)
fell into stage III and these latter cases will not be discussed.
The five year survival of stages I and II treated with an
A.V.R.U.E.L. operation are presented in table VI.
As can be seen, better results were obtained in stage I (86.2
percent) than in stage II (74.2 percent). Also evident from
table VI is that the relatively better results were obtained
in both stages of the disease after treatment during the last
period (1970-1974) under study; 92.0 percent in stage I and
80.0 percent in stage II.

TABLE V

The involvement of parametrium in 376 A.V.R.U.E.L. operation specimens in relation to the stage of disease (1961-1979 incl.)

	total	Involvement of the parametrium					
		Bilateral		Unilateral		Total	
	No	No	%	No	%	No	%
Stage I	255	15	5,9	22	8,7	37	14,6
Stage II	119	13	10,9	15	12,6	28	23,5
Stage III	2	0		0		0	

Table VI

The five year survival of patients with invasive carcinoma of the uterine cervix, treated with the A.V.R.U.E.L.-procedure from 1957 through 1974.

	stage I		stage II	
	No.	percent	No.	percent
1957-1960	54/64	84.4	55/74	74.3
1961-1969	33/42	78.6	29/42	69.0
1970-1974	69/75	92.0	28/35	80.0
1957-1974	156/181	86.2	112/151	74.2

The operative deaths and patients lost-sight-of were included as died from cancer; patients who died from intercurrent disease were excluded entirely.

The differences between stage I and stage II were statistically significant ($p<0.01$), the differences between the different periods within the stages were not.

The five year survival rates after treatment with the
A.V.R.U.E.L. procedure in relation to the histological type
of tumour are given in table VII.

As shown, the overall five year survival in stages I and II
combined was 77.3% for adenocarcinoma and 81.3% for squamous
cell carcinoma. In our review of thirty years treatment of
patients with invasive cancer of the uterine cervix, 5 year
survival of all patients treated (including A.V.R.U.E.L. and
other methods) was significantly lower in adenocarcinomas
than in squamous cell carcinomas (6). From the data given in
Table VII (where no such statistically significant difference
between the two types of carcinoma was demonstrated) we may
possibly assume that treatment of invasive adenocarcinoma of
the cervix using the A.V.R.U.E.L. operation does improve the
results.

Table VII

The five-year survival of patients with invasive carcinoma of the uterine cervix, treated
with the A.V.R.U.E.L.-procedure from 1957 through 1974, in relation to the histological type of tumour.

	squamous cell carcinoma		adenocarcinoma		others	
	No.	%	No.	%	No.	%
Stage I of disease negative lymph nodes	130/142	91.5	11/12	91	7/8	-
Stage I of disease positive lymph nodes	8/16	50.0	0/2	-	0/1	..
Stage I, all patients	138/158	87.3	11/14	78	7/9	-
Stage II of disease negative lymph nodes	79/97	81.4	5/7	-	8/9	-
Stage II of disease positive lymph nodes	18/34	52.9	1/1	-	1/3	--
Stage II , all patients	97/131	74.0	6/8	-	9/12	--
Stages I and II all patients together	235/289	81.3	17/22	77.3	16/21	76

The differences between squamous cell carcinoma and adenocarcinoma (stages I and II)
were statistically not significant.

In Figures 17 and 18 the cumulative survival rates in relation
to the involvement of lymph nodes are shown in stages I and
II. Figure 17 demonstrates that, during a follow-up period

lasting up to ten years death occurs mainly in the first five years after treatment. From 225 patients (stages I and II) with a follow-up of ten years, 4 were lost-sight of in the first five years (1.8 percent) and 9 in the second five year period (4 percent). Of interest in both Figures 17 and 18, and already apparent during the first five years of. follow-up, is the lower five year survival found in stage I with involvement of the lymph nodes when compared to stage II with lymph node involvement. It is possible that tumours in stage I cases of invasive carcinoma of the uterine cervix with involvement of the lymph nodes, are relatively more agressive. In these cases, at the time of localised primary tumour formation there is already involvement of the lymph nodes and spread of tumour above the pelvic region, resulting in relatively lower survival rates.

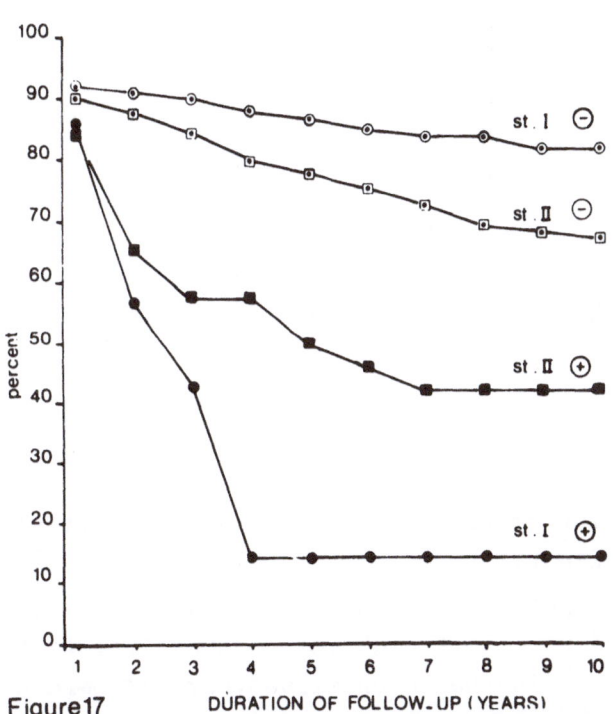

Figure 17   DURATION OF FOLLOW-UP (YEARS)

The cumulative survival of patients with invasive carcinoma of the uterine cervix, stages I and II, treated in the Wilhelmina Gasthuis with the A.V.R.U.E.L.-procedure from 1957 through 1969, in relation to the involvement of the lymph nodes

138

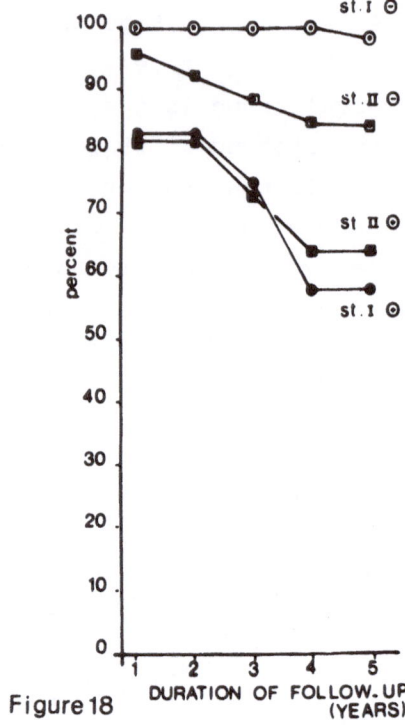

Figure 18 DURATION OF FOLLOW-UP (YEARS)

The cumulative survival of patients with invasive carcinoma of the uterine cervix, stages I and II, treated in the Wilhelmina Gasthuis with the A.V.R.U.E.L.-procedure from 1970 through 1974, in relation to the involvement of the lymph nodes.

Additional information on the cumulative survival rates is given in table VIII.

From the 225 patients (stages I and II) with a follow-up of ten years, 4 were lost-sight-of in the first five years (1.8 percent) and 9 in the second five years (4 percent), the incidence of lost-sight-of during the second five years being higher than the incidence of death from cancer (3.1%). Survival rates calculated after a follow-up of more than five years are, therefore, to a relatively important extent, in-

fluenced by the number of patients, lost-sight-of. This should
be borne in mind when considering Figure 17.

Table VIII

The number of patients who died from cancer, were lost-sight-of and died from intercurrent disease, after treatment for invasive carcinoma of the uterine cervix with the
A.V.R.U.E.L.-procedure from 1957 through 1974; a follow-up of five and ten years.

Stages I and II of disease, with or without involvement of the lymph nodes

Total number of patients	139		86		116
died from cancer	27	6	21	1	14
Lost-sight-of	3	6	1	3	0
Died of interc.disease	1	3	2	0	5

During 10 years follow-up 48 out of 55 patients, who died from cancer, died during the
first five years (87.3 percent), 9 out of 13 patients, who were lost-sight-of, were lost
during the second five years (69 percent).

Discussion

The meticulous study of 517 A.V.R.U.E.L. operation specimens
by the pathologist gave an excellent opportunity to study the
metastatic involvement of the pelvic lymph nodes. A correlation between higher stages of the disease and a greater degree
of lymph node involvement was found (none in stage IA, 19%
in stage IB, 22.7% in stage IIA and 5 out of 9 in stage IIB).
The high correlation between lymph node involvement and the
prognosis of the patient is most important. In stage IB the
five year survival rate after treatment with an A.V.R.U.E.L.
operation in patients without lymph node involvement was 91.4%
and with lymph node involvement 42.1%. The corresponding figures
for stage IIA were 79.1% and 54.0% respectively.
These differences become even more important if we take into
account the fact that the majority of patients without lymph
node involvement underwent no post-operative radiotherapy,

whereas almost all patients with lymph node involvement were
irradiated post-operatively. It is interesting to note that
lymph node involvement in stage IB caused greater deteriora-
tion in prognosis than in stage IIA (91.4 - 42.1 = 49.3%
against 79.1 - 54.0 = 25.1% in 5 year survival).

It is not unlikely, that a carcinoma, leading to lymph node
involvement in stage I, is more malignant than a carcinoma producing lymph node involvement in stage II.

Removal of positive pelvic lymph nodes leads to recovery in
less than 50% of all cases. "Radical" methods of treatment,
which remain limited to the pelvic region are inadequate in
a considerable number of stage IB and IIA cases, and can be
explained by the fact, that in early stages, involvement of
the para-aortic lymph nodes may already have occurred.

The microscopic infiltration of the parametria was also found
to be related to the stage of disease; none in stage IA, 14.6%
in stage IB and 21.8% in stage IIA. These findings demonstrate
the possibility of clinical understaging before commencement
of treatment and provide a strong argument in favour of extended radical surgery.

No other factor however, showed such a striking connection
with the prognosis as did the clinical stage.

Since between 5 and 10 years after treatment, the number of
lost-sight-of patients and the number of patients dying from
intercurrent diseases rises, whereas the number of patients
dying from cancer during that period is very small, the five
year survival rate seems to be the best yardstick for comparison of different forms of treatment. During the last decade our aim has been to employ operative treatment in those
patients who, in all probability, can be cured by surgery
alone and to treat all others with radiotherapy.

Therefore, we selected the stages IIB, III and IV for primary
treatment with radiotherapy. Only stages IB and IIA were selected for extended surgery, almost always using the A.V.R.U.E.L.
procedure. If examination of the lymph nodes failed to reveal
involvement, no radiotherapy was given. In the period 1970-
1974 this was the case in 65 patients with stage IB. Of this

group only one patient died from cancer within 5 years of operation. In the same period 12 patients appeared to have positive lymph nodes. Although these patients were irradiated post-operatively, 5 of them died from cancer within 5 years. In stage IIA these figures were 4 out of 28, and 4 out of 11 respectively. These figures show that the great majority of patients in stage IB and IIA (84% in IB and 72% in IIA) can be treated by surgery without radiotherapy with good results (98.4% cure-rate in IB and 84.0% in IIA). The overall results for stages IB and IIA were 92% and 80% during the period 1970-1974. Although our results, especially in the last decade, have been encouriging and provide a strong argument for proceding with our scheme of management, it cannot, at present, be proved beyond doubt that the A.V.R.U.E.L. operation surpasses all other forms of treatment.

References

1. Aartsen, E.J. 1978. An Atlas of Drawings of the A.V.R.U.E.L. procedure.
2. Averette, H.E., Jobson, V.W., Belinson, J.L., Girtanner, R.E. 1979. Selective Therapy of Cervical Carcinoma Based Upon Surgical Staging. In: Advances in medical oncology, research and education; proc. 12th int. cancer congress, Buenos Aires, 1978; vol. 8: gynecological cancer, Thatcher, N. Editor: Oxford, Pergamon, p. 263-269.
3. Baltzer, J., Kaufmann, C., Ober, K.G., Zander, J. 1980. Komplikationen bei 1092 erweiterten abdominalen Krebs-operationen mit oblegatorischer Lymphonodektomie. Geburtshilfe und Frauenheilkunde, 40, 1-5.
4. Christensen, A., Folgmann, R. 1976. Cervical Carcinoma Stage I and II, treated by primary Radical Hysterectomy and Pelvic Lymphadenectomy. Acta Obstetrica et Gynecologica Scandinavica, Supplement 58, 3-44.
5. Ederer, F., Axtell, L.M., Cutler, S.J. 1961. The relative survival rate: A statistical methodology. In: Endresults and mortality trends in cancer. U.S. Department of Health, education and Welfare; Public Health Service: National Cancer Institute. (Monograph, 6, p. 101-104).
6. Ketting, B.W. 1981. Surgical Treatment of Invasive Carcinoma of the Uterine Cervix. Thesis, University of Amsterdam.
7. Mitra, S. 1960. Mitra Operation for Cancer of the Cervix. Editor E.C. Hamblen. Charles C. Thomas, Publisher. Springfield, Illinois, U.S.A.

8. Morris, J.M., Meigs, J.V. 1950. Carcinoma of the Cervix. Statistical evaluation of 1938 Cases and Results of Treatment. Surgery, Gunecology and Obstetrics, 90, 135-150.
9. Schauta, F. 1908. Die erweiterte vaginale Totalextirpation des Uterus beim Kollumkarzinoms. Verlag von Josef Safár, Wien.
10. Sindram, I.S. 1959. A New Combined Approach in the Treatment of Cancer of the Uterine Cervix. Extrat de Acta Union Internationale Contre le Cancer, XV, 403-405.
11. Sindram,I.S. 1960. Twee jaren ervaring met de abdomino-vaginale hysterectomie. Nederlands Tijdschrift voor Verloskunde en Gynaecologie, 238, 252-260.
12. Symmonds, R.A. and Pratt, J.H. 1961. Prevention of Fistulas and Lymphocysts in Radical Hysterectomy. Preliminary Report of a New Technic. Obstetrics and Gynecology, 17, 57-64.
13. Taussig, F.J., St. Louis, Mo. 1943. Iliac Lymphadenectomy for Group II Cancer of the Cervix. American Journal of Obstetrics and Gynecology, 45, 733-748.
14. Wertheim, E. 1911. Die erweiterte Abdominale Operation bei Carcinoma Colli Uteri (auf Grund von 500 Fällen). Urban & Schwarzenberg, Berlin, Wien.

13. URODYNAMICS AFTER RADICAL SURGERY FOR CARCINOMA OF THE UTERINE CERVIX

Mogens Asmussen, M.D.

"By all means cure them of their cancer but don't do it by making them into urological cripples."

This well-known saying draws a vivid picture of the quandary in which the gynecological cancer surgeon finds himself when performing radical hysterectomy with lymph node dissection for carcinoma of the uterine cervix. He must be radical without compromise if there is to be a success in curing this disease. At the same time he must avoid complications, especially urinary tract complications, which can very easily make the patients life a misery or become so serious, that the threat to her lift makes the whole exercise valueless. Speaking generally, the frequency of complications varies with the extent of the operation. If extensive surgery is combined with radiotherapy, the complication rates of both forms of treatment must be added to one another.
It is out of place to discuss here the pros and cons of radical cancer treatment. Suffice it to say, that radical surgery has been proven to achieve results which can compete successfully with radiotherapy in early stage carcinoma of the cervix.
Urological complications following surgical treatment of cervical cancer have mainly concerned ureteric obstruction with hydronephrosis and deteriorated renal function as well as different types of fistulas. Although the frequencies of these severe complications today have decreased considerably, the urinary tract must still be considered to be at particular risk in radical hysterectomy with lymph node dissection. Disturbances of micturition with residual urine and accompanying

infection as well as urinary incontinece are often reported.
The explanation for these urologic dysfunctions differs from
one author to another. It is reasonable to state, however,
that the disorders generally depend on the extent and method
of tissue removal around the cervix, whereby the nerve supply
to the lower urinary tract is damaged. The immediate changes
post-operatively have most often been described as a hyperactive bladder which later became hypoactive.

The explanation for these findings have not been fully under-
stood but Forney (10) clearly demonstrated, that if the extent
of the operation was limited in that only the upper part of
the cardinal ligament was removed, dysfunction of the bladder
and urethra could be diminished.

In this presentation a new surgical procedure for primary radical hysterectomy with lymph node dissection will be described.
It has been developed as a clinical research project and is
specially designed to preserve the nerve and blood supply to
the bladder and urethra. In a group of patients undergoing
this procedure, lower urinary tract function has been evaluated before and after surgery with simultaneous urethrocystometry and urethral pressure profile measurement. Furthermore,
the effect of this procedure on ureteric function has been
estimated by isotope renography and effective renal plasma
flow (ERPF).

Twentyfive patients age 27 to 56 (average 43) years with stage
I and II cancer of the cervix were studied. All patients underwent a thorough urological examination before and after surgery including intravenous pyelography, urethrocystoscopy,
urethrocystography and urine culture.

Urodynamic investigations

The urodynamic investigations were performed immediately before surgery and 14 days and 11 months post-operatively. All
patients but two had normal preoperative urological findings.
One patient had suffered from mild urge-incontinence, and the
other patient from stress-incontinence.

The measuring technique for simultaneous urethrocystometry

is shown in Fig. 1, and is performed as described by Asmussen
in 1975 (1). The bladder is initially filled to a volume of
100 ml, and urethral pressure profiles taken every 100 ml's
while the bladder is been filled at a slow rate of approximately 20-30 ml/min. Between the profile measurements the proximal transducer is placed at the maximum urethral pressure.
First sensation and maximum bladder capacity are noted and
the pressure variations in the bladder and urethra recorded
when the desire to void is so strong, that the patient cannot
prevent initiation of micturition.
When micturition starts, the urine flow is recorded and after
micturition is complete the amount of residual urine is measured.

Renal function test

If renography using 131 J-Hippuran is combined with a series
of blood tests to estimate the concentration of isotope after
various time intervals, it is possible to work out the so-
called effective renal plasmaflow (ERPF) and thereby estimate
the amount of functioning tissue in each kidney. This new
method is being increasingly used and may indeed come to play
a major part in the pre- and post-operative assessment of renal function where either the disease process or the treatment may result in renal damage. All 25 patients underwent
this examination procedure.

Surgical procedure

The relevant stept in the standarized lateral procedure which
the author has described(in "Clinical Gynecological Urology",
Asmussen, Blackwell Scientific Publications, 1982) is as follows: After ligating the round ligaments and the infundibulopelvic ligaments the paravesical and pararectal spaces are
opened by blunt dissection down to the pelvic floor (Fig. 2).
The structure running from the pelvic wall into the uterus
and vagina separating these two spaces is "the lateral retinaculum" (the cardinal ligament, the web, Mackenrodt's ligament,

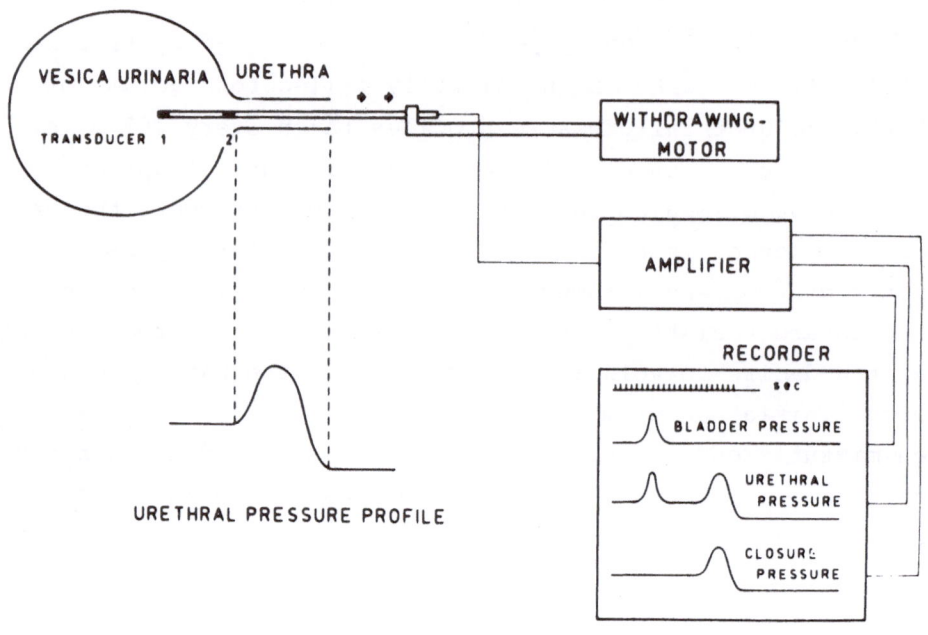

URETHRAL PRESSURE PROFILE

Fig. 1.

Principles of simultaneous urethrocystometry using double microtip transducer technique.

parametrium). When the common iliac, internal iliac, obturator and external iliac lymph nodes have been removed the uterine artery and obliterated umbilical arteries are identified where they originate from the internal iliac (hypogastric) artery (Fig. 3). As much fat as possible is then removed, normally exposing some smaller veins running from the pelvic wall to the vagina and bladder (Fig. 4). These veins are ligated individually as laterally as possible.

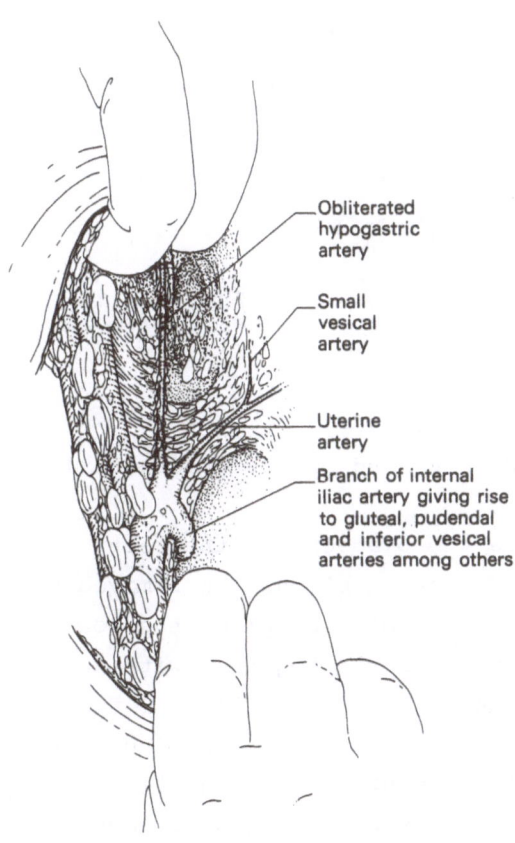

Obliterated
hypogastric
artery

Small
vesical
artery

Uterine
artery

Branch of internal
iliac artery giving rise
to gluteal, pudendal
and inferior vesical
arteries among others

Fig. 2.
Blunt finger dissection of the perivesical and perirectal spaces.

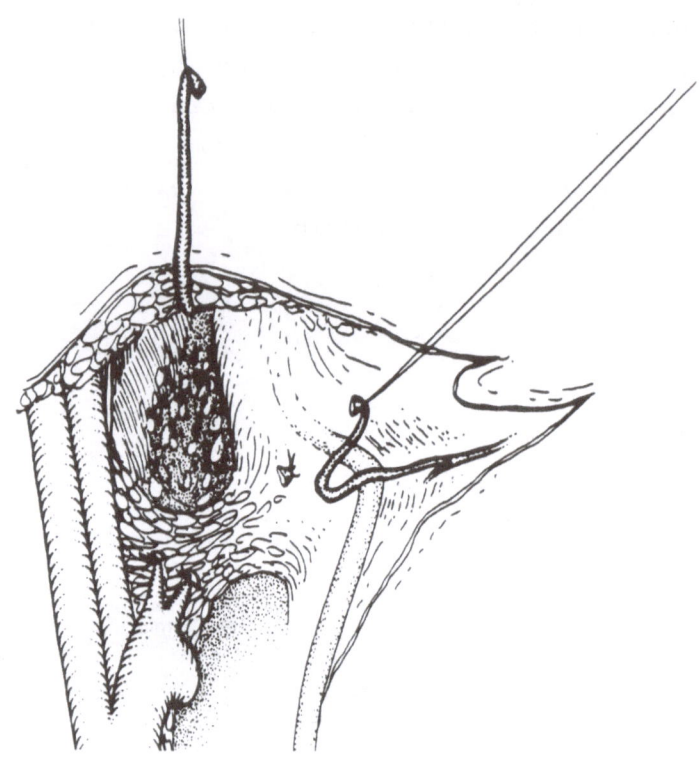

Fig. 3.
Uterine and obliterated arteries divided.

All fat beside the bladder and the rectum and on the rest of
"the lateral retinaculum" must be removed and that part of the
hypogastric plexus which supplies the lower urinary tract with
sensory and motor fibres together with the inferior vesical
artery are then exposed (Fig. 5).
The surgical procedure is then continued by tunnelling and
free-dissecting the ureteres (Fig. 6). Finally the specimen
is removed with as good a margin as required (Fig. 7).
The technique outlined here spares the major part of the nerve
and blood supply to the bladder base and urethra without in-
terfering with the radicality of the surgical procedure. Bilateral well functioning extraperitoneal drainage is used

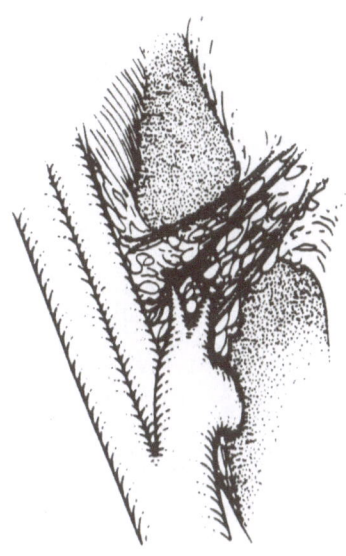

Fig. 4   Some smaller veins identified

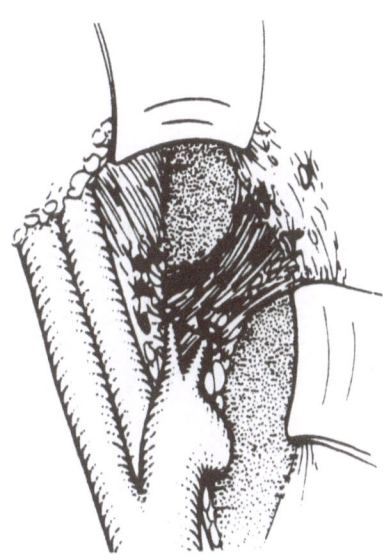

Fig. 5   The hypogastric plexus exposed

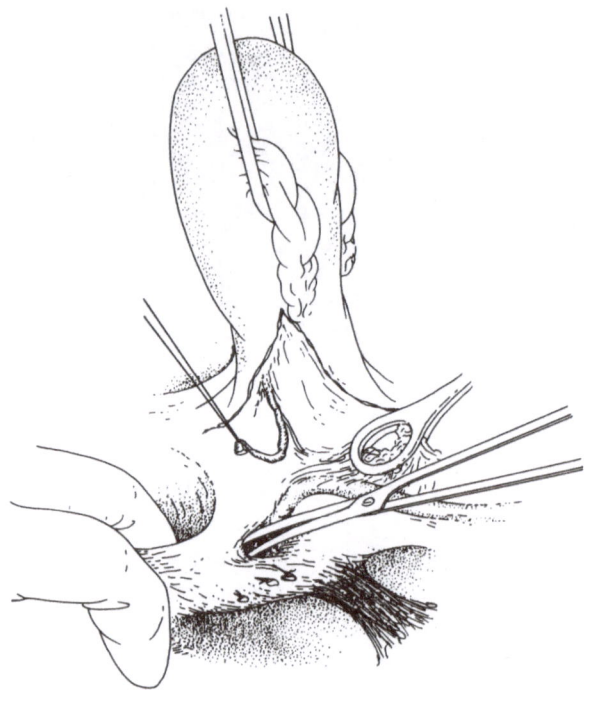

Fig. 6   Tunnelling and free-dissecting
          the left ureter

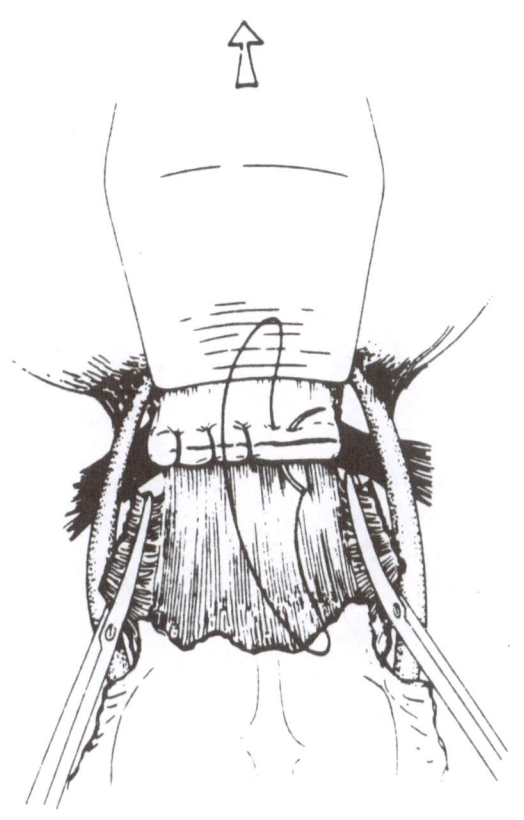

Fig. 7 Uterus removed. Vagina closed.

normally between 5-10 days after the operation. These are
first removed when lymph production has ceased to a few ml's
daily (Fig. 8). A catheter à demeure is kept for about 10-14
days after the operation.

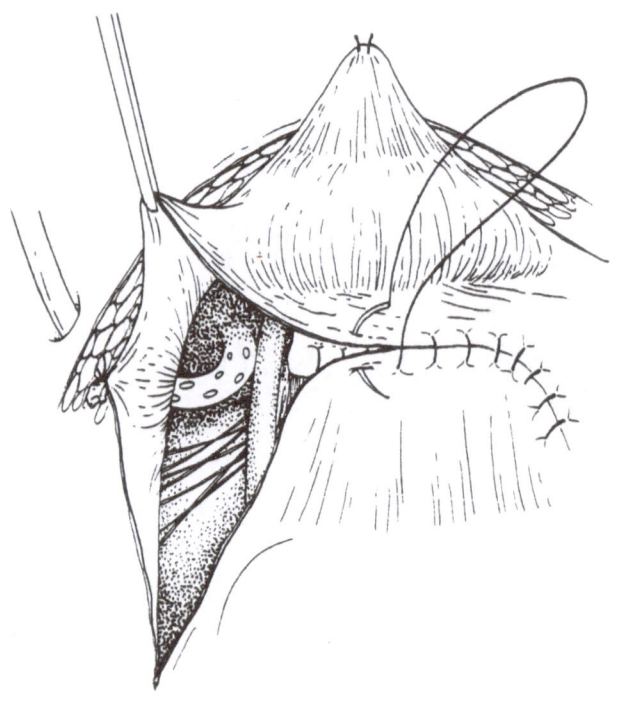

Fig. 8.
Peritonealisation and application of extraperitoneal drainage in each obturator fossa.

Results

Bladder and urethra

Before operation, 24 patients showed normal initiation of micturition with a fall of urethral pressure followed by an increase of bladder pressure intil leakage occurred. One patient could not initiate micturition and used additional Valsalva manoevre, which made the initiation pattern uncertain (Figs 9, 10). Residual urine was less than 10 ml in all patients.

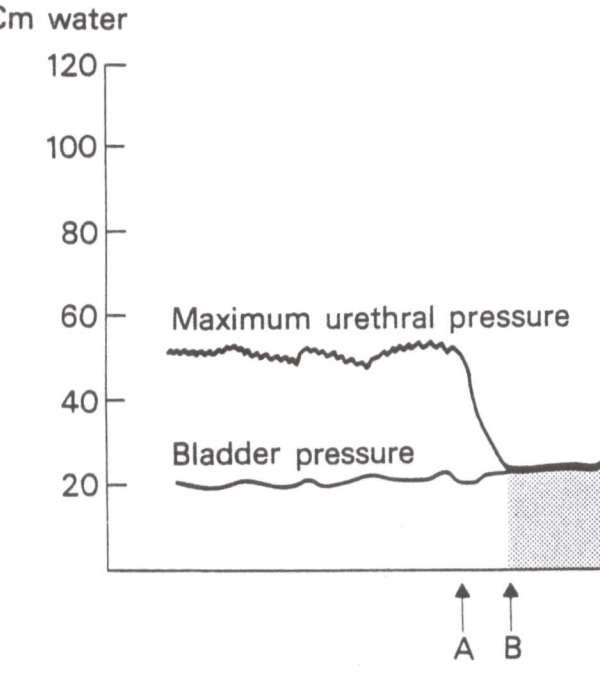

Fig. 9.
Normal interplay between intraurethral and intravesical pressure during initiation of micturition.

Post-operatively 7 patients showed a normal micturition pattern at 14 days, 2 of these showed a relaxation of the urethral pressure without demonstrable detrusor contraction. The residual urine in these 7 was 0-45 (average 21). Seventeen

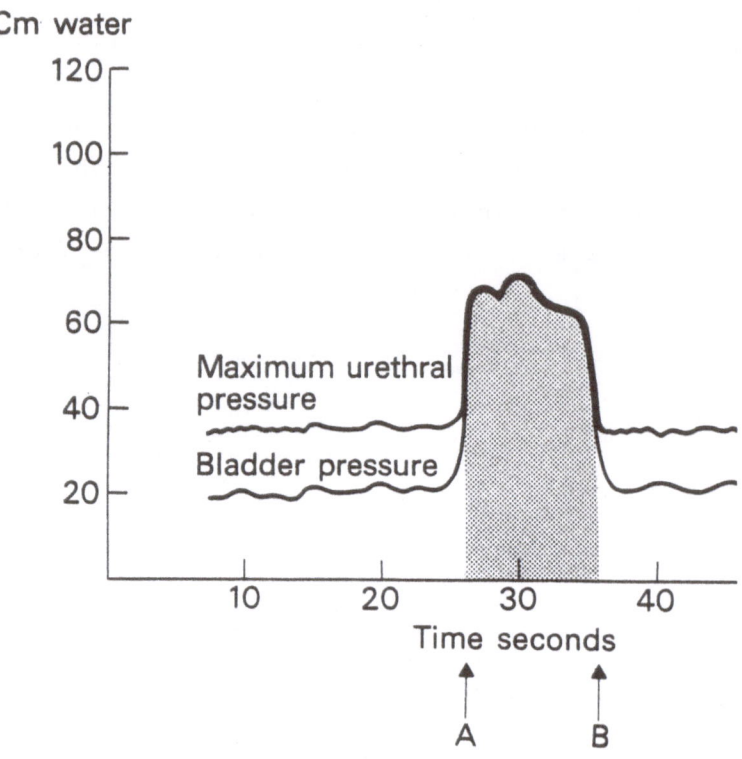

Fig. 10.
Valsalva micturition.

patients could not initiate micturition and 1 was doubtful.
None of these 18 patients showed any sign of detrusor hyperactivity düring filling with 20-30 ml/min., but developed a
typical overflowing incontinence (Fig. 11). Especially the
infusion of the last ml's produced a marked increase in bladder pressure so that it exceeded the maximum urethral pressure
and caused urine leakage. If the filling was stopped just before incontinence occurred as shown in Fig. 12, the intravesical pressure decreased somewhat and if just a few ml's were
emptied out of the bladder, the intravesical pressure decreased
markedly indicating that the increase in bladder pressure was

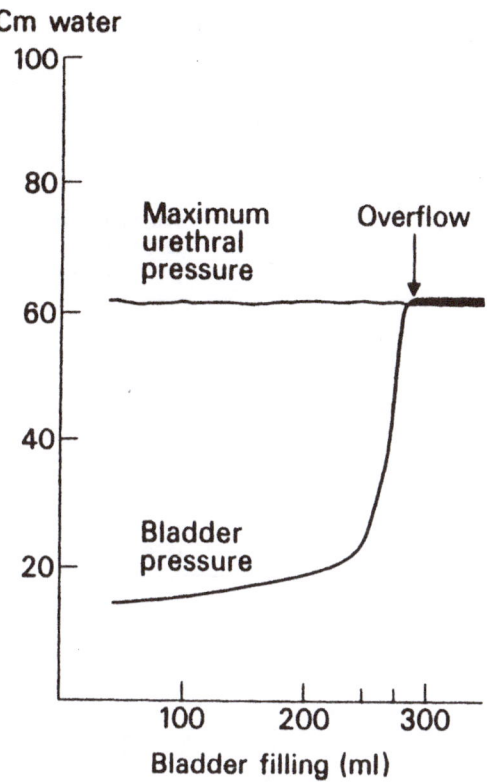

Fig. 11.
Immediate changes in urethrocystometrogram.
Changes in bladder compliance leads to over-
flow incontinence without detrusorcontraction.

due to stiffness of the bladder wall (change in compliance)
and not detrusor contraction.
These patients attempted to empty their bladder by a Valsalva
manoevre and had an average residual urine of 110 ml (10-230).
About 1 year post-operatively 22 patients initiated micturition normally. Three (2 new) could not initiate micturition
normally, but used a Valsalva manoevre. None developed stress
incontinence. The patient with pre-operative urgency, was
cured of the symptoms and the one patient with stress incontinence still had her symptoms and was later operated upon

156

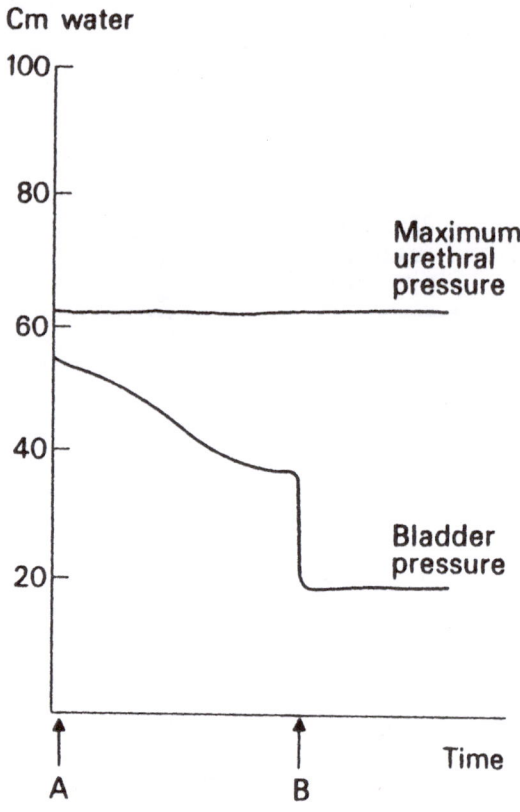

Fig. 12.
Same patient as fig. 11.
A. infusion stopped.
B. 10 ml emptied from the bladder.

with a colposuspension. No urinary infection could be demonstrated in any of the patients using either midstream specimen or suprapubic bladder puncture. Residual urine was less
than 10 ml in all patients.

The changes in urethral pressure profile measurements, first
sensation, and maximal bladder capacity is presented in table
1. As seen bladder sensation was only little affected.
Although, marked changes could be demonstrated shortly after
this operation the urethral pressure profile was only slightly

affected about one year later.

Table 1.

Examination	Pre-operative		After 14 days		After 1 year	
First sensation: ml	299 ml		(299 ml)		348 ml	
Maximal bladder capacity ml	598 ml		463 ml		600 ml	
Bladder volume ml (average)	200	484	200	416	200	472
Total urethral length mm "	35.0	34.5	33.8	31.4	35.1	33.8
Functional urethral length "	28.1	26.5	26.4	21.7	27.5	25.5
Maximum urethral pressure cm H_2O "	93.2	91.5	77.9	78.4	84.3	84.0
Bladder pressure cm H_2O "	21.0	26.2	22.1	37.4	23.0	27.1

In 2 patients only a certain change of micturition could be demonstrated but they emptied their bladder sufficiently using a Valsalva manouevre. The postoperative hyperactive bladder which has been described by several authors could not be con-firmed in these cases. The lower urinary tract in these pa-tients is not hyperactive immediately postoperatively. If blad-der hyperactivity was presented catheter drainage would not have been necessary in these postoperative patients. As is well known, catheter drainage is a necessity in all patients imme-diately after radical hysterectomy since the patients actually cannot void.
It has been argued by Hohenfellner that postoperative bladder drainage is necessary because of increased urethral resistance.

Nevertheless, this dysfunction could not be demonstrated in
this study. The most likely explanation is, that the nervous
control over micturition reflex is temporarily disturbed so
that the lowering of the urethra, a pressure followed by a
detrusor contraction, cannot be produced. This together with
perivesical adhaesions, oedema, exsudate, and haematoma formation in the surrounding tissues cause marked alteration in
bladder elasticity. The cystometrogram especially when using
high filling rate can easily be misinterpreted, so that the
increased bladder pressure is taken as a detrusor contraction.
In the authors opinion the Carbacholin or Nor-adrenalin test
offers little practical help in daily clinics.

In a recently performed study, where 5 patients underwent the
same procedure, but with total transection of the nerve supply
to the bladder and urethra and thereby probably also transsection of the main blood supply to the bladder base and the
urethra, the inferior vesical artery, the same immediate postoperative changes were noted. None of these patients however,
regained normal bladder sensation or micturition pattern one
year after surgery. Bladder filling did not result in the normal desire to void but more an unpleasant feeling in the pelvis and on simultaneous urethro-cystometry the urethra could
not relax and overflow incontinence occurred although not as
dramatically as immediately postoperatively. These patients
however, could empty their bladder completely by Valsalva manouevre. The urethral pressure profiles in these patients
seemed to be somewhat lower one year after operation than in
the group where the nerve- and blood supply has been saved.
However, the number is too small to draw any valid conclusion
and the interpretation of such an observation is difficult
since not only the nerve supply to the urethra seems to be
important, but recent studies have shown that the blood supply
to the urethra is also of utmost importance in maintaining
intraurethral pressure. The conclusion, which has been drawn
by Low (15), that the decreased urethral pressure is caused
by a defect sympathic innervation of the lower urinary tract
is probably too simplified. Recent anatomical studies by the

Dutch anatomist Huisman (14) have shown, that the anatomy of
the bladder base and urethra is much more complex than thought
earlier and that new thinking is necessary to explain the
function of this delicate organ.

Fig. 13 shows the different flow pattern about one year after
operation. If the hypogastric plexus has been preserved intact,
as described above, the detrusor muscle can contract and empty
the bladder almost completely. However, the last few ml's
often remain, probably because of persisted perivesical adhesions and rigidity in the bladder wall, and are expressed
by a Valsalva manouevre.

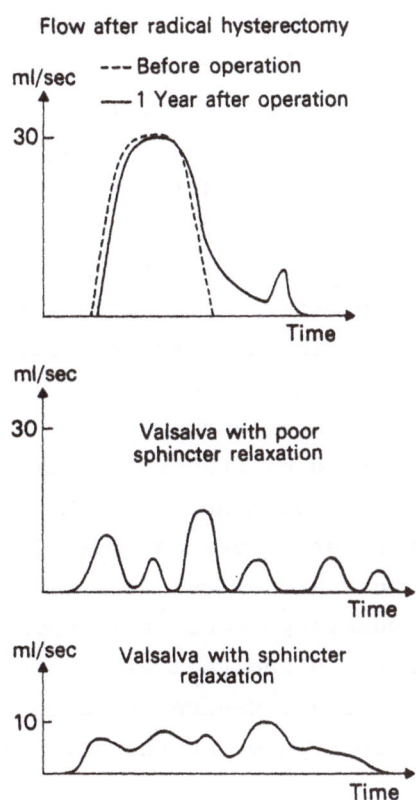

Fig. 13   Different types of flowpattern after radical hysterectomy. The upper curve shows that although the flowcurve
is almost normalized 1 year after operation, many patients have to squeeze out the last few ml's, probably
due to stiffness in the bladderwall.

The ureteres

As a final remark the author will not only emphasize the need
of extremely careful dissection of the ureteres during operation, but also stress the importance of well functioning retroperitoneal suction drains in each obturator fossa. The author strongly believes that postoperative hematoma and lymphcyst formation can and should be prevented by efficient suction drainage, which should be maintained until nothing more
comes out.
The considerable amount of lymph will drain out simply because
the lymphatic drainage system from the femoral and inguinal
nodes has been removed. If this is allowed to form a large
collection in the pelvis the danger of infection is great.
These lymph cysts can even produce bilateral ureteric obstruction with uremia whether they are infected or not (fig. 14).
Lymph leakage usually ceases after 3 - 7 days. Bleeding in the
form of oozing from the wound surfaces stops within a few
hours, but can nevertheless amount to several hundred ml's.
Infection, hematoma formation, lymphcyst formation with com-
pression and kinking of the ureteres are all serious complications which may result in hydronephrosis. They can lead to
uretric necrosis, stricture, and fistula formation.
Although, the lower third of the ureters are completely dissected peristalsis still continues. In the standard operation
described above the superior vesical arteries, which send
branches to the ureters are always sacrificed but as seen
in table 2, the immediate postoperative changes in the reno-
grams has all disappeared one year after. These immediate
changes did not lead to any severe hydronephrosis and kidney
damage, which can also be seen on the effective renal plasma
flow values.

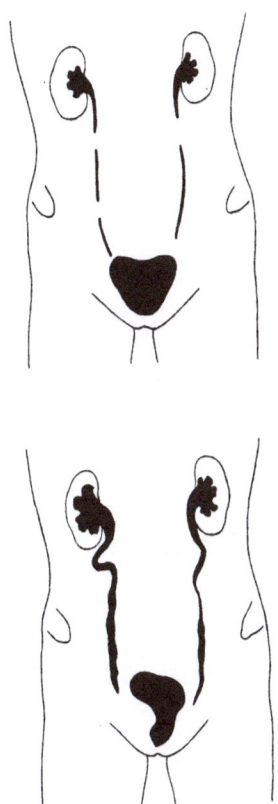

Fig. 14 Urograms before and after radical hysterectomy.
A lymphcyst in the right obtorator fossa produces
hydronephrosis and impression in the bladder.

Table 2.

Renography and ERPF

Examination	Pre-operative		After 14 days		After 11 months	
average	right	left	right	left	right	left
t min.	3.9	4.0	7.0	6.3	3.9	3.9
t½ min.	7.1	6.1*)	13.9	10.5	5.5	5.3
ERPF ml	479 ml		527 ml		489 ml	
ERPF %	50.8%	49.2%	49.7%	50.3%	52.3%	47.7%

*) In 1 ptt. t½ 30 min. was normalised after 1 year.

Table 3.   Urograms

	Normal		Dilatation					
			Mild		Moderate		Extensive	
	right	left	right	left	right	left	right	left
Pre-op.	24	25	1					
14 days postop.	22	20		3		1	3	
11 months postop.	24	25	1*)					

*) Same ptt. as pre-op.

Table 3 shows the urograms in the same group of patients.
Severe complications and dysfunction of the lower urinary tract
can, and must be kept to a low level if radical hysterectomy
with lymph node dissection is performed. The many advantages
of surgical treatment must not be sacrificed because of an un-
acceptably high rate of urological complications compared to
radiotherapy. Radical hysterectomy with lymph node dissection

is an exciting surgical procedure which still should be in the field of surgical gynecology.

REFERENCES

1. Asmussen, M. 1975. Urethro-cysteometry in women. M.D. Thesis. University of Lund.
2. Asmussen, M. & Ulmsten, U. 1976. Simultaneous urethro-cystometry a new technique. Scand. J. Urol. Nephrol. 10:7.
3. Asmussen, M. 1980. Aspects of continence, incontinence and micturition in women. In Gynecologic Urology & Urodynamics, Ed. D. Ostergard. Williams & Wilkins, Baltimore.
4. Asmussen, M. 1981. Radical hysterectomy without denervating the lower urinary tract. Proc. I.U.G.A. Meeting, Stockholm.
5. Asmussen, M. 1981. Bladder & urethral function after radical hysterectomy. Proc. International Continence Society, Annual Meeting, p. 99.
6. Asmussen, M. & Ulmsten, U. 1982. Immediate bladder dysfunction after radical hysterectomy (in press).
7. Bates, P. et al. 1979. Standardisation of terminology of lower urinary tract funciton. J. Urol. 121:554.
8. Bonney, V. 1974. In: Bonney's Gynecological Surgery, 9th edn. Ed. Howkins J. and Stallworthy J. Bailliere Tindall, London.
9. Curtis, A.H. et al. 1952. Anatomy of the pelvic Autonomic nerves in relation to gynecology. Surg. Gyn. Obstet. 75: 743.
10. Forney, J.P. 1980. Effect of radical hysterectomy on bladder physiology. Am. J. Obstet. Gynecol. 138:374.
11. Glahn, B.E. 1970. The neurogenic factor in vesical dysfunction following radical hysterectomy for carcinoma of cervix. Scand. J. Urol. Nephrol. 4:107.
12. Green, T.H., Meigs, J.V., Ulfelder, H., Curtin, R.R. 1962. Urologic complications of radical Wertheim hysterectomy. Obstet. & Gynecol. 20:293.
13. Hohenfellner, R. 1965. Die urologischen Komplicationen des Collum-Carcinoms. Springer Verlag, Heidelberg.
14. Huisman, A.B. 1979. Morfologie van de vrouwelijke urethra. M.D. Thesis, Univ. of Groningen.
15. Low, J.A., Mauger, G.M., Carmichael, J.A. 1981. The effect of Wertheim hysterectomy upon bladder and urethral function. Am. J. Obstet. Gynecol. 139:826.
16. Mackenrodt, A. 1905. Ergebnisse der abdominalen Radikaloperation des Gebärmutterscheiden Krebses. Zeits. f. Geburtshilfe und Gynäkologie 54:514.
17. Martius, H. 1971. Die gynäkologischen Operationen. Georg Thieme Verlag. Stuttgart.
18. Meigs, J.V. 1954. Surgical Treatment of cancer of the cervix. Grune and Stratton. New York.
19. Nakano, R. 1981. The Okabayashi operation and its modifications. Gynecol. Obstet. Invest. 12. 281.

20. Nelson, J.H.jr. 1977. Atlas of radical pelvic surgery. 2nd ed. Appleton, Century Crofts. New York.
21. Novak, F. 1956. Procedure for the reduction of the number of uretero-vaginal fistulas after Wertheims operation. Gynecol. 72:506.
22. Palm, L., and Ronnike, F. 1977. Bladder function following either radiotherapy or radical operation ad modum Okabayashi for cervical cancer. Danish Med. Bull. 17:113.
23. Rud, T. et al. 1980. Factors maintaining the intraurethral pressure in women. Invest. Urol. 17:343.
24. Seski, J.C.,Dioko, A.C. 1977. Bladder dysfunction after radical abdominal hysterectomy. Am. J. Obstet. Gynecol. 128:643.
25. Ulmsten, U. 1974. Studies on urethral function in women. M.D. Thesis, Univ. of Lund.
26. Wertheim, E. 1911. Die erweiterte Operation bei Carcinoma Colli Uteri. Urban Schwarzenberg, Berlin.
27. Yagi, H. 1955. Extended abdominal hysterectomy with pelvic lymphadenectomy for carcinoma of the cervix - the Okabayashi operation. Am. J. Obstet. Gynecol. 69:33.

14. RADIOTHERAPY IN CONJUNCTION WITH SURGERY IN THE TREATMENT
OF PATIENTS WITH EARLY CERVICAL CANCER

Kjell E. Kjoerstad, Oslo, Norway.

Early cervical cancer may be defined as clinical Stages IA,
IB and IIA. Prognostically a border exists between Stage IIA
and IIB, also setting the limit between cases suited for surgery and cases in which full reliance is placed upon radiotherapy. Preoperative and postoperative irradiation is widely
used as an adjunct to surgical treatment, and from the latest
issue of the "Annual Report" published by FIGO it is evident
that in more than 4000 cases, treated surgically, preoperative
irradiation was given to at least 1/3 of the patients. The
rationale for the use of two treatment modalities, each of
which is potentially curative, is that the two methods together
will give better treatment results than either one used alone.
To the author's knowledge, no randomized series are published
that can substantiate this idea and to compare results from
one institution to another is virtually impossible because
surgical series are always selected. Preoperative irradiation
is usually delivered by means of intracavitary deposits of
radium or other isotopes and the objective of this treatment
is to achieve primary cure of the local tumor. Because of the
enormous doses that can be delivered by radium, this objective is usually fulfilled. Postoperative, external irradiation
in most cases is used when the primary treatment has either
failed as when tumor has been transsected, or when the operation cannot be expected to give optimal results, as in the
case of pelvic lymph node involvement.
The addition of irradiation to the surgical trauma has been
accused of producing prohibitive complication rates without
adding anything positive to the final treatment results. This

is uncritically used in all high-risk cases in order to try
to achieve results that realistically are unachievable. When
one modality alone is known to produce acceptable results,
there is no reason to superimpose the other as the only effect is liable to be an increase in the complication rate.
At the Norwegian Radium Hospital combined treatment schedules
have been in use for the last 30 years. The following is a
brief presentation of some of the patient materials recently
analyzed. The objective of this presentation is to show that
irradiation can be combined with surgery without undue complications.

Stage IA

Due to earlier detection the number of patients presenting
with this stage of disease is steadily increasing.
In Norway Stage IA accounts for approximately 15% of all cases.
Numerous definitions of this entity are in use, but the common
denominator of most of these definitions is the depth of
stromal invasion. Local treatment (conisation or conservative
hysterectomy) will give excellent results with 5-year survival as high as 99% (1). When the depth of the lesion is less
than 5 mm, these cancers will have a very limited potential
for dissemination and if there is no evidence of lymphatic invasion, we have failed to find pelvic lymph node involvement.
(Table I). These relatively superficial lesions will always

Table I. Stage IA. - Patients treated with local tumour excision, subsequently observed from 5-15
years; maximum depth of tumour: 5 mm.

	No.	Metastases
No lymphatic involvement	108	0
lymphatic involvement	10	3

easily be eradicated by surgery and thus there is no place
for radiotherapy in addition to surgery in these patients. In
the Norwegian Radium Hospital series no notice was taken of
the surface or growth pattern of the tumor, and the only criterion for the diagnosis was the depth of infiltration. This
lesion, with a very favorable prognosis should be carefully
sought for, because cure can be achieved with very simple
means. Therefore, we advocate conisation in all patients with
small tumors merely upon the visual impression that the tumor
is likely to be superficially infiltrating (Table II).

Table II. Treatment schedule, Norwegian Radium Hospital.

Small tumors:		Diagnostic conization
Stage IA :		Conservative
	Less than 5 mm infil-tration. No lymph vessel invasion:	Hysterectomy
Stage IB :		
	All patients:	Preoperative radium followed by modified radical hysterectomy and pelvic lymphaden-ectomy
	Patients with lymph node metastases:	Postoperative external beam. Total dose 4000-5000 rad given in 20-30 fractions.

Stage IB

Extensive use of diagnostic conisation leads to a less favorable stratification of the IB cases. A high metastasic rate
must be expected and in our hospital routine sectioning of

surgical removed pelvic lymph nodes has revealed a high and
constant rate of 25-30%. In these cases one is clearly dealing with a high risk group of patients within Stage I, and
the rational for combined treatment becomes evident. What
then can be achieved with preoperative treatment with radium?
If 6000-7000 rad is delivered to Point A, only 10% of the
patients will have residual tumor in the hysterectomy specimen, and of these 10% only a small fraction will actually
have viable tumor. Thus the objective of the preoperative
treatment in this stage of the disease, namely primary cure
of the tumor, can be achieved in perhaps 95-98% of the patients. Taking the number of patients with pelvic lymph node
involvement into account, the surgeon will be operating in a
tumor free field in approximately 79% of the cases. This will
allow a less radical dissection of the ureters and reduce the
risk of complications from the urinary tract. Further, the
vaginal cuff can be kept minimal with subsequent little impairment of the sexual function. Lastly, but also very importantly, is that the often found concommitant vaginal infection will be cured together with the tumor, minimizing
the risk of postoperative bacterial complications. The benefits of preoperative irradiation must be weighed against the
possible draw-backs (Tabel III). After radium treatment a
very pronounced hyperaemia will take place and surgery must
be delayed until this reaction has subsided, usually 4-6 weeks.
After this time, fibrosis will start to develop and surgery
may become impossible if for any reason the operation is
postponed beyond this period. The intracavitary treatment
delivers very modes doses to the pelvic walls, and no effect
from this irradiation can be expected on involved pelvic
lymph nodes. Therefore, for such patients the delay in treatment may, at least in theory, increase the risk of further
dissemination of disease. The validity of this argument is
extremely difficult to evaluate, but from extensive studies
of lymphangiography in conjunction with primary treatment of
cervical cancer, it is permissible to conclude that this phe-
nomenon must at least be very rare (2, 3). The second argument

against combination therapy is that prohibitive complication
rates will result from such treatment schedules.

Table III. Cancer of the cervix.

Pro: Reduced need for extensive surgery,
vaginal cuff small,
sexual functions less disturbed.

Less radical dissection of the ureters.

Reduced risk of urinary tract complications.

Few central recurrences.

75% of the patients will not need external irradiation.

Contra: Requires two hospitalization periods.

In case of metastases to the pelvic lymph nodes a
heavy radiation load in addition to surgical trauma.

Increased risk of complications?

Dissemination of disease between radium and surgery?

Analysis of 612 cases treated with a combination of intracavitary irradiation and radical surgery in our department
shows that in only 2 out of 12 cases of fistula formation in
the urinary and/or gastrointestinal tract, the intracavitary
treatment could be held chiefly responsible for the complication (Table IV) (4). We feel able to conclude that preoperative irradiation with radium can safely be conducted in
Stage IB.
In some large exophytic and bulky tumors the dose distribution from intracavitary implants cannot be expected to be optimal. In these cases the chances of primary cure are much
reduced and the 4-6 weeks necessary to accomplish the radiation treatment can only be considered a waste of time. External irradiation can sometimes reduce the tumor volume, but
tumoricidal doses given to the whole of the pelvis will

seriously influence the complication rates after surgery.

Table IV. "Etiology" of complications (fistulae).
          Combined therapy series, Norwegian Radium Hospital,
          1968-1977.

	No. of patients	No of permanent fistulae
Surgery	612	1
Intracavitary treatment	612	2
External irradiation, 4000-5000 rad	138	9

These tumors also have a higher incidence of pelvic lymph
node metastases than the average tumor in stage IB, and regardless of treatment modality the treatment results will be
inferior. Primary surgery is often difficult in these cases
and the risk of tumor involvement of resection borders substantial. Many of these tumors are perhaps better treated by
pure radiotherapy. In a series of 39 very large Stage IB tumors treated by primary surgery the resection borders were
involved in 11 and the recurrence rate was 65% over a three
year period.

Stage II

Residual tumor after intracavitary irradiation increases
with tumor volume. In Stage IIA a local, or central recurrence rate can be reduced by addition of radical surgery. In
a series of 119 patients with Stage IIA disease, randomized
to either full course of radiotherapy, or to a combined treatment schedule with preoperative radium followed by radical
surgery, the local recurrence rate was 9% in the radiotherapy
group and 1.5% in the combined treatment group (5). The number

of patients with residual tumor in the hysterectomy specimen
was twice as high as for Stage IB patients. This series il-
lustrates the benefit of local preoperative irradiation as
all 62 patients in the surgery group had resection borders
free of disease, despite the fact that they all had vaginal
tumor involvement prior to treatment. The incidence of pelvic lymph node metastases was high, 32%.

Postoperative irradiation

Postoperative external beam treatment is much more common
than preoperative intracavitary treatment with isotopes. It
is used as an adjunct to surgery when this treatment modality
has clearly failed or when the prognosis is poor despite radical surgery as is the case when metastases are found in the
pelvic lymph nodes. After radical surgery in Stage IB the
presence or absence of lymph node involvement has a drastic
effect on prognosis. Without metastases the 5-year survival
rate is 90-95%, opposed to 40-50% when metastases are found.
Postoperative external treatment is widely used in such cases,
but its effectiveness remains to be proven (6). Used alone,
there is conclusive evidence that radiotherapy can cure lymph
node metastases, even when the disease has progressed to involve the para-aortic nodes. In hte Norwegian Radium Hospital
series (7) two patients with proven para-aortic lymph node
involvement were alive and well after five years of observation following radiotherapy only. However, there is little
evidence that external irradiation improves 5-year survival
after surgical removal of cancerous lymph nodes (6, 8). Extended fields and higher doses have not improved survival
rates, but may well have contributed to increased morbidity
and mortality from complications (9). In Stage IB, para-aortic metastases will be found in a few per cent of the patients
and of all patients with pelvic lymph node involvement, distant metastases will be the first site of recurrence in a
substantial percentage (7). Local or regional irradiation
will not cure these patients and in the remaining the anticipated effect of extended fields and doses approaching max-

imum tolerance is so small that this kind of treatment cannot be accepted in view of the induced morbidity (4). In patients treated with 5000 rad to pelvic fields postoperatively because of metastases in the pelvic lymph nodes, the incidence of fistulae was 12% (Table IV). The presidential Panel of the Society of Gynecologic Oncology reported at the 1979 annual meeting that distant metastases are more common in patients treated by external irradiation for pelvic lymph node metastases than in patients who did not receive such treatment. From the same report it is evident that postoperative irradiation gives a better control of the disease in the pelvis. It is hard to accept that radiotherapy, which can cure squamous cell cancer of the cervix to the same extent as surgery, regardless of whether metastases are present or not, at the same time can induce dissemination of the disease. However, there are some experimental evidence in animal models that support this possibility (10). In conclusion, the benefit of external irradiation as an adjunct to surgery in this stage of disease remains to be conclusively proven, but as the primary goal of such treatment is a better pelvic control of the disease, and this seems to be possible, we find external radiotherapy justified and necessary. Extended fields and very high doses should be avoided, because when superimposed upon the surgical trauma the tissue tolerance is easily violated.

References

1. Iversen, T., Abeler, V. and Kjørstad, K.E. 1979. Factors influencing the Treatment of Patients with Stage IA Carcinoma of the Cervix. Br. J. Obstet. Gynaecol. 86:593.
2. Kjørstad, K.E., Drevvatne, T., Kobenstvedt, A. and Ørjasaeter, H. 1980. Lymphography and CEA in the Diagnosis of Metastases in Patients with Stage IB Cancer of the Cervix. Diagnost. Gynecol. Obstet. 2:71.
3. Kjørstad, K.E. and Kolbenstvedt, A. Ten Year Follow-up of 300 Patients with cervical Cancer, Stage IB. An Evaluation of the Role of complete Lymphadenectomy. In preparation.
4. Kjørstad, K.E. Marimbeau, P.W. and Iversen, T. Stage IB Carcinoma of the Cervix, The Norwegian Radium Hospital. Results and Complications III. Gynec. Oncol. In press.

5. Kjørstad, K.E. Surgery and Radiotherapy in Cancer of the Cervix, Stage IIA. A randomized Study of 119 Cases. In press.
6. Morrow, C.P. et al. 1980. Is pelvic Radiation beneficial in the postoperative Management of Stage IB Squamous Cell Carcinoma of the Cervix with pelvic Lymph Node Metastases treated by radical Hysterectomy and pelvic Lymphaden-ectomy? Gynec. Oncol. 10:105.
7. Martimbeau, P.W., Kjorstad, K.E. and Iversen, T. Stage IB Carcinoma of the Cervix, The Norwegian Radium Hospital. Results and Complications II, Results when Pelvic Nodes are involved. Obstet. Gynecol. In press.
8. Fuller, A.F., Elliot, N. et al. 1982. Lymph Node Meta-stases from Carcinoma of the Cervix, Stages IB and IIA: Implications for Prognosis and Treatment. Gynec. Oncol. 13:165.
9. Rutledge, F.M., Wharton, J.T. and Fletcher, G.H. 1976. Clinical Studies with adjunctive Surgery and Irradiation Therapy in the Treatment of Carcinoma of the Cervix. Cancer. 38:596.
10. Baker, D., Elkon, D. et al. 1981. Does Local X-irradiation of a Tumor Increase the Incidence of Metastases? Cancer. 48:2394.

15. PELVIC EXENTERATION IN THE TREATMENT OF RECURRENT CERVI-
CAL CANCER.

George W. Morley, M.D.

Ever since 1948, when Brunschwig (1) described the principles
and methods of pelvic exenteration as a therapeutic approach
to certain forms of pelvic malignancy, several technical changes have been advanced and many guidelines have been established in the over-all care of these patients. This has resulted
in a significant improvement in survival. To maintain excel-
lence in over-all survival, the established criteria must be
adhered to when considering patients as candidates for pelvic
exenteration therapy.
During the 16 year period from June 1, 1965 to June 1, 1981,
approximately 90 patients have been treated with some type of
pelvic exenteration at the University of Michigan Medical Center, Ann Arbor, Michigan. Our over-all survival rate has made
this radical surgical procedure an acceptable approach to the
treatment of recurrent carcinoma of the cervix. It also must
be remembered that the primary goal of every surgeon performing
this procedure is the control and cure of the existing disease, with palliation seldom an indication. Of the patients
treated with this form of radical pelvic surgery, over 75%
were treated with total pelvic exenteration; the remainder
being treated with either resection of the bladder anteriorly
or excision of the bowel posteriorly, depending on the location of the tumor. One must not be too conservative, however,
in selecting the type of pelvic exenteration to be performed
while trying to avoid more than one diversionary procedure.
Such conservatism may not only lead to fistulous complications
but may unfavorably affect survival, since microscopically
extended disease cannot be seen by the naked eye or palpated
by the examining finger.

Type of disease

The lesions most suitable for pelvic exenterative surgery are
those of squamous cell variety since spread of this type of
tumor beyond the primary organ often occurs in continuity and
in contiguity during the earlier stages of recurrence. For
this reason, then, patients with recurrent squamous cell carcinoma of the cervix are the most ideal candidate for this
treatment. Patients with carcinoma of the ovary are not to be
considered candidates for this type of radical pelvic surgery
since the pattern of recurrent growth in this disease is one
of disorganized abdominal dissemination. Carcinoma of the endometrium, on the other hand, is a more favorable lesion than
is carcinoma of the ovary; however, its pattern of growth is
also unpredictable. A patient with primary squamous cell carcinoma of the vulva may very well be a candidate for some
type of pelvic exenteration, primarily because of the geo-
graphic location of the primary lesion.

Extent of disease

Since it is our goal to perform a curative procedure - not a
palliative one - the criteria used to determine whether or
not a patient is a candidate for pelvic exenteration must be
strictly adhered to with a thorough clinical evaluation and
investigative work-up of the patient.
Whereas, (1) an abnormal pyelogram; (2) lower extremity edema;
and (3) sciatic distribution of pain have often been referred
to as the "Triad of Trouble", they cannot always determine
the candidacy of a patient for pelvic exenterative therapy.
They suggest, however, that the recurrent lesion is inoperable.
The presence of any one of these abnormalities suggests that
there is pelvic lymph node or lateral pelvic wall involvement
with tumor extending away from the central recurrent area.
Again, whenever one is in doubt as to the resectability of
a lesion and the curability of the disease, then exploratory
laparotomy is indicated irrespective of the results of these
studies. The court of last resort is in the operating room!

More recently, a number of investigative techniques have been
introduced into the preoperative evaluation period of these
patients. (1) The Tru-Cut biopsy needle has been used very
effectively in evaluating pelvic masses extending out toward
the lateral pelvic wall. These biopsies are obtained trans-
vaginally and are most helpful in determining the lateral
extent of the disease. (2) Computerized axial tomographic
scanning also adds additional information in the preoperative
work-up of these patients. (3) Lymphangiography is considered
somewhat unreliable in many institutions; however, with improved techniques and better interpretation, this diagnostic
evaluation can be of immeasurable assistance. Once the
lymphangiographic study is reported as suspicious or abnormal,
then a confirmatory biopsy can be performed utilizing the
transcutaneous fine-needle aspiration technique. To date,
over 50 fine-needle aspirations have been performed at the
University of Michigan Hospital with an approximate 75%
accuracy on the first aspiration and 85% accuracy rate can
be expected if one employs a second aspiration should the
first one be reported negative for metastatic disease. (5)
These specialized studies are coupled with the routine physical examination, thorough pelvic examination and basic laboratory and roentgenologic studies. In our institution, approximately 2/3 of all patients explored with recurrent disease
are treated with pelvic exenterative surgery as planned.
Over 90% of the patients who were not candidates for pelvic
exenterative therapy after intra-operative exploration were
dead of their disease within 24 months.

Technical advances

(a) Transverse abdominal incision. (Figure 1) The transverse
abdominal incision with transsection of the rectus muscles
bilaterally is the incision of choice in our performance of
pelvic exenteration. This incision allows free access to the
pelvic and abdominal contents and provides good exposure for
surgery in the pelvic lymph node area. Surgery in the upper
abdomen is not contemplated at the time of this exploration.

(b) Uretero-sigmoid conduit. (Figure 2 & 3) The utero-sigmoid
conduit for urinary diversion has been utilized in over 80%
of the patients who were treated with total pelvic exenteration and to date, we have been pleased with the results.
Acute urinary tract infection has been a post-operative complication; however, these incisions have responded satisfactorily to appropriate chemotherapy. Ureteral stricture,
ascending pyelonephritis and hyperchloremic-hypokalemic
acidosis is rarely encountered. (c) Sigmoid colostomy. A sigmoid colostomy prepared with a segment of bowel usually located above the previously irradiated field is used in preparation for fecal diversion. No major difficulties have been encountered with this procedure. (d) Inferior vena caval stapling.
As a prophylactic measure against major pulmonary embolization,
the inferior vena cava is compartmentalized by staples. This
then divides the inferior vena cava into four compartments
of decreased caliber. No major pulmonary embolus has occured
since this technique was adopted.

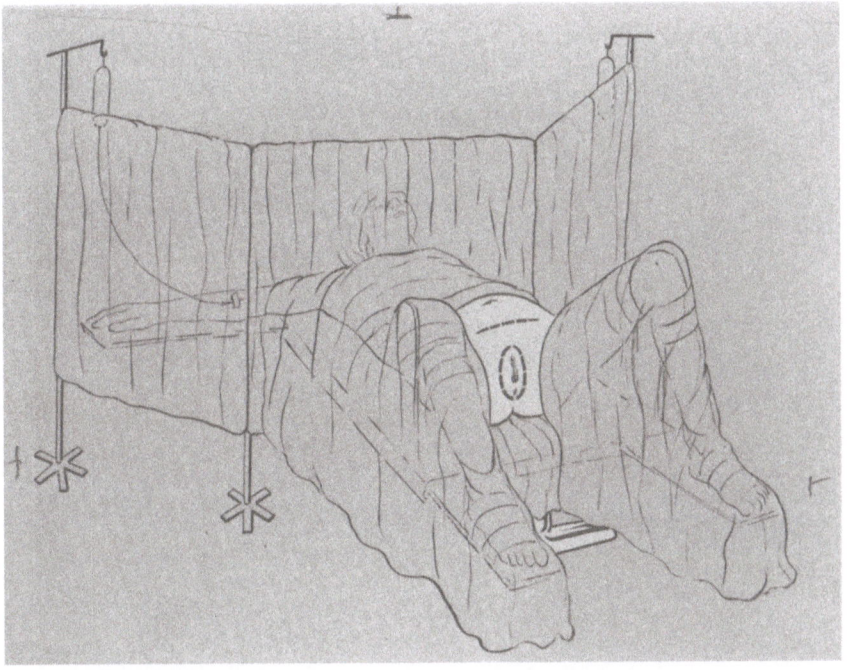

Fig. 1 "Ski Position" for performance of pelvic exenteration.

178

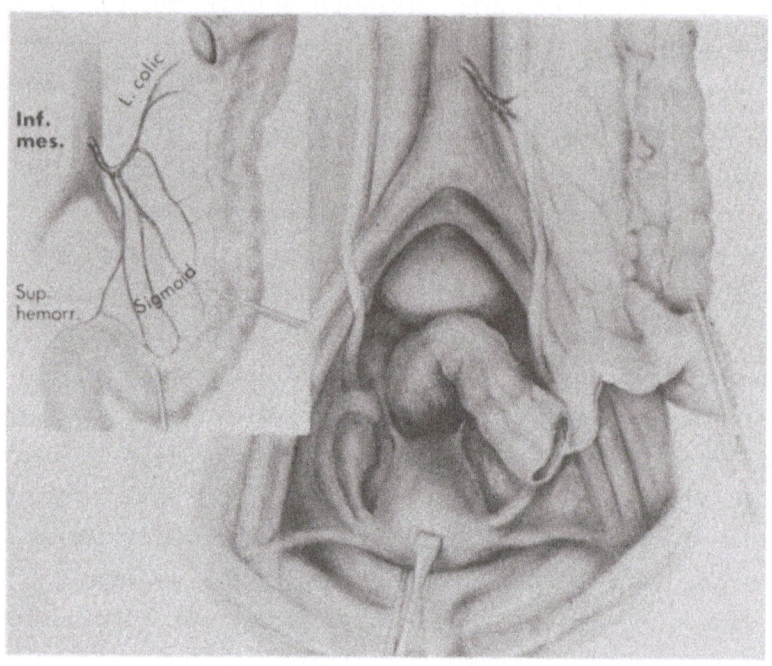

Fig. 2. Isolation of segment of sigmoid in preparation for
utero-sigmoid conduit.

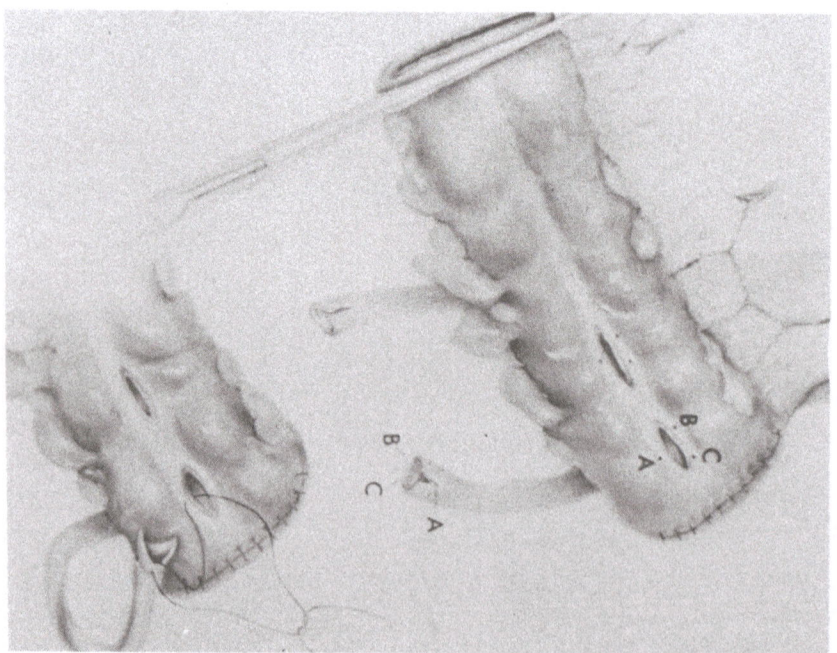

Fig. 3. Diagnostic drawing of utero-sigmoid conduit.

(5) Peritoneal graft. (Figure 4 & 5) Most surgeons involved
in total pelvic exenterative therapy have been somewhat dis-
couraged with the high incidence of post-operative complications directly related to the handling of the pelvic aperture.
Many techniques have been employed; however, we have been
most satisfied with the use of an isolated 12x12 cm. peritoneal graft. (4) This graft is taken from the anterior peritoneal wall and is positioned over the pelvic aperture at the
level of the pelvic diaphragm and levator ani muscles. This
graft acts as a floor for the pelvic contents and as a roof
for the vaginal vault. Post-operative complications have been
at a minimum in the 65 patients treated in this fashion.

Rehabilitation

The post-operative rehabilitation is significantly important
for these individuals. Certainly not all patients subjected
to exenterative therapy are candidates for vaginoplasty, for
reasons of age, marital status and personal inclination.
Split-thickness skin graft vaginoplasty; isolation and trans-
plantation of sigmoid colon; and the William's type vaginoplasty are possible techniques. (3-6-7)

Results

The over-all five-year survival rate for this series is 57%.
(5) The rate of five-year survival for recurrent carcinoma
of the cervix is 63%. There were ten patients on whom pelvic
exenterative therapy was performed even though frozen section
examination reported the presence of positive regional pelvic
lymph nodes with metastatic disease. All ten patients were
dead with disease at two years. Therefore, metastatic regional
lymph nodes are considered a contraindication to this ultra-
radical surgery.

Summary

Over the past 30 years, pelvic exenterative therapy has become
increasingly successful in the control of gynecologic malignancy when the lesion was centrally located in the female genital

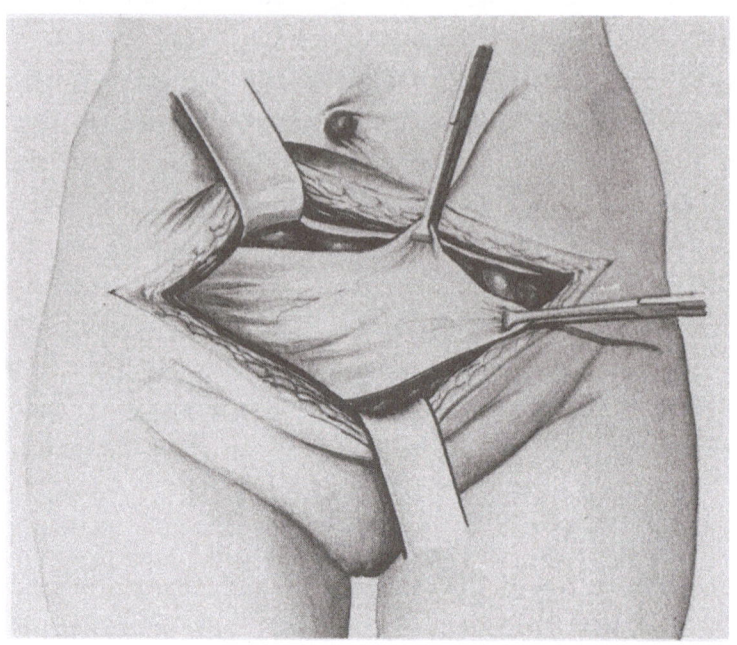

Fig. 4. Preparation of peritoneal graft from anterior peritoneu

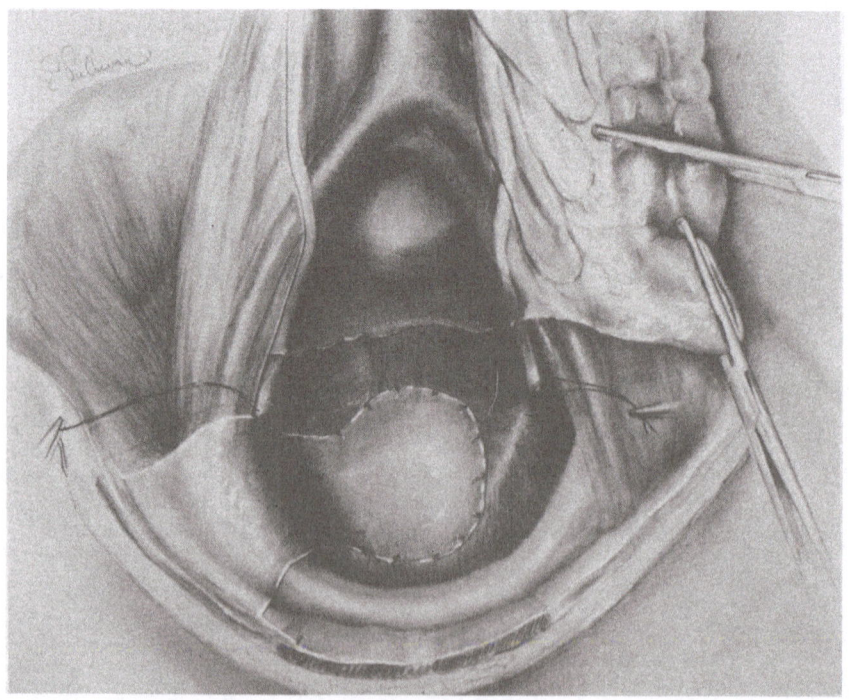

Fig. 5 Placement of peritoneal graft at level of pelvic diaphra

tract. It is believed that when all of the criteria are met, the over-all five-year survival of patients so treated should approximate 60%. The surgeon who embarks on a program of pelvic exenterative therapy must be ready to accept increased responsibility, not only for the significant operative risk, the critical and extensive problems of post-operative care, but also for the long-term rehabilitation of the patient. On the other hand, the rewards are gratifying - - - pelvic exenteration does afford the patient a second chance of survival and those who have been cured are able to lead active and rewarding lives.

REFERENCES

1. Brunschwig, A. 1948. Complete excision of pelvic viscera for advanced carcinoma. Cancer 1:177-183.
2. Brunschwig, A. 1965. Pelvic Exenteration. JAMA 194:160
3. McIndoe, A.H. and Barrister, J.B. 1938. Operations for cure of congenital absence of vagina. J. Obstet. Gynecol. Brit. Emp. 45:490.
4. Morley, G.W. and Lindenauer, S.M. 1971. Peritoneal graft in total pelvic exenteration. Am. J. Obstet. Gynecol. 110: 696-702.
5. Morley, G.W., Lindenauer, S.M. and Cerny, J.C. 1971. Pelvic exenterative therapy in recurrent pelvic carcinoma. Am. J. Obstet. Gynecol. 109:1175.
6. Morley, G.W., Lindenauer, S.M. and Youngs, D.D. 1973. Vaginal reconstruction following pelvic exenteration. Surgical and psychological considerations. Am. J. Obstet. Gynecol. 116:996-1002.
7. Williams, E.A. 1964. Use of vulvar pouch in creation of neo-vagina. J. Obstet. Gunecol. Brit. Comm. 71:511.

16. PELVIC RECONTRUCTION

L.D. Lagasse

Introduction

The management of patients with serious complications resulting from the treatment of gynecologic cancer is complex and
requires care and foresight. Prevention and management of disability resulting from intensive radiotherapy or extended
surgery require an understanding of the operative techniques
of pelvic reconstruction. Techniques now exist to restore
vaginal and rectal function and to reconstruct the pelvic
floor. A coordinated plan for surgical management of patients
who are disabled by the treatment of gynecologic cancer is
discussed.

Vaginal Reconstruction

Loss of adequate vaginal function can be seen following treatment for pelvic malignancy because of scarring associated
with intensive radiation or after extended operative procedures. A careful, individualized approach can restore vaginal
function in many of these patients. A functional and anatomic
reconstruction of the vagina ideally results in a moist, smooth
surface of normal depth and caliber that covers soft and un-
infected surrounding tissues. All of these criteria cannot
be met in every patient. If a suitable anatomic space is
lined with an adequate cover of grafted skin, the resulting
neovagina still may become scarred and rigid. Nevertheless,
attempts to restore sexual function should be made, and in
many instances, such efforts will enable the motivated patient to achieve sexual gratification.
Vaginal reconstruction often is indicated following vaginect-

omy for localized vaginal neoplasia, when there is radiation damage to the vagina or after pelvic exenteration. The optimal reconstructive procedure and its timing should reflect the needs of the individual patient, the antecedent disease process, and the treatment that necessitated vaginal reconstruction.

Following Vaginectomy with Removal of Bladder and Rectum

Vaginal reconstruction using a split-thickness skin graft is satisfactory and may be performed at the time of vaginectomy in patients with superficial vaginal cancer. The technique is simple to perform and is similar to that emplyed in patients with vaginal agenesis (1, 2). In addition to preserving sexual function, vaginal reconstruction permits pelvic examination that can aid in the early diagnosis of recurrence. It supports the base of the bladder and thereby helps prevent bladder dysfunction that can follow vaginectomy. Management of patients with vaginal stenosis secondary to radiation therapy presents a more difficult problem. Extensive fibrosis and absence of normal tissue planes make elimination of the scar tissue difficult. At operation, the scar must be excised and the cavity enlarged maximally (3). In some patient an adequate cavity can be developed by incision of the levator muscles. A split thickness skin graft then is placed and supported for 7 days by a soft vaginal pack. It is likely that the grafted skin will survive, but varying degrees of rigidity often remain. No attempt should be made to reconstruct the vagina damaged by radiation until all acute reaction has subsided. At UCLA we have reviewed our experience of vaginal reconstruction after severe pelvic fibrosis in 12 patients.

After Pelvic Exenteration

McGraw et al (4) have developed a technique using gracilis myocutaneous flaps for vaginal reconstruction at the time of pelvic exenteration. The gracilis muscle and overlying skin

are brought from the thigh to the perineum through a subcutaneous tunnel. The vascular pedicle to the muscle which also
supplies the overlying skin is preserved. Bilateral myocutaneous flaps are dissected and sewn together to form a vaginal
tube that is inserted into the open pelvic cavity. The procedure provides a fatty, musculocutaneous tissue mass that serves
as a functional vagina. In addition, the neovagina has sufficient bulk to fill a large part of the empty pelvic cavity
following pelvic exenteration thereby decreasing the risk of
complications related to the raw pelvic floor. The major disadvantage of the procedure is the increase in operative time
for the pelvic exenteration. The resulting lower limb scars
have not been debilitating, but may limit early postoperative
ambulation. The results of the procedure are promising but
further trial is needed.

It is often difficult to establish a functional vagina after
extensive treatment of a pelvic malignancy. Successful restor-
ation of anatomy is not always possible, and when accomplished
is not always associated with complete sexual rehabilitation.
Surgical techniques are sufficiently advanced to offer vaginal
reconstruction to most of these patients; however, the levels
of emotional and sexual adjustment that existed before treatment also are reflected in the final result.

Vulva reconstruction

Rotational pedicle flaps

Rotational pedicle flaps can be used to cover moderate size
vulva defects. Flaps are mobilized from the periphery of the
vulva defects and rotated medially. They should be broad at
the base to preserve blood supply and the length should not
be more than two times the width of the base. Defects created
by mobilization of flaps can usually be closed without tension.

The gracilis myocutaneous flap

The gracilis myocutaneous flap described for vaginal reconstruction can be used to cover larger tissue defects of the

vulva or perineum.

The anterior border of the flap lies on a line drawn between the proximal adductor longus tendon and the distal semitendonosis tendon. The flap extends 6 cm posterior to this line and can be as long as 25 cm. A skin incision is made and elevation of the flap begins at the posterior margin of the adductor longus tendon. The proximal vascular pedicle of the gracilis muscle is identified between the fascia which separates the adductor longus and brevis muscles.. The gracilis muscle with attached skin and subcutaneous tissues then is elevated and freed from all attachments except its vascular pedicle. The flap is then rotated into position to cover the defect in the vulva. Redundant subcutaneous tissue may be trimmed from the graft, but care must be taken to preserve all mobilized muscle or loss of blood supply to the skin could result. The edges of the graft are sewn to the edges of the defect with 2-0 nylon sutures. The defect in the leg then is closed with 3-0 chromic subcutaneous sutures and 2-0 nylon sutures reapproximate the skin. Suction catheters are placed in the donor site and the grafted site through separate stab incisions.

Restoration of Rectal Function

The disability resulting from a permanent colostomy is a major obstacle to the rehabilitation of patients undergoing total or posterior pelvic exenteration. Bacon (5), Swenson and Bill (6) and others have shown that normal rectal function can be achieved by substituting a segment of sigmoid colon for the resected rectum. The reconstruction can be attempted only if the rectal sphincter can be preserved while providing wide surgical clearance of the tumor. In suitable candidates, rectal substitution, which is performed at the time of pelvic exenteration, can obviate the need for permanent colostomy and decrease the disability that otherwise would result. The extent of the operative procedure with preservation of the rectal sphincter is outlined in the figure. Total exenteration involves the en bloc removal of the tumor

and adjacent organs, including the rectum, vagina, adnexae
and bladder (7-10) (Fig. 1).

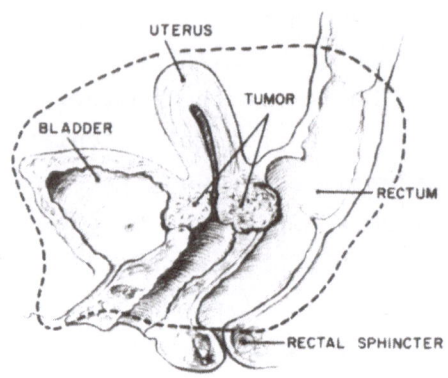

Fig. 1   Total exenteration to include removal of all structures within the broken line.

The colon is transected superiorly at the recto-sigmoid function and inferiorly at the rectal sphincter. The descending
colon and splenic flexure are freed from their lateral peritoneal attachments. The most critical portion of the operative procedure is the preservation of adequate blood supply
while mobilizing the sigmoid colon. To allow the distal sig·
moid to reach the level of the rectal sphincter without tension, the remaining sigmoid colon is mobilized by ligating
all but the most superior branches of the inferior mesenteric
artery. A wide cuff of mesentary must be mobilized with the
sigmoid colon to preserve the blood supply provided by the
marginal artery of Drummond. Interruption of this arterial
segment usually results in ischemic necrosis of the distal
colon.

The transverse colon is transected near the mobilized splenic
flexure and the distal segment is brought out through the
abdominal wall as a mucous fistula. The functioning transverse
colostomy then must be placed immediately adjacent to the
mucous fistula (Fig. 2). The intervening segment of transverse
colon is isolated for use as a urinary conduit as noted in

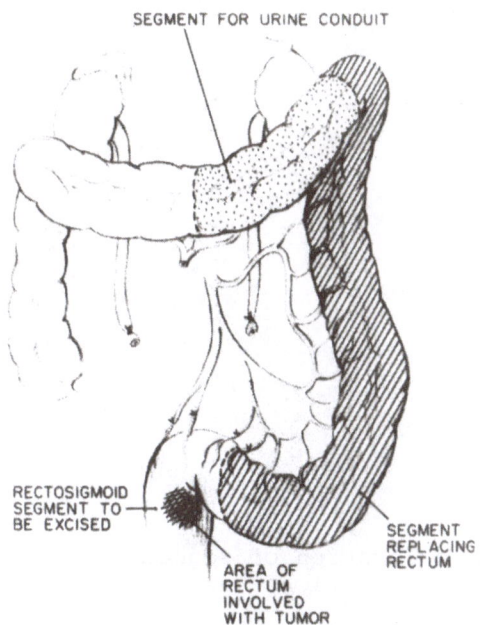

SEGMENT FOR URINE CONDUIT

RECTOSIGMOID SEGMENT TO BE EXCISED

SEGMENT REPLACING RECTUM

AREA OF RECTUM INVOLVED WITH TUMOR

Fig. 2   Alternate choice of colon segments to be used for
urine conduit and rectal substitution. Transverse
colon is used for urinary conduit.

the figure. The distal portion of the bowel segment to be
used as the urinary conduit is closed with a double layer of
polyglycolic acid sutures after which the ureters are implanted
The base of the conduit is anchored to the posterior peritoneum and the proximal portion is brought through the anterior
abdominal wall as a stoma (Fig. 3).

The anastomosis of the sigmoid colon to the rectal stump is
carried out through a perineal approach. We now chose to employ a stapling technique using the end to end EEA Stapler.
Closure of the colostomy should be considered four to six
months after rectal substitution following evaluation of the
colorectal anastomosis and rectal sphincter. A radiopaque
contrast medium is instilled in the distal segment to assess
the integrity of the anastomosis. Sphinter function is evalu-

188

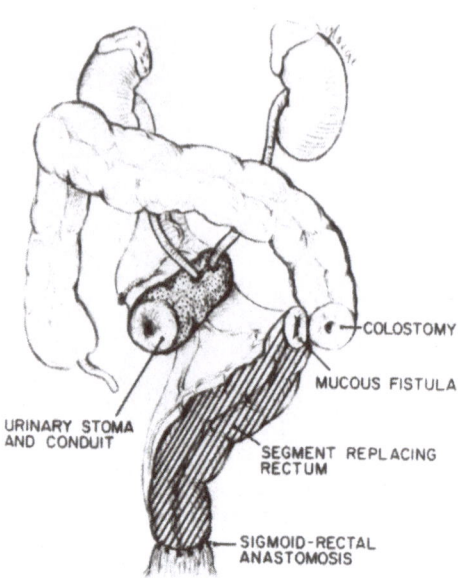

Fig. 3   Postoperative location of segment replacing rectum.
Mucous fistula positioned next to colostomy stoma.

ated by instilling saline and then injecting air into the neo-
rectum. The colostomy may be closed after demonstration of a
satisfactory sphincteric mechanism and a healed anastomosis
(Fig. 4).

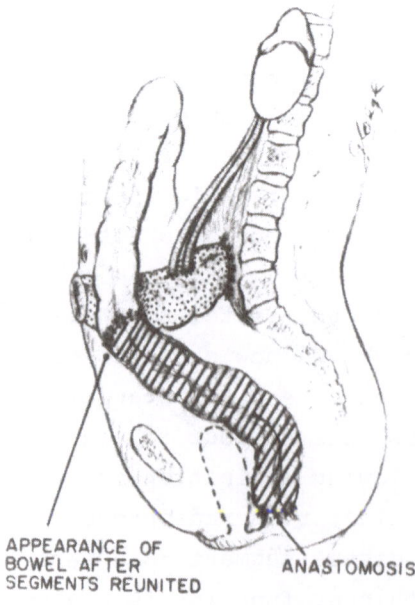

Fig. 4   Appearance of colon after
closure of colostomy and
re-establishment of conti
nuity. The broken line in
dicates area of possible
vaginal reconstruction us
ing the sigmoid segment a
a floor for the new vagin

Rectal reconstruction demands increased attention to surgical detail and additional operating time. While not suitable for all patients undergoing exenteration, it can help to restore selected individuals to a more normal life.

REFERENCES

1. McIndoe, A.H., Banister, J.B. 1938. An operation for the care of congenital absence of the vagina. J. Obst. Gynaec. Brit. Emo. 45:490.
2. Whitely, J.M., Parrott, M.H., Rowland, W. 1964. Split-thickness skin graft tehcnique in the correction of congenital or acquired vaginal stresia. Am. J. Obst. Gynec. 89:377.
3. Watring, W.G., Lagasse, L.D., Smith, M.L., et al. 1976. Vaginal reconstruction following extensive treatment for pelvic cancer. Am. J. Obst. Gynec. 125:809.
4. McGraw, J.B., Massey, F.M., Shanklin, K.D. 1976. Vaginal reconstruction with gracilis myocutaneous flaps. Plastic. Reconst. Surg. 58:176.
5. Bacon, H.E. 1945. Evaluation of sphincter muscle preservation and re-establishment of continuity in the operative treatment of rectal and sigmoidal cancer. Surg. Gynec. Obst. 81:113.
6. Swenson, O., Bill, A.H., Jr. 1948. Resection of rectum and rectosigmoid with preservation of the sphincter for benign spastic lesions producing megacolon. Surgery 24:212.
7. Bricker, E.M., Butcher, H.R., Jr, Lawler, W.H., Jr, McAfee, C.A. 1960. Surgical treatment of advanced and recurrent cancer of the pelvic viccera: An evaluation of ten years experience. Ann. Surg. 152:388.
8. Brunschwig, A. 1967. Surgical treatment of carcinoma of the cervix recurrent after irradiation or combination of irradiation and surgery. Am. J. Roent. 99:365.
9. Rutledge, F.M. Burns, B.C., Jr. 1965. Pelvic exenteration. Am. J. Obst. Gynec. 91:692.
10. Symmonds, R.E., Pratt, J.H., Webb, M.J. 1975. Exenterative operations: Experience with 198 patients. Am. J. Obst. Gynec. 121:907.

17. THE MORPHOLOGICAL BASIS FOR THE TREATMENT OF ENDOMETRIAL
CARCINOMA IN SITU

H. Fox

In this contribution the relationships between the various
forms of endometrial hyperplasia and the subsequent development of endometrial adenocarcinoma are evaluated. The current
uncertainties about this relationship reflect the extraordi-
nary variations in terminology and definitions, the differing
conceptual approaches, the methodological flaws in most prospective and retrospective studies and the lack of agreement
amongst pathologists as to the criteria for distinguishing
between some forms of hyperplasia and adenocarcinoma which
cloud this whole topic.

Classification of endometrial hyperplasia

Endometrial hyperplasia is not a single entity and to use this
term without any qualification not only denies the existence
of a variety of hyperplastic conditions of the endometrium but
also conceals their independent, and vastly different, relationships to the subsequent development of an endometrial adenocarcinoma.

A useful histological classification of endometrial hyperplasia, based largely on that of Welch and Scully (30), allows
for the recognition of four forms:-

      1. Cystic glandular hyperplasia.

      2. Adenomatoid hyperplasia.

      3. Glandular hyperplasia with architectural atypia.

      4. Glandular hyperplasia with cellular atypia.

The term "cystic glandular hyperplasia" is retained largely
because it has become hallowed by long usage in the litera-

ture: it is, however, a somewhat misleading form of nomenclature for the glands in this form of hyperplasia are not necessarily cystic and the hyperplastic process is, furthermore,
not confined to the glands but also involves the stroma.
Glandular hyperplasia with cellular atypia is synonymous with
"atypical hyperplasia" and there is no real objection to the
use of this terminology except that it implies that there is
such an entity as "typical" hyperplasia and, more importantly,
this name is also often applied to glandular hyperplasia with
architectural atypia, an abnormality which is probably of much
lesser importance. A notable absentee from this classification is "adenomatous hyperplasia", a form of nomenclature
which has not only been used in an indiscriminate and pro-
miscous fashion but also is indefensible in both semantic and
conceptual terms in so far as a lesion can not be both neoplastic and hyperplastic in nature at one and the same time.
The term "adenomatoid hyperplasia" is, on the other hand,
quite acceptable for it is perfectly possible for a hyperplastic condition to resemble a neoplasm: this diagnosis is,
however, restricted here to an uncommon, but specific, form
of endometrial hyperplasia and is not used as a synonym for
"adenomatous hyperplasia".

Pathology of endometrial hyperplasia
Cystic glandular hyperplasia: This involves the whole endometrium which is thickened and not infrequently polypoid, often having a velvety appearance: tiny custs may be seen even
with the naked eye. The myometrium is also usually hypertro-
phied and the uterus bulky. Histologically there is a diffuse
involvement of the endometrium and the distinction between
functional and basal zones is lost. The glands are characterised by their marked variability in size, some being unduly
large, others being of normal calibre and yet others being
unusually small. The glands usually have a regular, smooth
rounded outline but occasionally a minor degree of epithelial
budding into the endometrial stroma is seen. The epithelium
lining the glands is formed of plump, regular, tall cuboidal

or columnar cells which have strongly basophilic cytoplasm and round, basally or centrally placed nuclei. There is commonly a minor or moderate degree of multilayering but intraluminal tufting, loss of polarity and cellular atypia are not seen. The ratio of stroma to glands is normal for the stroma shares in the hyperplastic process and usually appears markedly hypercellular, often showing the "naked nuclei" appearance characteristic of a proliferative phase endometrium. Mitotic figures may be common or sparse, are seen both in the glands and in the stroma and are invariably of normal form.

Adenomatoid hyperplasia: This is a rare form of hyperplasia and is invariably focal in nature: the lesion often appears to be localised to an endometrial polyp but whether this is because the glands in a polyp have undergone this form of hyperplastic change or whether this particular localised form of hyperplasia is characterised by a simple excess of glands which, whilst of somewhat variable calibre, are usually of approximately normal size: they have the rounded appearance characteristic of the endometrial glands during the normal proliferative phase. There is no multilayering, cellular atypia or intraluminal tufting and the overall appearance differs from that of a normal proliferative endometrium only by the marked excess of glands and the striking reduction, though never the complete disappearance, of the intervening stroma.

Glandular hyperplasia with architectural atypia: This form of hyperplasia is restricted to the glandular component of the endometrium and is usually focal rather than diffuse. The glands, though variable in size, are often rather larger than normal and are more numerous, the glands tending to be crowded and the intervening stroma reduced. There is an abnormal pattern of glandular growth with outpouchings, or buddings, of the glandular epithelium into the surrounding stroma to produce the so-called "finger in glove" appearance. Often the glands appear elongated and multiple outpouchings may impart a serrated appearance which may be confused with that of a

normal late secretory phase endometrium. Papillary projections
of epithelial cells, with connective tissue cores, into the
glandular lumens are not uncommon and sometimes solid buds
of cells project into the glands. The glandular epithelium
is regular and formed of tall cuboidal or columnar cells with
ovoid, or less rounded, basal or central nuclei: there is no
cellular or nuclear atypia, little multilayering and no loss
of nuclear polarity. Mitotic figures may be present in the
glands and are of normal type.

Glandular hyperplasia with cellular atypia: This form of hyperplasia is also restricted to the glands of the endometrium and
is always focal in nature, often very sharply so: not uncommonly, however, it is multifocal and this may give a false
impression of diffuse involvement which can only be dispelled
by careful topographic study which shows that the foci of
glands showing cellular atypia are separated from each other
either by normal or atrophic endometrium or by glands showing
another form of hyperplasia. In the affected areas of the
endometrium there is always some crowding of the glands with
a reduction in the amount of interglandular stroma and in the
more severe cases the stroma may be either reduced to a thin
wisp between the glands, often only detectable by a reticulin
stain, or completely obliterated with the glands assuming a
"back-to-back" appearance. The glands may have an outline similar to that seen in an architectural atypia but are often
markedly irregular in shape and size, showing a degree of
irregularity and deformity which goes beyond that explicable
solely in terms of multiple outbuddings. The cells lining the
hyperplastic glands tend to be larger than those seen in a
normal proliferative phase endometrium and show varying degrees of nuclear and cytoplasmic atypia. In the milder forms
of cellular atypia the nuleo-cytoplasmic ratio is either normal or only slightly increased, the nuclei are ovoid or sau-
sage-shaped, nuclear polarity is retained, there is no notice-
able enlargement of the nucleoli and the nuclear chromatin
pattern is normal. In more severe cases the nucleo-cytoplasmic

ratio is increased, the nuclei tend to be rounded, the nucleoli are enlarged, nuclear polarity is disturbed or lost and
the nuclear chromatin may be either clumped or cleared: if
clearing of nuclear chromatin occurs the nuclear membrane is
often very prominent.

In a mild cellular atypia there is commonly, but by no means
invariably, a degree of pseudostratification of the cells lining the glands and with progressing severity of atypia there
is an increasing degree of multilayering and of intraluminal
tufting and budding: the intraluminal tufting can, in severe
forms, be of a complex pattern and the tufts can fuse to give
a cribiform pattern within the glands: these apparent bridges
retain, however, a stromal support, albeit one which may only
be revealed by trichome or reticulin stains.

Mitotic figures are uncommon in mild cases of hyperplasia
with cellular atypia but tend to increase in number with increasing atypia: they are usually of normal form.

Interrelations of the various forms of endometrial hyperplasia

Although each form of endometrial hyperplasia has been described separately it is not uncommon to encounter various
forms of hyperplasia co-existing in the same endometrium. Cystic glandular hyperplasia may exist in a pure form but it is
not uncommonly seen in combination with glandular hyperplasia
with architectural atypia or cellular atypia or both.
Conversely, whilst a pure glandular hyperplasia with architectural atypia can be found in isolation there is often an
accompanying cystic glandular hyperplasia or a glandular hyperplasia with cellular atypia. Glandular hyperplasia with
cellular atypia is rarely, if ever, not accompanied by glands
showing only architectural atypia and may also be associated
with a cystic glandular hyperplasia. The only exception to
this general rule of frequent co-existence is adenomatoid
hyperplasia which, in our experience, appears always to develop in isolation.

These somewhat complex inter-relationships may suggest that
the various forms of hyperplasia are either different morpho-

logical expressions of a common basic abnormality of growth
or that they form a continuous spectrum. In fact, there is no
evidence that cystic glandular hyperplasia is a precursor of,
or evolves into, a purely glandular type of hyperplasia for
transitional forms between the two conditions are not seen,
even when both are present in the same endometrium: often
there is a very sharp and clear boundary between the two abnormal patterns. There is also no evidence that adenomatoid
hyperplasia is related in any way to cystic glandular hyperplasia or to the various forms of glandular hyperplasia with
atypia. On the other hand a glandular hyperplasia with architectural atypia does often appear to evolve into a glandular
hyperplasia with cellular atypia and transitional stages between the two varieties are commonly observed. It is not known
however, if glandular hyperplasia with architectural atypia
commonly, or even usually evolves into a glandular hyperplasia with cellular atypia or whether it is indeed a necessary
and inevitable precursor of cellular atypia.

Endometrial carcinoma in situ

Before discussing the distinction between glandular hyperplasia with severe cellular atypia and adenocarcinoma it is necessary to consider precisely what is meant, in this context,
by adenocarcinoma. It is perfectly clear that an adenocarcinoma which invading the myometrium is a true malignant neoplasm but there has been, and still is, considerable controversy as to the meaning of endometrial adenocarcinoma in situ
(8, 3, 11, 13, 28). The term "endometrial adenocarcinoma in
situ" has in fact been used in three quite different ways,
though this is not always clear in accounts of endometrial
pathology, some authors using the same term in two, or more,
different senses in the same account. Some equate adenocarcinoma in situ with glandular hyperplasia with severe cellular atypia whilst others, though drawing a distinction between these two entities, do not always elaborate as to whether
they consider an in situ adenocarcinoma to be one which is
not invading the endometrial stroma or which is not invading

the myometrium. An adenocarcinoma in situ is, however, by
definition a non-invasive lesion and therefore a true adenocarcinoma in situ of the endometrium is one in which the glands
have undergone neoplastic change but in which there is no
invasion of the endometrial stroma. It is doubtful if an adenocarcinoma of this type exists or if it could be recognised
even if it did exist. Therefore a form of nomenclature has
to be found to describe a lesion which, although thought to
be adenocarcinomatous in nature, is confined to the endometrium and not invading the myometrium. The term "Stage 0 carcinoma" has been applied to a lesion of this type but this
appears to be using a clinical staging to describe a histological finding. "Focal adenocarcinoma" is appropriate for
a tumour which is invading the myometrium may also be focal
whilst "early adenocarcinoma" is too imprecise. If it is in-
sisted upon that a form of adenocarcinoma localised to the
endometrium be recognised and distinguished from glandular
hyperplasia with severe cellular atypia then the term "intraendometrial adenocarcinoma" has much to recommend it though,
as discussed later, a case can be made out for classing both
these lesions as "intraendometrial neoplasia".

Histological distinction between hyperplasia and adenocarcinoma

One of the heaviest crosses which a histopathologist has to
bear is, however, tha task of differentiating histologically
between a glandular hyperplasia with severe cellular atypia
and a well differentiated adenocarcinoma. In a hysterectomy
specimen this burden is, of course, lightened for if there is
unequivocal myometrial invasion then the lesion is, irrespective of morphological niceties, an adenocarcinoma: if there
is no invasion of the myometrium then no practical necessity
for differentiating the two conditions arises in so far as
they both have the same excellent prognosis and are both cured
by the therapeutic measure which has already been performed.
The difficulty is therefore encountered in its most acute
form in curettage material and suggested criteria for indicating that the glands in such specimens are neoplastic rather

than hyperplastic include the formation of intraglandular
bridges without stromal support, the presence of nuclear debris and polymorphonuclear leucocytes within glandular lumens,
stratification of cells to form a "gland-within-gland" pattern,
loss of nuclear polarity, marked nuclear irregularity, rounding of the nuclei, nucleolar prominence, the presence of pale
eosinophilic cytoplasm, the finding of numerous mitotic figures,
the presence of abnormal mitotic figures, the complete absence of stroma between glands and the piling up of cells into random sheets or masses (12, 23, 26, 27). Features suggested
as indicating stromal invasion, and therefore implying the
malignant nature of the glands, include fibrosis of the interglandular stroma, focal stromal necrosis and a stromal accumulation of histiocytes (26).
Those who have attempted to draw up these lists of distinguishing characteristics have, however, rarely indicated whether
they are attempting to draw a distinction between hyperplasia
and intraendometrial adenocarcinoma or between hyperplasia
and an adenocarcinoma that is truly invasive, in so far as
it is penetrating into the myometrium. Only Hendrickson and
Kempson (12) have clearly defined their aim and have indicated that they are attempting to differentiate between hyperplasia and the best differentiated adenocarcinoma that are
behaving biologically as carcinomas, i.e. are invading the
myometrium. If this is taken as the acceptable aim then a
true guide to achieving it can only be gained by retrospective analysis of those features seen in curettage specimens
from patients in whom a subsequent hysterectomy revealed an
adenocarcinoma invading the myometrium. If this is done it
soon becomes clear that many of the distinguishing features
listed above (such as nuclear changes, the finding of mitotic
figures, the presence of eosinophilic cytoplasm, loss of nuclear polarity and nucleolar enlargement) are of dubious or
minimal value in the differential diagnosis. A number of findings do, however, stand out as being of real significance,
these being the presence of true intraglandular cellular
bridges which are devoid of stromal support, the finding of

polymorphonuclear leucocytes and nuclear debris within gland
lumens and cellular anarchy. This last term perhaps requires
some explanation: it is applied to the piling up of cells with
rounded, irregular nuclei and scanty cytoplasm into sheets
of cells and masses, this change sometimes being seen focally
within a gland which appears otherwise to have a fairly regular epithelium. A further valid differentiating point between
hyperplasia and invasive carcinoma, but unfortunately one
which is relatively rarely encountered, is the presence of
abnormal mitotic figures. It is virtually impossible to weight
each of these individual features though the presence of cellular anarchy is probably the single most important indicator
of an invasive neoplasm. Having said all this it must be admitted that cases are encountered in which an invasive adenocarcinoma of the endometrium shows _less_ cellular atypia and
in which all the above listed criteria of true malignancy are
absent: in such cases one can only resort to the platitude
that morphology does not always parallel biological behaviour.
It is therefore possible in most, though admittedly not all,
curettage specimens to draw a distinction between glandular
hyperplasia with severe atypia and an invasive adenocarcinoma.
Is it possible, however, to distinguish in such specimens
between a glandular hyperplasia of this type and an intraendometrial adenocarcinoma? This is only possible if definite,
as opposed to presumed, stromal invasion is seen and suggestive features of such invasion certainly include stromal fibrosis and stromal necrosis with polymorphonuclear leucocytic
infiltration: unfortunately such features are not commonly
present and it is therefore often a matter of opinion, rather
than of fact, as to whether one is dealing with a hyperplastic condition or an intraendometrial adenocarcinoma (21).

Endometrial hyperplasia as a precursor of endometrial adenocarcinoma

Attempts to establish the relationship, if any, between endometrial hyperplasia and the subsequent development of an endometrial adenocarcinoma have involved prospective follow-up
of cases of endometrial hyperplasia (1, 4, 5, 11, 17, 25),

retrospective analyses of curettings from women who have later developed an endometrial adenocarcinoma (2, 13, 24, 31),
and studies of the non-neoplastic portion of the endometrium
in which an adenocarcinoma is present (9, 10, 20, 22). The
number of prospective studies has been small and in many the
true natural history of the disorder has been obscured by the
administration of various forms of therapy, including irradiation, to a high proportion of patients. Retrospective
studies will of course give a highly biased, and unduly gloomy,
view of the risk of adenocarcinoma in hyperplastic conditions
in so far as they selectively pick out a group of women with
a preceding history of abnormal vaginal bleeding. The study
of the non-neoplastic portion of an endometrium harbouring
an adenocarcinoma can give valuable information if hyperplasia is absent but if hyperplasia is present it can be very
difficult to tell if there is a glandular hyperplasia with
severe cellular atypia or an intraendometrial adenocarcinoma.
Quite apart from these methodological difficulties which have
beset attempts to establish the malignant potential of the
various forms of endometrial hyperplasia the greatest problems
encountered in attempting to probe the relationship between
the two conditions are the terminological morass, which often
results in a complete uncertainty as to the type of hyperplasia being documented, and the common failure to state whether
the diagnosis of adenocarcinoma has been based upon the presence of myometrial invasion or not.
Within the obvious limitations imposed by these drawbacks
only a few conclusions can be drawn with any degree of certainty. The first of these is that women with a pure cystic
glandular hyperplasia of the endometrium appear to have only
a marginally increased risk of developing an invasive adenocarcinoma (17, 25). Indeed, it is doubtful if a pure cystic
glandular hyperplasia ever evolves into an adenocarcinoma,
cases of frank neoplasia usually being due to, or a consequence of, focal glandular hyperplasia with atypia occurring
in the setting of a cystic glandular hyperplasia. It is also
clear that glandular hyperplasia with cellular atypia can,

and does, progress to an invasive carcinoma: the quoted incidence of such progression has, however, varied widely and
there are few reliable guidelines for assessing the true malignant potential of this form of hyperplasia. Welch and
Scully (30), after reviewing the literature on this topic,
came to the depressing conclusion that it "is impossible to
render even a scientific estimate of the proportion of cases
of precancerous hyperplasia that are destined to progress to
cancer if untreated". Ferenczy (6) came to a similar conclusion but made an "educated guess" that approximately 10 per
cent of women with glandular hyperplasia and cellular atypia
will eventually develop an adenocarcinoma: it must be empha-
sised however, that this is a guess rather than a hard or
proven fact.

This still leaves unanswered the malignant potential of glandular hyperplasia with architectural, but not cellular atypia.
No figures are available to allow for an assessment of this
and, again, only a guess can be made that it is probable that
there is a very low risk of the eventual development of an
adenocarcinoma in such cases.

Aetiology, pathogenesis and nature of endometrial hyperplasia

It is generally accepted that cystic glandular hyperplasia is
usually the result of prolonged unopposed oestrogenic stimulation of the endometrium, whether this be the result of a
series of anovulatory cycles, an oestrogenic ovarian tumour
or administration of exogenous oestrogens. Indeed it is almost certainly the case that most women whose endometrium is
subjected to prolonged oestrogenic stimulation will eventually
develop some degree of cystic glandular hyperplasia and that
this form of hyperplasia does not occur in the absence of
oestrogenic stimulation. This, together with the diffuse involvement of glands, stroma and muometrium indicates that
this type of hyperplasia is the normal, almost physiological,
response to an abnormal degree of oestrogenic stimulation, a
view bolstered by the finding that chromosomal and microspec-
trophotometric DNA studies of the cells in this type of hyper-

plasia have shown patterns identical to those of normal proliferative endometrium (15, 29). If cystic glandular hyperplasia is therefore a normal tissue response it is perhaps not
surprising that the risk of evolution into an adenocarcinoma
is so low.

By contrast, glandular hyperplasia with atypia, either architectural or cellular, involves only the endometrial glands:
nevertheless this form of hyperplasia also often develops
against a background of prolonged oestrogenic stimulation
and in such cases usually co-exists with a cystic glandular
hyperplasia. Glandular hyperplasia with cellular atypia is
however always focal rather than diffuse and can develop in
an otherwise normal, or atrophic, endometrium. It seems reasonable to suggest therefore that this form of hyperplasia
represents a local tissue abnormality which is commonly oestrogen induced but which can also develop in the absence of any
obvious abnormal oestrogenic stimulation of the endometrium.
The implication of this is that glandular hyperplasia with
cellular atypia is biologically fundamentally different from
cystic glandular hyperplasia and, indeed, we would suggest
that there are grounds for believing that this endometrial abnormality should be considered as a neoplastic process, albeit
one which is capable of spontaneous arrest or regression,
rather than as a form of hyperplasia. This view is based on
the following considerations:

1. The lesion is focal in nature and involves only the glands.
2. Some cases, e.g. those arising in an atrophic endometrium,
   are independent of oestrogenic stimulation.
3. A proportion of cases evolve into an invasive adenocarcinoma.
   Morphologically, there is a continuous spectrum between
   cases with mild cellular atypia and those with severe
   cellular atypia; in histological terms the latter merge
   imperceptively into intraendometrial adenocarcinoma.
4. It is probable that intraendometrial adenocarcinoma is a
   common, possibly almost inevitable, precursor of invasive
   adenocarcinoma though progression to this stage is proba-

bly not inevitable and may be relatively uncommon.

5. Exfoliated cells from cases of hyperplasia with cellular atypia have cytological characteristics which are similar to those of cells exfoliated from an endometrial adenocarcinoma (19).

6. Microspectrophtometric analysis of DNA in hyperplasia with cellular atypia has shown patterns similar to those found in adenocarcinomas (29).

7. Experimental endometrial carcinogenesis e.g. the administration of methylcholanthrene to rabbits, results in a lesion which initially resembles a glandular hyperplasia with cellular atypia and eventually progresses to an invasive adenocarcinoma (18).

Implicit in this concept is the theme of a continuous spectrum of abnormality and this has been challenged by Ferenczy's (6) observation that, at the ultrastructural level, the cells in a glandular hyperplasia with cellular atypia differ from those in an intraendometrial adenocarcinoma by showing a lack of oestrogen-induced morphological features, such as microvilli and cilia. This has however, not been everyone's experience (16) and would, even if proved correct, not represent an impregnable bar to the concept of a continuous process.

Belief in the fundamentally neoplastic nature of glandular hyperplasia with cellular atypia still leaves unanswered the nosological status of glandular hyperplasia with architectural atypia and adenomatoid hyperplasia. The former appears to lie somewhere in that grey hinterland between hyperplasia and neoplasia whilst the latter has to us many of the features of a true adenoma of the endometrium: it has always appeared strange that non-malignant neoplasms of the endometrium do not exist and it is possible that this deficiency is repaired by the recognition of adenomatoid hyperplasia as a form of endometrial adenoma.

Nomenclature of endometrial hyperplasia

Much of the confusion surrounding the topic of endometrial hyperplasia is due to the existence of a bewildering medley

of nomenclatures. It may therefore appear to be making a far-
rago still worse by suggesting yet another system of nomenclature. It appears, however, that the terminologies currently in use tend to ignore the basic biological nature of the
various processes they are describing.

It would appear reasonable, therefore, to propose the following:

1. Cystic glandular hyperplasia should be known as "simple
   endometrial hyperplasia".

2. A belief in the neoplastic nature of glandular hyperplasia
   with cellular atypia leads ineluctably to a comparison
   with cervical intraepithelial neoplasia and it is probable
   that a similar terminology could, with advantage, be a-
   dopted for the endometrium. Thus glandular hyperplasia with
   mild cellular atypia could be classed as intraendometrial
   neoplasia (IEN) Grade I, cases with moderate atypia as IEN
   Grade II and both glandular hyperplasia with severe cellular atypia and intraendometrial adenocarcinoma could be
   classed IEN Grade III.

   This concept of intraendometrial neoplasia has been opposed
   before (24) and not received with any great enthusiasm.
   All the disadvantages that have been claimed for the use
   of the term cervical intraepithelial neoplasia also apply
   with equal force to the use of intraendometrial neoplasia,
   these including the application of the term "neoplasia" to
   a non-malignant process, the possibility of spontaneous
   arrest or regression of the lesion, the risk of overtreat-
   ment of relatively innocuous abnormalities and the possible
   psychological ill effects of a diagnosis of neoplastic
   disease. On the other hand it could be argued that these
   would be outweighed by the possible benefits of a more
   realistic view of the basic biological nature of the process and, certainly, pathologists would benefit by not
   being forced to make an often subjective and possibly unnecessary, distinction between hyperplasia with severe
   cellular atypia and intraendometrial adenocarcinoma.

3. Glandular hyperplasia with architectural atypia would not

be included under the heading of intraendometrial neoplasia: a term such as "simple glandular hyperplasia" would
probably suffice to cover this condition.

Therapeutic considerations

Currently it is recognised that intraendometrial neoplasia,
of any degree, carries a risk of eventual development of an
invasive adenocarcinom. Unfortunately the magnitude of this
risk, the identification of those lesions which will progress
and those which will not and the time scale of the process
of frankly malignant evolution are still unknown. It is probable, however, that the therapeutic problem to be faced is
one of a relatively slowly evolving neoplastic process with
a probably quite low risk of eventual overtly malignant adenocarcinoma. It would therefore appear fully justifiable to
accept that a hysterectomy is not, in young women desirous
of having further pregnancies, necessarily the first treatment of choice and that a trial of hormonal therapy is indicated. In such patients a 4-6 weeks course of a progestational
agent should be followed by a repeat curettage. If the endometrium has reverted to normal no further treatment is required: if there has been partial improvement a further course
of hormonal therapy is indicated whilst if there has been no
improvement a simple hysterectomy should be considered: this
latter course may seem a little extreme in a young woman but
it would seem improbable that a young patient with such an
abnormal endometrium would ever be able to have a normal pregnancy. The rate of successful pregnancies in those women who
have responded satisfactorily is by no means established
whilst no information is available about possible recurrences
of the endometrial abnormality after hormonal therapy.
In older women, who have completed their families, it may
be felt that there is less justification for hormonal therapy
and that simple hysterectomy could be proceeded to with relative alacrity.

REFERENCES

1. Arfwedson, H. & Winblad, S. 1953. Endometrial changes presumably malignant. Acta Obstet. et Gynecol. 32:190-210.
2. Beutler, H.K., Dockerty, M.B. & Randall, L.M. 1963. Precancerous lesions of the endometrium. Amer. J. Obstet. Gynecol. 86:433-443.
3. Buehl, I.A., Vellios, F., Carter, J.E. & Hubner, C.P. 1964. Carcinoma in situ of the endometrium. Amer. J. Clin. Pathol. 42:594-601
4. Campbell, P.E. & Barter, R.A. 1961. The significance of atypical endometrial hyperplasia. J. Obstet. Gynaecol. Brit. Emp. 68:668-672.
5. Chamlian, D.L. & Taylor, H.B. 1970. Endometrial hyperplasia in houng women. Obstet. Gynecol. 36:659-666.
6. Ferenczy, A. 1980. The ultrastructural dynamics of endometrial hyperplasia and neoplasia. In: Advances in Clinical Cytology, edited by L.G. Koss and D.V. Coleman, pp. 1-43, Butterworths, London.
7. Gore, H. 1973. Hyperplasia of the endometrium.In: The Uterus, edited by H.J. Norris, A.T. Hertig and M.T. Abell, pp. 255-275, Williams and Wilkins, Baltimore.
8. Gore, H. & Hertig, A.T. 1966. Carcinoma in situ of the endometrium. Amer. J. Obstet. Gynecol. 94:134-155.
9. Gray, L.A., Robertson, R.W. & Christopherson, W.M. 1974. Atypical endometrial changes associated with carcinoma. Gynecol. Oncol. 2:93-100.
10. Greene, R.R., Roddick, J.W. Jr. & Milligan, M. 1958. Estrogens, endometrial hyperplasia and endometrial cancer. Annals N.Y. Acad. Sci. 75:586-599.
11. Gusberg, S.B. & Kaplan, A.L. 1963. Precursors of corpus cancer, IV. Adenomatous hyperplasia as stage 0 carcinoma of the endometrium. Amer. J. Obstet. Gynecol. 87:662-676.
12. Hendrickson, M.R. & Kempson, R.L. 1980. Surgical Pathology of the Uterine corpus. W.B. Saunders, Philadelphia.
13. Hertig, A.T. & Sommers, S.C. 1949. Genesis of endometrial carcinoma. I. Study of prior biopsies. Cancer 2:946-956.
14. Hertig, A.T., Sommers, S.C. & Bengloff, H. 1949. Genesis of endometrial carcinoma. III. Carcinoma in situ. Cancer 2:964-971.
15. Katayama, K.P. & Jones, H.W. 1967. Chromosomes of atypical (adenomatous) hyperplasia and carcinoma of the endometrium. Amer. J. Obstet. Gynecol. 97:978-983.
16. Klemi, P.M., Grönroos, M., Rayramo, L. & Punnonen, R. 1980. Ultrastructural features of endometrial atypical adenomatous hyperplasia and adenocarcinomas and the plasma level of estrogens. Gynecol. Oncol. 9:162-169.
17. McBride, J.M. 1959. Premenopausal cystic hyperplasia and endometrial carcinoma. J. Obstet. Gynaecol. Brit. Emp. 66:288-296.
18. Merriam, J.C. Jr., Easterday, C.L., McKay, O.G. & Hergig, A.T. 1960. Experimental production of endometrial carcinoma in the rabbit. Obstet. Gynecol. 16:253-262.
19. Ng, A.B.P. 1974. The cellular detection of endometrial carcinoma and its precursors. Gunecol. Oncol. 2:162-179.

20. Ober, W.B. 1973. Adenocarcinoma of the endometrium: a pathologist's view. In: Endometrial Cancer (Eds.) Brush, M.G., Taylor, R.W. and Williams, D.C. pp. 73-81, Heinemann, London.
21. Ober, W.B. 1978. Recent ideas in the pathology of endometrial carcinoma. In: Endometrial Cancer (Eds.) Brush, M.G., King, R.J.B. & Taylor, R.W. pp. 111-117, Bailliere Tindall, London.
22. Ritzmann, H. 1978 Types of endometrial hyperplasia and their relationship to carcinoma of the endometrium. In: Endometrial Cancer edited by Brush, M.G., King, R.J.B. & Taylor, R.W. pp. 119-123, Bailliere Tindall, London.
23. Robertson, W.B. 1981. The Endometrium, Butterworths, London.
24. Sherman, A.I. & Brown, S. 1979. The precursors of endometrial carcinoma. Amer. J. Obstet. Gynecol. 135:947-954.
25. Schröder, R. 1954. Endometrial hyperplasia in relation to genital function. Amer. J. Obstet. Gynecol. 68:294-309.
26. Silverberg, S.G. 1977. Surgical Pathology of the Uterus, John Wiley, New York.
27. Tavassoli, F. & Kraus, F.T. 1978. Endometrial lesions in uteri resected for atypical endometrial hyperplasia. Amer. J. Clin. Pathol. 70:776-779.
28. Vellios, F. 1972. Endometrial hyperplasia, precursors of endometrial carcinoma. Pathol. Ann. 7:201-229.
29. Wagner, D., Richart, R.M. & Terner, J.Y. 1967. Deoxyribonucleic acid content of presumed precursors of endometrial carcinoma. Cancer 20:2067-2077.
30. Welch, W.R. and Scully, R.E. 1977. Precancerous lesions of the endometrium. Hum. Pathol. 8:503-512.
31. Wentz, B.D. 1974. Progestin therapy in endometrial hyperplasia. Gynecol. Oncol. 2:362-367.

18. NEW TECHNIQUES FOR OUT-PATIENT DIAGNOSIS OF ENDOMETRIAL
CARCINOMA

A.P.M. Heintz & J.B. Trimbos

Introduction

Increased attention has been given to cytologic and histologic
techniques for the detection of endometrial lesions because of
an increasing incidence of endometrial malignancy. The mortality rate of endometrial cancer has remained unchanged in recent years. One effective way to reduce this mortality rate
is the screening of women who are at risk with respect to endometrial carcinoma. Although out-patient procedures for the
diagnosis of endometrial carcinoma have been advocated for 50
years, conventional dilatation and curettage under general anaesthesia has remained the prime diagnostic procedure. In recent years new diagnostic procedures have been developed, many
of them easy to perform and with a high degree of accuracy.
Creasman (5) formulated criteria for acceptable diagnostic
procedures for endometrial cancer:
1. the procedure must be easy to perform;
2. the procedure must be acceptable to the patient and not
   give too much discomfort;
3. the apparatus must be narrow and easily introduced into
   the endometrial cavity;
4. the equipment must be inexpensive;
5. the technique must not be time consuming;
6. the processing and evaluation of specimens must be easy
   to perform and subject to a minimum of error.

Techniques for the detection of endometrial carcinoma

In general the available techniques for the detection of endometrial carcinoma fall into one of two categories, i.e.,

cytological or histological (Table 1). These techniques are listed and their diagnostic accuracy indicated in Table 1.

Table 1

Cytological techniques	Diagnostic accuracy
Cervico-vaginal smears	45 - 55%
Endocervical aspiration	64 - 83%
Lavage of endometrial cavity	80 - 95%
Brush	75 - 90%
Jet wash	75 - 95%
Histological techniques	**Diagnostic accuracy**
Sponge biopsy	75 - 97%
Endometrial biopsy	62 - 96%
Vabra aspirator	74 - 97%

Cytological techniques

Papanicolaou cervical/vaginal pool smears:
For the detection of endometrial carcinoma the results with the routine cervical smear collected with cottonwool swabs or cervix scrapers are poor. An accuracy of no more than 30-55% is reported (19). The results are not much better when material is taken from the posterior vaginal vault, for which an accuracy of 75% is reported (16).
Excellent diagnostic results obtained with endocervical aspiration smears, including the discovery of adenocarcinoma and hyperplasia in asymptomatic patients, have been reported by Reagan (21) but could not be confirmed by others.
To obtain an aspiration smear the following can be used:
Isaacs cell sampler. A small perforated cannula with a diameter of 2.9 mm is inserted directly into the endometrial cavity through the cervix. A syringe is attached to the end of the cannula for aspiration. The material is drawn through the per-

foration by gentle suction and then smeared on a glass slide.
The accuracy of this technique ranges from 75 to 92% (16). The
rate of detection of precursors of endometrial cancer is much
lower.

Lavage of the endometrial cavity was first described by Morton et
al. (19), who used saline and collected the fluid from the
posterior vaginal fornix. This technique has been modified by
several other authors and an accuracy of 80-95% has been reported (14).

The endometrial brush technique was developed by Ayre (2), who
rotated a thin brush to collect material within the endometrial
cavity. A number of modifications of Ayre's system are now
available (18). The objections to the technique are its awkward-
ness, the relatively high incidence of increased bleeding, and
the occasional retention of bristles. The technique is reported to have an accuracy of 75-90% and can be performed as an
out-patient procedure without analgesia.

Histological techniques

Sponge biopsy

Chatfield and Watson (3) introduced the technique of sponge
biopsy for endometrial tissue sampling. An abrasive polyvinyl
sponge is passed into the uterus in an IUCD-introducer; when
the sponge is withdrawn from the uterus, it abrades and col-
lects tissue. The entire sponge is processed as a routine
histologic specimen. Analysis of 250 sponge biopsy specimens
showed good correlation with curettage material. The method
can be performed as an out-patient procedure, but because the
outer diameter of the introducer is 5 mm, prior dilatation
and local anesthaesia are required.

Adequate biopsy specimens were obtained in 97.6% of the cases.
The endocervix and ectocervix were sampled in 32%. No carcinomas were missed by these authors (3).

Endometrial biopsy

The most commonly employed histologic sampling technique is
based on endometrial biopsy (4, 5, 9, 10, 19). Most of the
cannulas range in diameter from 4 to 6 mm. One of the modifi-

cations of the metal and plastic cannulas used for this purpose is the Novak curette.

Insertion of the curette is performed through the cervical
canal without dilatation and without anesthaesia. The endometrial cavity is scraped. Suction is performed with a syringe
applied to the end of the curette. The accuracy of this method
for cancer detection ranges in the literature from 62 to 96 per
cent (3).

Hofmeister reported an accuracy of 94% in his series of 20,000
cases (9).

The Vabra aspirator

Vacuum aspiration curettage is not new. It was devised in Den-
mark by Jensen & Jensen (11). The instrument consists of a
16 cm long metal cannula which is attached to a hollow plastic
filter basket to which a negative pressure source can be connected. The same principle was used for a polythene aspirator
for cervical curettage.

The Gravlee Jet washer consists of a reservoir, a syringe, and
a double cannula with perforations. Saline is drawn by negative pressure from the reservoir through the lower cannula,
flushed around the cavity of the uterus, and drawn back into
the syringe. The outer diameter of the cannula is 4.6 mm. The
negative pressure makes it unnecessary to force fluid out of
the cannulas into the peritoneal cavity. However, Hofmeister
(9, 10, 13) found that spillage can occur during the procedure.
There have been numerous reports describing the use of the Jet
wash technique (1, 4, 5, 8, 15). The report by some authors
(2) that 20% of all Jet-washing specimens are unsatisfactory
for interpretation is disturbing. The Jet washing method is
realtively painless, easy to perform, and can be applied as
an out-patient procedure without analgesia or anaesthesia. The
diagnostic accuracy of this method is reported to be 75-90%.
According to most authors, the tissue specimens are of the
same quality as those obtained by conventional curettage and
permit a histological diagnosis (4, 5, 6, 11, 15, 16). The procedure can be performed on an out-patient basis. Local anaesthesia and dilatation of the cervical canal are not necessary. The

diagnostic accuracy of the Vabra method reported in the literature ranges from 74 to 97.8%.

In most of the studies on out-patient diagnosis of endometrial
carcinoma in symptomatic women reported in the literature, the
method in question was compared with dilatation and curettage
(D & C) performed in the same patient under general anaesthesia or was not compared with any other method. A randomized
study comparing any new method with D & C has not been reported. In the Department of Obstetrics and Gynecology of the
Leiden University Hospital, we undertook a randomized study
to compare Vabra suction curettage with the conventional D & C.

Material and methods

Both Vabra curettage and conventional D & C were performed
under general anaesthesia. In all cases a hysteroscopy was
then performed to identify any lesions which had been missed.
If much tissue was left in the endometrial cavity or if there
were structures which were difficult to interpret, a biopsy
specimen of the remaining tissue was taken. The hysteroscopy
was performed under Hyskon[R] distention (32% dextran - 70). Of
the total screen of 198 patients, 98 underwent curettage of
both the cervix and the uterine cavity and in 100 a Vabra
suction curettage of cervix and corpus was performed.
The characteristics of these two groups of patients are shown
in Table 2.

Table 2

	D & C	Vabra
Number of patients	98	100
No. pre-menopausal	51 (52%)	55 (55%)
No. post-menopausal	47 (48%)	45 (45%)
Mean age	53,2	51,0
Mean parity	2,4	2,7

Both groups were divided into two sub-groups to distinguish

pre- and post-menopausal women. The similarity of the characteristics in these groups shows clearly that the randomization procedure was adequate.

Results

Pre-menopausal women

The indications for curettage in this sub-group are listed in
Table 3. There were no significant differences in the number

Table 3

Pre-menopausal women
Indications for curettage

	D & C	Vabra
Meno-metrorrhagia	50	54
Control hyperplasia	-	1
Analysis amenorrhoea	1	-
Total	51	55

of diagnoses made between the D & C and the Vabra groups (Tables 4 and 5). In this sub-group we took biopsy specimens of

Table 4

Histological diagnosis cervix
in the pre-menopausal group

	D & C		Vabra	
	N	%	N	%
Normal endocervical epith.	30	58.8	27	49.1
Endocervical polyps	4	7.8	3	5.5
Cervicitis	16	31.4	21	38.2
Dysplasia	1	2.0	1	1.8
Adenocarcinoma	0	-	1	1.8
Inadequate material	0	-	2	3.6
Total	51	100	55	100

the tissue left in the uterus in 19 patients. In all of these cases the histological findings were identical to those made in the tissue obtained by curettage. In the D & C group we per-

Table 5

Histological diagnosis endometrium in the pre-menopausal group

	D & C		Vabra	
	N	%	N	%
Atrophic endometrium	2	3.9	2	3.6
Secretion phase	9	17.7	8	14.5
Proliferation phase	29	57.1	36	65.6 (N.S.)
Endometrium polyps	3	5.9	5	9.1
Cystic glandular hyperplasia	0	-	1	1.8
Adenomatous hyperplasia	2	3.9	1	1.8
Atypical hyperplasia	1	1.9	0	-
Adenocarcinoma	1	1.9	1	1.8
Decidual endometrium	1	1.9	0	-
Others	1	1.9	0	-
Inadequate material	2	3.9	1	1.8
Total	51	100	55	100

formed biopsies in five patients, and here too the histology was in agreement with the histology of the tissue obtained by D & C. The amount of endometrial tissue was too small for diagnosis in two patients in the D & C group and in one patient in the Vabra group. In these patients hysteroscopy showed empty uterine cavities and normal endocervical canals (no ridges, no ulcers).

Post-menopausal women
In the post-menopausal sub-group there were no significant differences in the number of diagnoses between the two procedures (Tables 6 and 7). In the D & C group we performed a separate biopsy in seven cases. In six of these patients the histology of the biopt was in agreement with that of the tissue obtained by D & C. In the seventh at hysteroscopic control we removed

an endometrial polyp which was missed at D & C. In the post-
menopausal Vabra group additional biopts were taken in 22
cases. In 21 of these patients the histological pictures of
the biopt and the Vabra material were similar. In one patient
we removed at hysteroscopy an endocervical polyp which had been
missed at curettage. In the post-menopausal D & C group too
little material was obtained for diagnosis in six patients
(12.8%); in the Vabra group this problem arose in 15 cases
(33.3%). This difference is statistically significant (p = 0.034)

Table 6

Histological diagnosis of the cervix in the post-menopausal group

	D & C		Vabra	
	N	%	N	%
Normal epithelium	31	65.9	23	51.2
Endocervical polyps	2	4.3	5	11.1
Cervicitis	7	14.9	6	13.3
Dysplasia	2	4.3	1	2.2
Endocervical carcinoma	0	−	1	2.2
Endometrium carcinoma	0	−	1	2.2
Metastasis mammacarcinoma	0	−	1	2.2
Inadequate material	5	10.6	7	15.6
Total	47	100	45	100

In all of these patients hysteroscopy showed an atrophic and
empty uterine cavity with little endometrial tissue. Biopsy
findings confirmed the atrophic state of the endometrium. Diagnoses missed at curettage and detected by hysteroscopy are
listed in Table 8. No carcinomas were missed, but the number
of patients with cancer is small.

Complications

We perforated the uterus on five occasions, i.e., two patients
in the D & C group (2%) and three patients in the Vabra group

(3%). No pelvic inflammatory diseases were seen after either of the procedures.

Table 7

Histological diagnosis of the endometrium in the post-menopausal group

	D & C		Vabra	
	N	%	N	%
Atrophic endometrium	22	46.8	15	22.3 (N.S.)
Secretion phase	1	2.1	0	-
(Irregular) proliferation	11	23.4	8	17.8 (N.S.)
Endometriumpolyps	3	6.4	2	4.5
Cystic glandular hyperplasia	0	-	1	2.2
Adenomatous hyperplasia	0	-	0	-
Atypical hyperplasia	0	-	0	-
Adenocarcinoma	4	8.5	4	8.9
Inadequate material	6	12.8	15	33.3 (S.: p=0.034)
Total	47	100	45	100

Table 8

Diagnoses missed at curettage

	D & C	Vabra
Pre-menopausal		
Submucous myoma	1	4
Perforation	1	0
Carcinomas	0	0
Post-menopausal		
Submucous myoma	1	2
Perforation	1	2
Uterine septum	-	1
Cervical polyps	-	1
Endometrium polyp	1	-
Carcinomas	0	0

Carcinomas

We diagnosed endometrial carcinoma in ten patients (5.1%), 2
of them in the pre-menopausal sub-group (1.9%) and eight in
the post-menopausal sub-group (8.7%). No endocervical carcinomas were diagnosed in the pre-menopausal sub-group. In the
post-menopausal sub-group, however, we diagnosed three endocervical carcinomas: one case of adenocarcinoma of the endocervical epithelium, one case of adenocarcinoma of the endometrium with tumor growth into the cervical canal, and one
case of metastasis of a mamma carcinoma to the endocervical
canal. These three (3.3%) tumors were all diagnosed in material obtained by Vabra suction curettage (6.7%).

We had four patients (2.8%) with intra-endometrial neoplasia;
three of these patients had adenomatous hyperplasia, in two
of them diagnosed by D & C and in one by Vabra, and the fourth
had atypical hyperplasia which was diagnosed in material obtained by D & C. In the entire series we did not miss a single
case of carcinoma. During the follow-up, which now covers a
four-year period, no new diagnosis of malignancy has been made
in any of these patients.

Discussion

The larger number of hysteroscopic biopsy specimens taken in
the Vabra group reflects the fact that more endometrium is
left in the uterine body after a Vabra curettage than after
D & C. Endometrial carcinomas or endocervical carcinomas were
not missed in either the D & C or the Vabra group. Our findings in the pre-menopausal sub-group are in agreement with the
results in the literature. In this sub-group Vabra curettage
seems to provide accurate information for diagnosis of the
cause of abnormal uterine bleeding and thus for the detection
of endometrial carcinoma.

In the post-menopausal group, however, we had a high percentage of patients in whom we could not obtain sufficient material to reach a diagnosis (Table 9). In the literature the main
reason for failure of the Vabra technique is inability to enter

Table 9

Inadequate material

Vabra

Pre-menopausal	:	1/55	
Post-menopausal	:	15/45	S: p < 0.01

D & C

Pre-menopausal	:	6/47	
Post-menopausal	:	2/51	N.S.

a stenotic cervical canal. We did not encounter this problem.
The combination of curettage with hysteroscopy gave satisfactory results because it permitted visualization of the endocervical canal and the uterine cavity, especially in cases where
we could not obtain enough appropriate material for diagnosis.
The conclusion based on the hysteroscopic findings is that in
patients with an atrophic endometrium it is easier to obtain
material for diagnosis by D & C than by the Vabra method. The
diagnostic accuracy of many histological and cytological techniques varies widely between the series reported in the literature. Creasman & Weed (5) reported that diagnostic accuracy
in the detection of endometrial carcinoma increased when several techniques were combined (Table 10). If the patients with
a prior D & C are excluded the accuracy of their combined technique approaches 100%. The present results suggest that it is
possible to reach the same accuracy with the combination of
Vabra curettage and hysteroscopy.
Critics of the use of hysteroscopy in the routine evaluation of
patients with abnormal uterine bleeding are concerned about
transtubal spillage of viable tumor cells and subsequent tumor
dissemination in patients with endometrial cancer.Johnson's
(12) report is the most complete on this subject. He found
that patients in whom hysterography was performed did not show
more distant metastasis or local tumor spread than patients

without hysterography. Sugimoto (23), who found 53 endometrial

Table 10

Diagnostic accuracy of combination of techniques

Creasman & Weed, 1976

Brush + jet	91%	Brush	74%
Brush + biopsy	91%	Biopsy	74%
Brush + Vabra	89%	Vabra	74%

Heintz & Trimbos, 1982 (this study)

Vabra + hysteroscopy	100%
D & C + hysteroscopy	100%

---

cancers among 4000 patients investigated hysteroscopically, was unable to demonstrate tumor implantation outside of the uterus at subsequent laparotomy.

Follow-up of patients in whom hysterography was performed for the diagnosis of endometrial cancer showed no increase in the incidence of intra-abdominal metastases. It is known that spill-age of tumor cells into the peritoneal cavity can occur during any intrauterine manipulation. The ability of these cells to establish metastatic growth is not known but seems to very low. In our hands Vabra suction curettage is now easily performed as an out-patient procedure without anesthesia or premedication. Others have, however, reported moderate or severe pain in 20% of the patients.

Hysteroscopy performed in the classical way required cervical dilatation and local anesthesia, but it is often possible to pass the modern smaller hysteroscopes through the cervical canal with minimal dilatation.

Most cytological techniques require highly specialized labora-tory methods and experienced cytopathologists, and also have the disadvantage that their diagnostic accuracy is lower in the precursor states.

The advantage of histological out-patient techniques, is that

the findings in material treated with routine laboratory
techniques are easy to interpret. Our conclusion based on
the literature and our own experience is that the Vabra suction curettage is a satisfactory technique for the accurate
diagnosis of abnormal uterine bleeding and for the detection
of endometrial carcinoma. This method fulfills all of the
criteria stipulated by Creasman (5). Combination with hysteroscopy makes it possible to reach a diagnosis in cases in which
no tissue can be obtained.

Since the information yielded by hysteroscopy, like that obtained by colposcopy, is dependent on individual experience,
we do not consider this technique suitable as a routine method
for the diagnosis of abnormal uterine bleeding or for screening
for endometrial carcinoma. For general gynecological practice,
we advise the performance of a Vabra curettage on an out-patient basis in cases where endometrium sampling is indicated.
If insufficient material is obtained for diagnosis or if abnormal uterine bleeding recurs after Vabra curettage, a conventional D & C under general anesthesia is indicated. Once
the technique is mastered, hysteroscopy offers a rapid and
efficient method to combine with Vabra curettage, especially
in cases where it is impossible to reach a histological diagnosis on the basis of Vabra specimens alone.

Conclusion

Many different techniques are available for the out-patient
diagnosis of endometrial abnormalities. In our opinion, the
histological techniques are preferable to the cytological, because the former do not require highly specialized laboratory
processing. Vabra curettage has proved to be of value in cases
where endometrium sampling is indicated. Our results suggest
use of the Vabra method where appropriate would reduce the
use of the classical D & C with general anesthesia by about
70%. This means that the Vabra method is much more acceptable
socially as well as much less expensive.

References

1. Abate, S.D., Edwards, C.L., Vellios, F. 1979. A comparative study of the endometrial Jet washing technique and endometrial biopsy. J. Clin. Path. 58:118.
2. Ayre, J.R. 1955. Rotating endometrial brush: New technique for the diagnosis of fundal carcinoma. Obstet. Gynecol. 5:137.
3. Chatfield, W.R., Bremner, A.D. 1972. Intrauterine sponge biopsy. Obstet. Gynecol. 39:323.
4. Cohen, C.J., Gusberg, S.B. 1975. Screening for endometrial cancer. Clin. Obstet. Gynecol., 18:27.
5. Creasman, W.T., Weed, J.C. 1976. Screening techniques in endometrial cancer. Cancer 38:436.
6. Denis, R. Jr., Barnett, J.M., Forbes, S.E. 1973. Diagnostic suction curettage. Obstet. Gynecol. 42:301.
7. Fox, C.F., Turner, F.G., Johnson, W.L., Thornton, N.W. 1962. Endometrial cytology: A new technique. Am.J. Obstet. Gynecol. 83:1582.
8. Gravlee, L.C. 1969. Jet irrigation method for the diagnosis of endometrial adenocarcinoma. Obstet. Gynecol. 34:168.
9. Hofmeister, F.J. 1974. Endometrial biopsy: Another look. Am. J. Obstet. Gynecol. 15:773.
10. Hofmeister, F.J. 1974. Panel on endometrial cancer. Ann. Meeting of Am. College of Obstet. Gynecol., Las Vegas.
11. Jensen, J.G. 1970. Vacuum curettage. Out-patient curettage without anaesthesia. A report of 350 cases. Danish Med. Bull. 17:199.
12. Johnson, J.E. 1973. Hysterography and diagnostic curettage in carcinoma of the uterine body. Acta radiol. (suppl.) 326:1.
13. Kanbour, A., Klionsky, B., Dym, J. 1972. The Gravlee jet washer: Evaluation of the reflux into the fallopian tubes. Acta cytol. 16:199.
14. Koss, L.G., Schreiber, K., Moussouris, H., Oberlander, S.G. 1982. Endometrial carcinoma and its precursors: Detection and screening. Clinical Obstet. and Gynecol. 25, 1, 49.
15. Lewis, B.V., Melcher, D.H., Chapman, P.A. 1978. Out-patient diagnosis of endometrial carcinoma. In: Endometrial Cancer (ed. Brush, King, Taylor). Billière Tindall London.
16. Lubbers, J.A. Diagnostic suction curettage without anesthesia. Acta Obstet. Gynaecol. Scandinavica, suppl. 62.
17. McGowan, L. 1974. Cytologic methods for the detection of endometrial carcinoma. Gynecol. Oncol. 2:272.
18. Milan, A.R., Markley, R.L., Fisher, R.S., Linthicum, C.M., Witherspoon, B., Eidschun, A.G. 1976. Obstet. Gynecol. 48:111.
19. Morton, D.G., More, J.G., Chang, N. 1959. Lavage of the endometrial cavity, an aid in the diagnosis of carcinoma of the uterine corpus. J. Int. Coll. Surg. 31:520.
20. Ng, A.B.P., Reagan, J.W., Hawliczek, S., Wentz, B.W. 1974. Significance of endometrial cells in the detection of endometrial carcinoma and its precursors. Acta Cytol. 18: 356.

21. Reagan, J.W., Ng, A.B.P., 1973. The cells of uterine adeno-
    carcinoma, 2nd ed. Baltimore, Wiliams & Wilkins.
22. Schwartz, P.E., Kohorn, E.I., Knowlton, A.H., Morris, J.M.
    1975. Routine use of hysterography in endometrial carci-
    noma and postmenopausal bleeding. Obstet. Gynecol. 45:378.
23. Sugimoto, O. 1975. Hysteroscopic diagnosis of endometrial
    carcinoma. Am. J. Obstet. Gynecol. 121:105.
24. Wamsteker, K. 1977. Hysteroscopy. Dissertation Leiden
    University.

19. SURGICAL TREATMENT OF ENDOMETRIAL CANCER

Robert C. Knapp

Historical background

Surgery was introduced as the method of therapy for endometrial cancer soon after the malignancy was defined as a specific entity. In 1900, Cullen described the treatment of endometrial cancer by abdominal hysterectomy and bilateral salpingo-oophorectomy (1). He recommended the vaginal hysterectomy only in the very obese or medically indigent patient. Satisfactory results were obtained without surgery, with the advent of radium and later external radiation. William Healy was the first to describe the combination of radiation therapy with surgery for the treatment of endometrial cancer (2). The early use of combination therapy, however, did not lead to significantly better results than hysterectomy alone. Advances in radiation therapy and surgery began to show improved survival with combined therapy. Arneson compared radiation plus surgery, surgery alone, and radiation alone, and found that the combination therapy did yield improvement in five-year survival as compared to the other groups (3). However, the results were not statistically significant. Brunschwig, in the late 1940's, popularized the use of radical hysterectomy for endometrial cancer (4). His rational was to remove possible lymph node metastasis, paravaginal tissue and the upper portion of the vagina. Although the results were good, the morbidity was high. The radical hysterectomy is still being used in some institutions for Stage II endometrial cancer.

Staging

Clinical diagnostic staging. The clinical stage is determined

under anesthesia and a careful pelvic examination and fraction-
al dilation and curettage must be performed. The endocervical
canal must be vigorously curetted without sounding or dilatation and the curettings placed in a separate container for
pathologic interpretation. The uterus is then sounded, preferably in centimeters and the cervix dilated. The endometrium
is then curetted noting, if possible, the particular location
of the tumor. The operator should evaluate by bimanual examination, benign uterine pathology, adnexal disease and parametrial infiltration. A metastatic workup is permitted in
determining the clinical stage, but not laparotomy.

Staging of carcinoma of the corpus uteri:

Stage 0   Carcinoma in situ
              Histologic findings suspicious of malignancy
              Cases of Stage 0 should not be included in any
              statistics of therapeutic results.
Stage I   Carcinoma is confined to the corpus
  Stage IA   The length of the uterine cavity is 8 cm or less
  Stage IB   The length of the uterine cavity is more than 8 cm
              The Stage I cases should be subgrouped as to the
              histologic grade of the adenocarcinoma as follows:
       G1   Highly differentiated adenocarcinomas
       G2   Differentiated adenocarcinomas with partially
              solid areas
       G3   Predominantly solid or entirely undifferentiated
              carcinomas
Stage II   The carcinoma has involved the corpus and cervix
Stage III   The carcinoma has extended outside the uterus, but
              not outside the true pelvis
Stage IV   The carcinoma has extended outside the true pelvis
              or has obviously involved the mucosa of the blad-
              der or rectum. A bullous edema of the bladder does
              not permit allotment of the case to Stage IV.
The clinical diagnostic stage should not include the surgical-
valuative staging or the post-surgical-treatment-pathologic
staging. Many papers in the literature incorporate these lat-

ter stages with the clinical diagnostic staging making interpretation of results from the particular report difficult
for interpretation.

The prognostic significance of uterine size has been of considerable controversy. Jones, in a careful review of the literature evaluated the relationship between uterine size and
five-year survival and found an 85.4% survival in the normal
size uterus as compared to a 66.6% if the uterus sounded to
greater than 8 cm (5). The size of the uterus may be related
to the volume of tumor present in the corpus and tumors of
large volume have been shown to have a poorer prognosis than
those with small tumor volume (6).

Natural history

Spread of endometrial cancer is dependent upon stage, histology and the degree of myometrial penetration. Approximately
85% of patients with endometrial cancer have their disease
clinically confined to the uterine corpus at initial diagnosis and are clinically staged as Stage I. Stage I disease
comprises a broad spectrum of neoplasms with varying propens-
ities for metastasis and recurrence. Stage I is, therefore,
subdivided into six categories, based on the depth of the
endometrial cavity and the histologic differentiation of the
tumor. The incidence of pelvic lymph node metastasis in Stage
I disease is approximately 10.6%, while in Stage II it is
36.5%. The five-year survival by stage in collected series
is 80% in Stage I, 60% in Stage II, 35% in Stage III and 10%
in stage IV. When one looks at survival rates for Stage I by
FIGO substages, there is a progressively decreasing survival
dependent upon histology and uterine size (Tabel 1) (7).

The histologic grade of endometrial cancer is a critical determinant of its biological behavior. Poorly differentiated
lesions are associated with a greater frequency of deep myometrial invasion and lymph node metastasis then well differentiated lesions resulting in a negative impact on survival
(8). Lewis evaluated pelvic nodes in patients with Stage I
endometrial cancer (9). In 36 patients with well different-

TABLE 1

Stage 1 Survival Rates for Endometrial
Adenocarcinoma by FIGO Substages

Stage	No. of Patients	Distribution by Substage (%)	5-year Survival Rates	
			Gross (%)	Corrected (%)
IaG1	18	5	94	94
IaG2	87	23	82	82
IaG3	41	11	66	71
IbG1	40	11	85	85
IbG2	143	38	70	75
IbG3	48	12	48	51
Totals	377*	100	72	77

*Only 377 patients of 538 patients in Stage I had sufficient data to allow retrospective substaging.

Source: Homesley, et al.: Obstet & Gynecol 47:102, 1976.

iated cancer, 2 (5.5%) had positive pelvic nodes; in moderately well differentiated, 5 (10%) of 50 had positive pelvic
nodes and in poorly differentiated, 5 (26%) of 19 had positive
nodes. In reviewing combined series for Stage I, the effect
of histologic grading correlates with the five-year outcome.
The survival with a grade I tumor was 84%; grade 2, 75%; and
grade 3, 48%. The incidence of positive pelvic nodes correlates
with the depth of myometrial invasion. Lewis found negative
pelvic nodes with nomyometrial invasion; with superficial
invasion, 2.8% nodal metastasis; moderate depth 17%; and deep
invasion 30%. The cure rate will be dependent upon the depth
of invasion. Looking at combined series for Stage I with involvement of the epithelium only, the five-year survival is
90%; superficial involvement 85%; deep invasion 66%. The tumor may involve the lower uterine segment and extend into the
endocervical canal (5-10% of patients). The cervix may have
either gross or microscopic spread of the cancer. There is
a statistically significantly lower survival with gross cervical involvement than with microscopic infiltration of the
cervix (10).

Piver correlated aortic lymph node metastasis and grade and
depth of myometrial invasion (11). This study revealed no
aortic node involvement with grade I carcinoma, but over 35%
of grade 3 carcinomas were associated with aortic lymph node
metastasis. A similar correlation was found with myometrial
penetration. When the tumor was limited to the endometrium
there was no lymph node metastases and with deep myometrial
invasion aortic lymph nodes were involved in 45.5%. Eighty
three percent of the patients who had aortic node metastasis,
had either grade 3 tumors or deep myometrial invasion.

The carcinoma may extend to the broad ligament and invade the
parametrium particularly with poorly differentiated tumors
and deep myometrial infiltration. Metastases to the tubes or
ovaries have been reported in 5-10% of patients, which also
correlates with grade and myometrial infiltration (12). The
incidence of vaginal metastases is dependent upon the stage
and degree of tumor differentiation. This type of recurrence

has been reported to be 5-10% without preoperative radiation, but can be reduced to 1-3% with adjuvant radiotherapy (13). Uterus and lung are considered the most common sites of local failure and distant metastases respectively. Endometrial cancer metastasis to the liver and lung in 6% and 8% of the cases respectively (14). Metastases in the upper peritoneal cavity and to the omentum is prevalent today as treatment has prevented local recurrences.

Surgical treatment

Integrated management of endometrial cancer by the gynecologist and radiation therapist is mandatory. No other gynecologic malignancy shows such clear cut evidence that combined therapy is the treatment of choice (Table 2). Consequently it is difficult to discuss the role of surgery without including adjuvant radiation therapy. The therapeutic approach will be determined by the stage of the tumor, size of the uterus, histologic type and degree of differentiation, and the medical condition and potential operability of the patient (15).

Exploratory laparotomy. It is preferable to perform an abdominal procedure rather than a vaginal operation for endometrial cancer in order to properly explore the abdomen. The external incision should extend above the umbilicus for adequate abdominal exploration (Table 3). Once the abdomen is open and prior to any intra-abdominal manipulation, cell washings should be obtained for cytologic interpretation of malignant cells. One hundred to 200 mls of saline is added to the peritoneal cavity and removed by suction and sent to the cytology laboratory. Creasman has found that 50% of his patients with positive cytologic findings died while only 7% with negative cytologic findings died (Table 4) (16). However, from most of the studies, including Creasman's, it is difficult to interpret the significance of positive cytologic findings as a sole prognostic factor. Patients with positive cytology are usually those with poorly differentiated tumors, deep myometrial involvement, extension of tumors to the endocervix or extrauterine spread. Whether the poor prognosis is related to the

TABLE II

Surgery Alone Versus Combined Therapy

Comparative 5-Year Survival Rates

	Surgery Alone			Combined Therapy		
	No. Pa-tients	Gross Cure	Corrected Cure	No. Pa-tients	Gross Cure	Corrected Cure
Stage I	68	81.2%	83.8%	45	86.7%	97.6%
Stage II	74	56.8%	66.9%	119	71.5%	83.0%
Stage III	35	25.7%	31.1%	53	49.1%	64.6%
Totals	178	60.1%	66.3%	217	69.1%	81.5%

Source: Gusberg & Yannopoulos: Am. J. Obstet. & Gynecol. 83:157, 1964.

TABLE III

ENDOMETRIAL CANCER LAPAROTOMY

External incision above umbilicus for adequate exploration

Peritoneal washings for cytology

Biopsy of any suspicious lesions in upper abdomen and biopsy
of omentum

Sample of pelvic and aortic nodes Grade III, deep myometrial
invasion, Stage II & Stage III

Total abdominal hysterectomy and bilateral salpingo-oophorectomy

TABLE IV

PERITONEAL CYTOLOGY IN ENDOMETRIAL CANCER

DEATHS FROM CANCER AND PERITONEAL FINDINGS

Cytologic findings	No. of patients	Deaths (%)
Positive	26	13 (50)
Negative	141	19 (7)

Other poor prognostic factors

Extrauterine spread   (14 of 26)
Grade, depth, cervix   (unknown)

(Creasman: Am. J. Obstet. & Gynecol. 1981).

positive cytology or these other prognostic factors is still
unanswered.

There must be careful exploration of the entire abdomen looking for any suspicious implants throughout the entire abdomen.
These implants may localize on the cul-de-sac, the bladder or
paracolic gutters. Tumor implants must be looked for on the
small and large bowel mesentery, and particularly near the
ligament of Treitz. Exploration of the upper abdomen is vital.
Attention should be directed to the diaphramatic surfaces and
omentum. Routine biopsy of the omental apron is adviseable.
There appears to be little justification for a total pelvic
lymphadenectomy at the time of surgical therapy for endometrial
cancer with the possible exception of stage II endometrial
cancer in which there is gross evidence of cervical involvement. In this latter situation, the tumor can spread similar
to cervical carcinoma. In most patients endometrial cancer
remains localized for a long period of time and when it
spreads it does so, not only to regional pelvic nodes, but to
the aortic nodes and occasionally to the inguinal nodes. It
can also be blood born. Pelvic and aortic nodal sampling is
of value in grade 3 lesions, deep myometrial invasion, the
enlarged uterus with large tumor volume, and Stage II and stage
III. The localization of the lymphatic dissection may be helped
by prior computerized axial tomography. Pelvic and aortic lymph
 node sampling is important in determining prognosis and as a
guide to treatment plan, particularly under protocol guidance.
A hysterectomy should always be extrafascial and the adnexa
removed because of the risk of ovarian metastases. The risk
of ovarian metastases is about 5% and correlates with the
grade of malignancy (12). It is advisable to have the pathologist cut the uterus in the operating room to note gross myometrial invasion. In an effort to prevent vaginal vault recurrences gynecologists have utilized a variety of techniques
to close the cervical os prior to hysterectomy (17). However,
there is no study that has demonstrated that these techniques
prevent vaginal recurrences or improves five-year survival.
It appears that vaginal vault recurrences are due to lymphatic

or vascular spread rather than spillage of tumor during surgery. Similarly, to prevent vaginal vault recurrences, the upper third of the vagina has often been excised with the hysterectomy specimen. However, the use of pre- or post-operative radium precludes the necessity for removal of the upper third of the vagina.

The vaginal hysterectomy for endometrial cancer has generally been selected for those patients who are obese or a poor medical risk. This procedure increases operability over the abdominal procedure. We have utilized the simple vaginal hysterectomy with bilateral salpingo-oophorectomy in selected cases with satisfactory results. However, due to the inability to explore the abdomen and the difficulty of removing the adnexa, the vaginal hysterectomy for endometrial cancer is not generally recommended.

Although it has been traditional to use preoperative external radiation, when indicated in Stage I, it is our policy to use post operative external radiation. Kinsella found no difference in survival whether the radiation was given pre- or postoperatively (10). Radiation therapy can be better planned if the extent of the disease has been defined prior to radiation. Limiting radiation to the pelvis only would be of little value with upper abdominal disease and therapy must be directed to the upper abdomen utilizing whole abdominal radiation or chemotherapy. Operating prior to radiation mitigates the delay in removing the primary tumor. Myometrial penetration of tumor can be best determined in the nonradiated uterus. Radiation administered postoperatively, in our institution, has not resulted in increased complications or morbidity, nor inability to administer the correct radiation dosages. The reported radiation complications following major surgery, such as bowel fistula and possibly diminished effectiveness of radiation due to a compromised blood supply has not occured in our series.

Management of Specific Stages

Stage IA. It is always preferable to have made the diagnosis of endometrial carcinoma prior to hospitalization. This can be performed as a simple outpatient procedure using suction

curettage*. At that time, the uterus can be adequately sounded
and an endocervical sample obtained. Patients with a Stage Ia,
G1 lesion may be treated directly by total abdominal hysterectomy and bilateral salpingo oophorectomy. Since the incidence of vault recurrence with a Stage IA, G1 lesion is less
than 1%, the use of either pre- or post-operative radium is
optional. However, with tumor involvement to the middle third
of the myometrium, post-operative vault radium and pelvic
external radiation is adviseable.

Stage IA, G2 and G3. Patients with these lesions are best treated
with pre-operative radium which can be administered using a
tandem and ovoid. At that time a formal D&C should be performed. The laparotomy and hysterectomy can be done soon after
the radium has been removed. The pathologist can determine
myometrial penetration better than if there has been a two
week delay. Post-operative external radiation is given in all
Grade 3 lesions and Grade 2 with deep myometrial invasion.

Stage IB. Radium by tandem and colpostat is given preoperative-
ly; total abdominal hysterectomy is performed as well as pelvic
and aortic node sampling. Post-operative pelvic radiation is
given if there is no demonstrable aortic node or upper abdominal metastasis.

Stage II. The radical hysterectomy and pelvic lymphadenectomy
has been utilized as treatment for stage II endometrial cancer
(18). In multiple series reporting the use of radical hysterectomy and pelvic lymphadenectomy for stage II disease, the
five-year survival rates vary from 9% to 70% (19). Kinsella,
et al evaluated combination radiation and total abdominal
hysterectomy for stage II endometrial cancer and found a disease-free survival of 83% at 10 years (10). Therefore, better
survival statistics with less morbidity can be obtained with
the use of combination radiation and total abdominal hysterectomy, than with the use of radical hysterectomy and pelvic
lymphadenectomy for stage II endometrial cancer. We employ
pelvic external radiation prior to the surgical procedure.
At the completion of the external radiation, one radium treatment is given using a colpostat and tandem. Four weeks after

* Editor's note: see also chapter 18.

the completion of the external radiation, a total abdominal
hysterectomy and bilateral salpingo-oophorectomy is performed
evaluating pelvic, aortic nodes and upper abdominal spread.
Stage III. In Stage III endometrial carcinoma the clinical stage
often does not exhibit the true extent of the cancer. Most
studies reflect the surgical-pathologic stage III endometrial
tumors. In a study by Bruckman reviewing stage III endometrial
cancer, only 31% were true clinical stage III (20). Therefore,
most stage III endometrial cancers are managed as either a
clinical stage I or II with additional therapy depending on
the operative and final pathologic findings. Stage III can
be divided into two grouds: one group in which the cancer has
spread to tube and ovary only, and the other group in which
the tumor has spread beyond these organs to other pelvic
structures. Most studies have shown a statistically significantly better survival in patients with spread limited to the
ovary and/or fallopian tubes than those who demonstrated
spread to other pelvic structures. In Bruckman's study, all
of the failures in patients whose spread was limited to ovary
or fallopian tube were in the upper abdomen or aortic lymph
nodes and 3 of 8 with spread to other pelvic structures re-
lapsed in the upper abdomen or aortic lymph nodes. In stage
III the assessment of metastasis to the upper abdomen and
aortic nodes is vital. Radium to the vault may be pre- or
post-operative. Preoperative radiation therapy is advisable
if there is obvious clinical pelvic spread. Postoperative
radiation is given in surgical-pathologic stage III. A total
abdominal hysterectomy, bilateral salpingo-oophorectomy,
nodal sampling and upper abdominal evaluation is the surgical
treatment of choice.
Stage IV. In this stage each patient must be individualized regarding the best method of treatment. With extension to bladder
or rectum, pelvic exenteration may be necessary providing there
is no demonstrable metastases to pelvic sidewall or upper abdomen and aortic lymph nodes. A patient can be considered
operable with central involvement only which may include
bladder and/or rectum. All other patients should be treated
by radiotherapy alone.

Recurrence. The manner of spread of endometrial cancer and the usual sites of recurrence precludes the use of the exenteration, except in rare instances. The exenteration is reserved for those patients who demonstrate central or vault recurrence without sidewall involvement and no upper abdominal or aortic lymph node spread. Usually ureteral obstruction or pelvic node involvement precludes the use of the exenteration. The exenteration for recurrent endometrial cancer has not been as successful as it has been for carcinoma of the cervix. Brunschwig reported only a 14.5% five-year survival (21). Recurrences must be central and limited to the pelvis if the exenteration is to be done. The manner of spread of endometrial cancer to peritoneum and upper abdomen limits this possibility to only a few selected cases.

References

1. Cullen, T.H. 1900. Cancer of the Uterus. Philadelphia, W.B. Saunders Co.
2. Healy, W. and Brons, R. 1939. Experience with surgical and radiation therapy in carcinoma of the corpus uteri. Am. J. Obstet. & Gynecol. 38:1.
3. Arneson, A. 1936. Clinical results and histologic changes following the radiation treatment of cancer of the corpus uteri. Am. J. Roentgenol. 36:461.
4. Brunschwig, A. and Murphy, A. 1954. The rationale for radical panhysterectomy and pelvic node excision in carcinoma of the corpus uteri. Am. J. Obstet. & Gynecol. 68: 1482.
5. Jones, H.W. III. 1975. Treatment of adenocarcinoma of the endometrium. Obstet. & Gynecol. Survey 30:147.
6. Johnsson, J.C. and Norman, O. 1979. Relation between prognosis in early carcinoma of the uterine body and hysterographically assessed localization and size of tumor. Gynecol. Oncol. 7:71.
7. Homesley, H.D., Boronow, R.C. and Lewis, J.L. 1976. Treatment of adenocarcinoma of the endometrium at Memorial-James Ewing Hospitals, 1949-1965. Obstet. & Gynecol. 47: 100.
8. Creasman, W.T., Boronow, R.C., Morrow, C.P., et al. 1976. Adenocarcinoma of the endometrium: Its metastatic lymph node potential. Gynecol. Oncol. 4:239.
9. Lewis, B.V., Stallworthy, J.A. and Cowdell, R. 1970. Adenocarcinoma of the body of the uterus. J. Obstet. Gynecol., Br. Commonw. 77:343.
10. Kinsella T.J., Bloomer, W.D., Lavin, P.T. and Knapp, R.C. 1980. Stage II endometrial carcinoma: ten year follow-up of combined radiation and surgical treatment. Gynecol. Oncol. 10-290.

11. Piver, M.S., Shaskikant, B.L., Barlow, J.J. and Blumenson, L. 1982. Para-aortic lymph node evaluation in Stage I endometrial carcinoma. Obstet. Gynecol. 59:97.
12. Berman, M.L., Ballon, S.C., Lagasse, L.D., et al. 1980. Prognosis and treatment of endometrial cancer. Am. J. Obstet & Gynecol. 136:679.
13. Ingersoll, F.M. 1971. Vaginal recurrences of carcinoma of the corpus. Management and prevention. Am. J. Surg. 121: 473.
14. Yoonessi, M., Anderson, D.G., Morley, G.W. 1979. Endometrial carcinoma: causes of death and sites of treatment failure. Cancer. 43:1944.
15. Malkasian, G.D. Jr. 1978. Carcinoma of the endometrium: Effect of stage and grade on survival. Cancer. 41:996.
16. Creasman, W.T., DiSaia, P.J., Blessing, J., et al. 1981. Prognostic significance of peritoneal cytology in patients with endometrial cancer and preliminary data concerning therapy with intraperitoneal radiopharmaceuticals. Am. J. Obstet. & Gynecol. 141:921.
17. Copenhauer, E.H. and Varsamin, M. 1967. Management of adenocarcinoma of the endometrium. Surg. Clin. North Amer. 47:723.
18. Homesley, D.H., Boronow, R.C. and Lewis, J.L. Jr. 1977. Stage II endometrial carcinoma - Memorial Hospital for Cancer, 1949-1965. Obstet. & Gynecol. 49:604.
19. Rutledge, F. 1974. The role of radical hysterectomy in adenocarcinoma of the endometrium. Gynecol. Oncol. 2:331.
20. Bruckman, J.E., Bloomer, W.D., Marck, A., et al. 1980. Stage III adenocarcinoma of the endometrium. Gynecol. Oncol. 9:12.
21. Brunschwig, A. 1970. Some reflections on pelvic exenterations after twenty years' experience. In: Sturgis, S.H. and Taymor, M.L. (eds.): Progress in Gynecology, Vol. 5 New York, Grune & Stratton, Inc.

20. THE ROLE OF RADIATION THERAPY IN CONJUNCTION WITH SURGERY
IN THE TREATMENT OF ENDOMETRIAL CARCINOMA

Tj. Kuipers

In the treatment of endometrial carcinoma adjuvant radiation
therapy can be applied in the preoperative or postoperative
phase or both. Until now, no clear difference in results has
been demonstrated between pre- and postoperative radiation
therapy, as stated in a recent report from Piver (1) and in
an earlier study from Graham (2). Figures from Graham's study
are presented (Table I).

Table I

Method of treatment (randomized)	5-years Survival	Vaginal Recurrence	Deaths from Carcinoma
	%	%	°c
Hysterectomy alone	64	12	12
Preoper.Rad.Th.+ Hyst.ect.	76	3	14
Hyst.ect.+ Postoper.Rad.Th.	81	0	3

John Graham, Buffalo, New York
Surg.Gyn.Obst.1971.132,855/860

In the group of European Curie Therapists a questionnaire was
used in 1976. The retrospective data from these non-randomised
patients treated at different institutions showed a somewhat
better 5-year survival rate of 83% for postoperative irradiat-

ion in comparison to 75% following preoperative radiation therapy.

Concerning preoperative irradiation, most authors feel that, "packing" of the uterus with radioactive sources is essential. In case of a bulky tumor, however, a heterogeneous dose distribution is obtained. The original Heyman method results in a high radiation exposure of the therapeutic staff. This is not the case if afterloading tubes are used: these also enable calculation of dosimetric data before irradiation is started. Together with measurement of the thickness of the myometrium by means of Ct-scan and methods for visualizing neighbouring organs, optimal dosimetry can be obtained. Preoperative external irradiation provides a more homogeneous dose distribution but a lower dose is delivered to the central part of the uterus. Both methods can be used in combination. In Rotterdam preoperative irradiation is not applied, but experience with the technical possibilities mentioned above, is obtained in the radiotherapy of inoperable patients. In this institution postoperative radiation therapy is preferred for different reasons.

1. The therapeutic indications are based on the operative findings and on the results of microscopic examination of the non-irradiated surgical specimen.

2. In contrast with preoperative intra-uterine applications no general anesthesia is necessary for vaginal brachytherapy.

The actuarial survival curves of 457 patients stratified by stage are presented (Fig. 1). Excluded were 3 patients in whom irradiation had to be stopped very early and 10 others who did not receive standard treatment. The 5-year survival rates are: Stage I 85%, Stage II 69%, Stage III 47% and Stage IV 29%.

The group of 350 stage I patients will be considered further in detail. All were treated with vaginal brachytherapy; the main criterium for additional external irradiation was infiltration of the growth to half or more of the thickness of the myometrial layer.

238

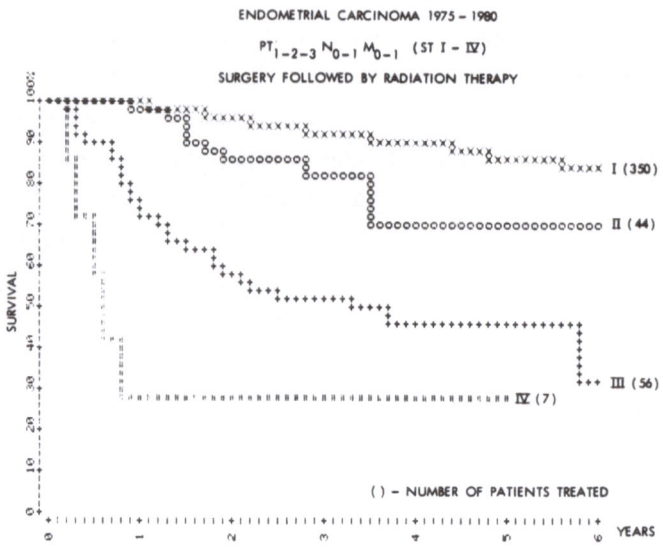

Fig. 1

If no deep infiltration occurred, postoperative treatment
was given by means of low dose rate brachytherapy: one vaginal application delivering 22.5 Gray (2250 rad) in 18 hours
at 5 mm depth in the vagina walls and at 10 mm depth in the
supravaginal tissues.

The 5-year survival rate was 94%; with such a high cure rate
one can ask whether in these patients a group can be defined
for which postoperative irradiation is not necessary. Piver
(1) and also Malkasian (3) feel that this is the case with
stage I endometrial carcinoma infiltrating less than half of
the myometrial thickness and with a high degree of differentiation.

Table 2 shows that the incidence of local recurrence was only
2% low with highly differentiated tumors. In this one case
the endometrial tumor was associated with endometrioid ovarian
carcinoma.

Table II

Endometrial Carcinoma 1975 – 1977

$PT_1N_0M_0$, (St I)

Depth of infiltration < half of myometrium

Surgery followed by

Low Dose Rate Brachytherapy, full regime

Degree of differentiation	Site of recurrent disease							Died			Living		Total number of patients
	L*	LR**	LRD***	LD	R	RD	D	With tumor	From treatment	Intercurrent, NED?	With tumor	NED	
High	–	1	–	–	–	–	2	2	–	2	1	41	46
Medium	–	–	–	1	–	–	–	1	–	2	–	18	21
Low	–	–	–	–	–	–	1	1	–	1	–	2	4
Not known	–	–	1	–	–	–	2	3	–	4	–	33	40
Total	–	1	1	1	–	–	5	7	–	9	1	94	111

* Local
** Regional
*** Distant
? No evidence of disease

Not a single further local recurrence was seen in the highly differentiated tumors, neither with other stage I patients (with deep infiltration) nor in such patients of other stage-groups. Therefore, the overall incidence of local recurrence of tumors with a high degree of differentiation in all patients referred for postoperative irradiation was 0.7%. Moreover, the results of treatment of a pure local recurrence show that 50% can be cured; these data are presented in Table III.

From these figures it appears that postoperative irradiation could be omitted following adequate surgery for a Stage I endometrial carcinoma infiltrating less than half of the myometrial thickness and with a high degree of differentiation. It must be emphasized that strict follow-up and centralized registration of such cases are imperative in order to ascertain as soon as possible whether the assumption stated above is true.

Table III

	Site of recurrence before treatment							Died			Living		Total number of patients
Degree of differentiation	L*	LR**	LRD***	LD	R	RD	D	With tumor	From treatment	Intercurrent, NED?	With tumor	NED	
High	2	–	–	1	–	–	–	2	–	–	–	1	3
Medium	2	2	1	–	–	–	1	5	–	–	–	1	6
Low	3	–	1	–	–	–	1	2	–	–	–	3	5
Not known	5	3	1	–	–	–	2	6	–	1	–	4	11
Total	12	5	3	1	–	–	4	15	–	1	–	9	25
Living NED	6	1	–	–	–	–	2						

Endometrial Carcinoma 1975 – 1980
Referred for Recurrent Disease
Following Surgery without Post–Operative Irradiation

* Local
** Regional
*** Distant
? No evidence of disease

Stage I carcinoma of the endometrium with infiltration of half or more of the myometrium was treated by surgery and postoperative external beam therapy combined with vaginal brachytherapy. The fields of external irradiation encompassed the surgical area and the pelvic nodes up to the aortic bifurcation. External irradiation was applied with megavoltage equipment to a total dose of 50 Gray delivered in 25 fractions during 5 weeks. The effective area of the vaginal application was shielded during different parts of the course of external irradiation, this practice resulted in 3 types of treatment:

1. Central shielding at 100% of the fractions of external irradiation combined with a full regimen of low dose rate brachytherapy: application time 16-20 hours.
2. Central shielding at 50% of the fractions of external irradiation combined with a 50% reduced regimen of low dose rate brachytherapy: application time 8-10 hours.

3. Central shielding at 30% of the fractions of external
   irradiation combined with an adapted regimen of high dose
   rate brachytherapy similar to the method applied by Joslin
   (4, 5): 2 x 8.0 Gray at 5 mm depth in the vagina walls. The
   short application times (15-30 minutes) improve reliability
   of dosimetric data and make admission to the hospital unnecessary. This means a great relief of the psychological
   burden which is inherent to the treatment of this malignant
   disease.

Neither the corresponding local recurrence rates: 3.1%, 2.3%
and 1.5% nor the actuarial survival curves showed significant
differences. The 5-year survival rates for treatment-types 1,
2 and 3 were respectively: 87%, 74% and 86% (Fig. 2).

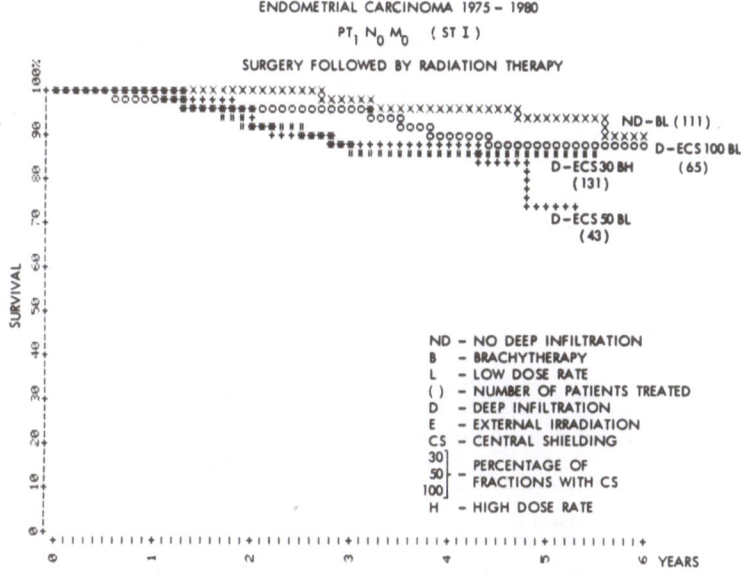

Fig. 2

More details are presented in the following tables (Table IV,
V and VI).

Table IV

Endometrial Carcinoma 1975 – 1977

$PT_1N_0M_0$, (St I)

Depth of infiltration $\geq$ half of myometrium

Surgery followed by

External Irradiation with 100 % central shielding

and Low Dose Rate Brachytherapy, full regime

Degree of differen-tiation	Site of recurrent disease							Died			Living		Total number of patients
	L°	LR°°	LRD°°°	LD	R	RD	D	With tumor	From treatment	Intercur-rent, NED?	With tumor	NED	
High	-	-	-	-	-	-	1	1	1	1	-	16	19
Medium	1	-	-	-	-	-	1	2	-	-	-	9	11
Low	-	-	-	-	-	-	3	3	-	-	-	7	10
Not known	1	-	-	-	-	-	-	1	1	2	-	21	25
Total	2	-	-	-	-	-	5	7	2	3	-	53	65

*   Local
**   Regional
***   Distant
?   No evidence of disease

Table V

Endometrial Carcinoma 1976 – 1977

$PT_1N_0M_0$, (St I)

Depth of infiltration $\geq$ half of myometrium

Surgery followed by

External Irradiation with 50 % central shielding

and Low Dose Rate Brachytherapy, half regime

Degree of differen-tiation	Site of recurrent disease							Died			Living		Total number of patients
	L°	LR°°	LRD°°°	LD	R	RD	D	With tumor	From treatment	Intercur-rent, NED?	With tumor	NED	
High	-	-	-	-	-	-	1	1	-	1	-	4	6
Medium	-	-	-	-	-	-	1	1	-	2	-	7	10
Low	1	-	-	-	-	-	3	4	-	1	-	3	8
Not known	-	-	-	-	-	-	1	-	-	3	1	15	19
Total	1	-	-	-	-	-	6	6	-	7	1	29	43

*   Local
**   Regional
***   Distant
?   No evidence of disease

Table VI

Endometrial Carcinoma 1976 – 1980

$PT_1N_0M_0$, (St I)

Depth of infiltration ≥ half of myometrium

Surgery followed by

External Irradiation with 30 % central shielding

and High Dose Rate Brachytherapy moderately reduced regime

Degree of differentiation	Site of recurrent disease							Died			Living		Total number of patients
	L*	LR**	LRD***	LD	R	RD	D	With tumor	From treatment	Intercurrent, NED?	With tumor	NED	
High	–	–	–	–	–	–	2	2	1	1	–	29	33
Medium	1	–	–	–	–	1	2	4	–	1	–	39	44
Low	–	–	–	1	–	–	2	3	–	2	–	12	17
Not known	–	–	–	–	–	–	3	3	–	–	–	34	37
Total	1	–	–	1	–	1	9	12	1	4	–	114	131

* Local
** Regional
*** Distant
? No evidence of disease

The tables show that distant metastases are a greater problem than local recurrence and that the incidence of intercurrent death was about half of that of death with tumor.

Death from radiation lesions of gut or sigmoid-colon was considered as a complication of brachytherapy. The incidence was 1.4% in all patients treated with external irradiation and low dose rate brachytherapy and 0.6% following external beam therapy and high dose rate brachytherapy.
At present gut and sigmoid-colon are localized by means of contrast medium and dose-determination is performed before treatment is started.

The question arises whether, following surgery for a stage I endometrial carcinoma with deep infiltration, it might be feasible to go further in the direction as previously started, by giving all fractions of external irradiation without shielding and omitting vaginal brachytherapy. In such cases the

244

full dose of 50 Gray is given to the whole bladder and to the
whole rectum. When calculating the radiobiological effect expressed in TDF units according to Orton (6, 7) the principle
proposed above might be accepted even with a 10% dose reduction: for 23 fractions of 2 Gray the TDF = 76.

This is indeed 30% lower than the combined treatment with
high dose rate brachytherapy but 20% higher than the first
regimen given with low dose rate brachytherapy and the survival curves of these both types of treatment were quite similar.

Substitution of low dose rate vaginal irradiation by high
dose rate brachytherapy in the postoperative treatment of
endometrial carcinoma stage II or stage III did not have an
impact on the survival rates (Fig. 3, 4).

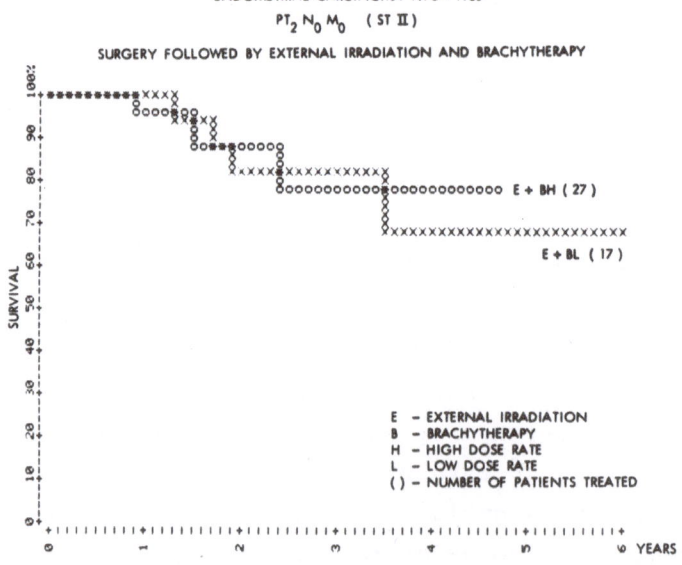

Fig. 3

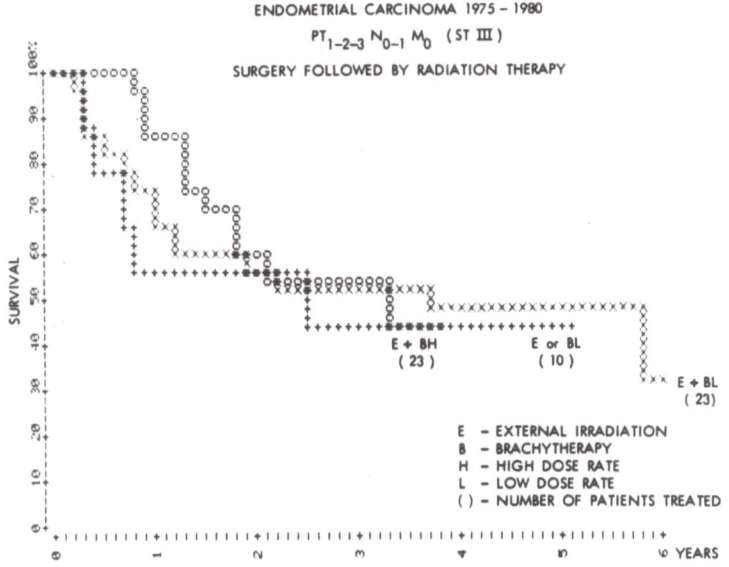

Fig. 4

Finally, actuarial survival curves related to degree of differentiation among patients with endometrial carcinoma stage
I with deep infiltration, are presented (Fig. 5).

Low degree of differentiation (grade 3) was associated with
a 5-year survival of 58%; for high and medium degree (grades
1 and 2) the curves were very similar: 86% was alive 5 years
after treatment which is a significant difference.
In the group with unknown degree of differentiation 88% sur-
vied 5 years. More information concerning these tumors will
be collected in the near future. At present pathologists always provide information concerning the degree of differentiation.

Conclusions

1. Stage I endometrial carcinoma infiltrating less than half
   of the thickness of the myometrium and with a high degree

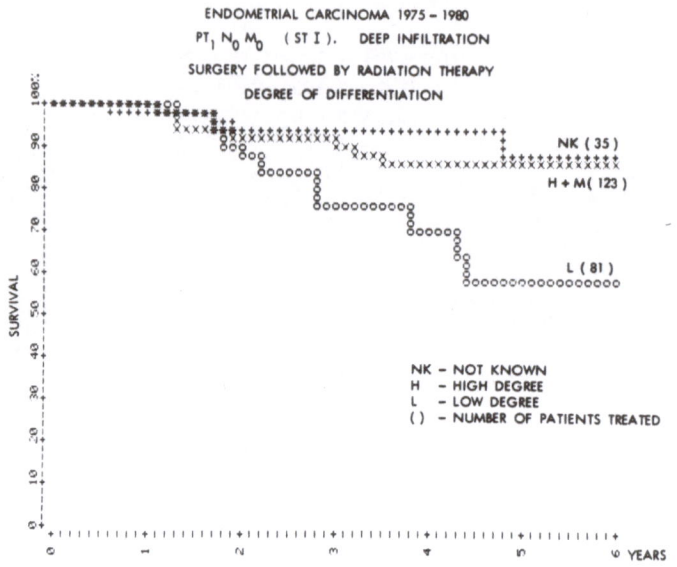

Fig. 5

of differentiation may adequately be treated by surgery
alone.

2. Stage I endometrial carcinoma with infiltration of half or
   more of the thickness of the myometrium, may be treated
   postoperatively with external irradiation without brachytherapy.

3. Replacement of low dose rate brachytherapy by high dose
   rate brachytherapy enables better dosimetry and treatment
   without admission to the hospital. This last fact is of
   great psychological value.

4. Strict follow-up and centralized registration are required
   for verification of the assumptions stated above.

References

1. Piver, M.S., Yazigi, R., Blumenson L. and Tsukada, Y. 1979.
   A prospective trial comparing hysterectomy, hysterectomy
   plus vaginal radium, and uterine radium plus hysterectomy
   in Stage I endometrial carcinoma. Obstet. Gvnec. 54:85-89.
2. Graham, J. 1971. The value of preoperative or postoperative
   treatment by radium for carcinoma of the uterine body. Surg.
   Gynec. Obstet. 132:855-860.
3. Malkasian, G.D., Annegers, J.F. and Fountain, K.S. 1980.
   Carcinoma of the endometrium; Stage I. Am. J. Obstet. Gynec. 136:872-888.
4. Joslin, C.A. and Wmith, C.W. 1971. Postoperative radiotherapy in the management of uterine corpus carcinoma.
   Clin. Radiol. 22:118-124.
5. Joslin, C.A., Vaishampayan, G.V. and Mallik, A. 1977. The
   treatment of early cancer of the corpus uteri. Brit. J.
   Radiol. 50:38-45.
6. Orton, C.G. and Ellis, F. 1973. A simplification in the
   use of the NSD concept. Br. J. Radiol. 56:529-537.
7. Orton, C.G. 1974. Time dose factors in Brachytherapy. Br.
   J. Radiol. 47:603-607.

21. THE MORPHOLOGICAL BASIS FOR THE TREATMENT OF BORDERLINE
TUMOURS OF THE OVARY

H. Fox

To many gynaecologists a histopathological diagnosis of "ovarian epithelial tumour of borderline malignancy" is taken as
being indicative of indecision on the part of the pathologist
as to whether a neoplasm is benign or malignant. If this were
indeed the case then the gynaecologist would have legitimate
grounds for complaint for little point would be served by
elevating pathological uncertainty into a nosological entity.
In fact, however, ovarian epithelial tumours of borderline
malignancy form, in pathological terms, a well delineated
and clearly defined group, the diagnosis of which is a positive one that is based on specific histological findings.
There is however, considerable justification for the gynaecological belief that a diagnosis of borderline malignancy
hints at uncertainty and irresolution for the term, although
recommended by WHO (22), is perhaps not the most suitable
and could, possibly with benefit, be replaced by a rather
less equivocal name such as "low grade adenocarcinoma".

Definition

In the WHO classification of ovarian tumours (22) a neoplasm
of borderline malignancy is defined as one "that has some,
but not all, of the morphological features of malignancy:
those present include in varying combinations, stratification
of epithelial cells, apparent detachment of cellular clusters
from their sites of origin and mitotic figures and nuclear
abnormalities intermediate between those of clearly benign
and unquestionably malignant tumours of a similar cell type:
on the other hand, obvious invasion of the stroma is lacking".

It will be noted that this definition is based solely upon
the histological features of the ovarian tumour and takes no
account of whether or not there is extra-ovarian spread.
The WHO definition does not sufficiently stress the prime
diagnostic importance of the lack of stromal invasion and
this, together with the difficulty which may be encountered
in deciding whether invasion is absent or not, has led to the
suggestion that some neoplasms, particularly those of mucinous type, can be classed as an adenocarcinoma even in the
absence of stromal invasion (8, 9). This view has not been
universally endorsed (20) and it is the practice in most centres in the United Kingdom to regard a tumour of borderline
malignancy as one in which the epithelium shows some, or all,
of the characteristics of malignancy but in which there is no
stromal invasion.
The insistence on lack of stromal invasion as a defining feature takes no account of whether the invasion is of a "destructive" nature or not and extensive sampling, coupled with
a readiness to resort to serial sectioning, is clearly necessary to establish a negative finding of this type.

Incidence

Tumours of borderline malignancy form a significant proportion of the overall group of ovarian epithelial neoplasms,
between 8 and 15 per cent of serous tumours and nearly 20 per
cent of mucinous tumours falling into this category (4, 20).
Endometrioid, Brenner and mesonephroid tumours of borderline
malignancy are uncommon.

Pathological features

Serous tumours

These are nearly always papillary and most resemble macros-
copically a benign papillary serous cystadenoma: a suspicion
that such neoplasms are not fully benign is, however, often
generated by the unusually luxuriant proliferation of fine
papillae and by the presence of exophytic papillary excresen-

ce on the outer surface of the cyst. A small proportion of
borderline serous tumours are grossly similar to a benign
papillary surface tumour but tend to have a rather more complex and dense papillary pattern.

Histologically these tumours are formed of rather fine branch-
ing papillae. In those with only minimal epithelial atypia
the cellular mantle of the papillae can be clearly recognised
as being of tubal type but in tumours with marked epithelial
abnormalities this resemblance tends to be lost and the cells
become predominantly rounded or cuboid. The epithelial component of the tumour shows a variable degree of multilayering
and has a marked tendency to form cellular buds or tufts:
those buds may break off to float freely within the cyst
whilst fusion of the tips of adjacent epithelial buds may
result in a honeycombed pattern. Nuclear crowding, atypia
and, hyperchromatism are of variable degree but the nucleoli
are often not particularly prominent: mitotic figures are
uncommon and rarely atypical whilst psammoma bodies are frequently present. In most of these neoplasms there is a sharp
junction between epithelium and stroma and the possibility of
stromal invasion can be excluded with relative ease: in others
there may be epithelial invaginations into the stroma and
these can cause a diagnostic difficulty which is, however,
often resolved by serial sectioning. By and large all borderline serous tumours have a strikingly similar and characteristic appearance: furthermore the borderline pattern tends to
be relatively consistent throughout the neoplasm and it is
unusual to find areas of clearly benign epithelium alternating,
or intermingled with, epithelium showing malignant characteristics.

A notable feature of serous tumours of borderline malignancy
is the high incidence, variously estimated as between 14 and
40 per cent, of bilaterality (11, 13, 16, 20): the bilateral
involvement is not always apparent to the naked eye and may
be only recognised on histological examination. It is, however, almost certain that the bilaterality is due to the concurrent development of two primary tumours rather than to me-

tastasis of a single primary lesion to the contralateral ovary. A further, and often disconcerting, aspect of these neoplasms is the frequency of apparent extraovarian spread at
the time of initial diagnosis, this usually taking the form
of multiple seedlings or implants on the pelvic peritoneum
and omentum. The presence of such implants has been noted in
between 16 en 47 per cent of cases (11, 13, 15, 16, 20) and
the fact that they are sometimes accompanied by ascites often
provokes a gloomy prognostic attitude. Histological examination shows, however, that many of these impoants are deep
to, rather than on the surface of, the peritoneum and that
some have a benign appearance and do not show any invasive
tendencies: most will show a borderline pattern and it is
uncommon for there to be an overtly malignant picture (20).
Some peritoneal implants do progress in a rather indolent and
leisurely fashion but many either remain stationary or regress
(5) and there are thus good grounds for believing that many
are not true implants or metastases but represent multiple
foci of neoplastic transformation, not necessarily or even
usually of a malignant nature, within peritoneal mesothelium
(20): indeed, in many instances the condition can be classed
as a form of endosalpingiosis.

Mucinous tumours

These usually present as large multilocular cysts. The lining
of the cyst is generally smooth but there may be focal areas
of thickening, nodularity or endophytic projections.
Borderline mucinous tumours differ significantly from their
serous counterparts in that there is no uniformity of histological appearances throughout the neoplasm, there commonly
being areas which have a fully benign epithelial pattern and
others in which there is a variable degree of epithelial irregularity and abnormality: the areas of borderline malignancy may be extremely focal. In borderline mucinous tumours
the epithelial component may show a complex glandular pattern
but is often characterised by short papillary infoldings which
give the epithelium a serrated appearance. There are varying

degrees of multilayering, loss of nuclear polarity, nuclear
hyperchromatism and cellular atypia whilst mitotic figures
tend to be seen with some frequency, albeit usually of normal
form. Because of outpouching of the epithelium and the formation of secondary cysts or glands in many borderline mucinous neoplasms the assessment of possible stromal invasion
is more difficult than is the case with serous tumours: this
is not, however, usually an impossible task for features such
as an irregular contour and arrangement of the glandular
structures, a focal chronic inflammatory cell infiltration
or the presence of immature type stroma all suggest invasion
rather than inclusion (20). Certainly there can be no doubt
that invasion is occurring if single cells, nests of cells
or cellular cords are seen infiltrating the stroma. Nevertheless, Hart and Norris (9) have maintained that, in the absence of definite stromal invasion a mucinous tumour should
be regarded as malignant, rather than borderline, if there
is marked overgrowth of atypical epithelial cells or striking
nuclear abnormalities: they also suggest that fingerlike papillary projections of solid cellular masses without a stromal
support should be regarded as diagnostic of adenocarcinoma
and regard as malignant those borderline tumours in which
stratification of atypical epithelial cells has exceeded three
layers in thickness. Russell (20) has commented that "these
supplementary criteria seem to add an unnecessary complication
to an already difficult area which is not justified by an increased precision of prognosis" and this is a sentiment which
my experience would lead me to endorse.
Borderline mucinous tumours occur bilaterally in only between
5 and 10 per cent of cases and are rarely accompanied by peritoneal or omental implats. A relatively common feature of
these neoplasms is, however, pseudomyxoma ovarii, which is
due to leakage of mucus into the ovarian stromal tissues: this
sometimes provokes a pseudosarcomatous reaction in the stromal
cells and progresses to pseudomyxoma peritoneii in a substantial proportion of cases.

Endometrioid tumours

Borderline forms of this type of epithelial neoplasm are uncommon and present two quite different pathological pictures.
One is seen in association with, and arising from, foci of
ovarian endometriosis, the histological features resembling
acutely those of an atypical hyperplasia of the endometrium
(3). It is, in fact, a moot point as to whether lesions of
this type should be regarded as neoplastic or hyperplastic
and all the difficulties which may be encountered in classi-
fying such lesions in the endometrium find their exact counter-
part in these ovarian lesions. The other type is the endometrioid adenofibroma of borderline malignancy in which endo-
metrial-type glands showing irregular budding, stratification
and nuclear atypia are set in an abundant, dense stroma (12,
17): neoplasms of this latter type are usually less than 10 cm
in diameter and tend grossly to resemble a fibroma.

Brenner tumours

The Brenner tumour of borderline malignancy is a clear cut,
but far from common, entity (7, 19). They are usually unilateral, generally large, partly cystic neoplasms the cut surface of which shows multiple locules containing clear or watery fluid. In some areas the locular lining is smooth but
in others it is formed by papillary, velvety, friable tissue.
Histologically, areas of typical benign Brenner tumour are
often, but not invariably, present whilst in the papillary
areas of the tumour the epithelium is thrown up into multi-
layered folds which are supported by thin connective tissue
stalks: the appearances in these areas bear an unmistakable
resemblance to those of a Grade I transitional cell carcinoma
of the bladder. Focal cellular and nuclear atypia are usually
present and there is often a sprinkling of mitotic figures:
stromal invasion, which is easy to assess in these neoplasms,
is not seen.

Mesonephroid tumours

Mesonephroid neoplasms of borderline malignancy are rare and appear always to take the form of an adenofibroma in which glands lined by hob-nail or clear cells showing varying degrees of cellular and nuclear atypia are embedded in a fibrous stroma (18).

Prognosis in relation to tumour type

There is broad agreement that the short term prognosis for women with an epithelial ovarian neoplasm of borderline malignancy is generally good but there has been some disagreement about long term prognosis, a factor which is of particular importance because of the relative youth of many of the patients with neoplasms of this type. There is a consensus that the 5-year survival rate of patients with a serous tumour of borderline malignancy is in the region of 90 per cent (1, 11, 15, 16) but reported 10 year survival rates have varied from 75 to 90 per cent (1, 11, 15, 21). The reported 5-year survival rate for women with mucinous tumours of borderline malignancy has ranged from 81 per cent (15) to 95 per cent (19) whilst estimates of the 10-year survival rate have varied from 68 to 95 per cent (1, 9, 15, 21). Little information is available about survival rates for periods greater than 10 years but Nikrui (15) has reported 15-year survival rates of 73 per cent for women with borderline serous tumours and of 57 per cent for those with borderline mucinous tumours.

Too few cases of borderline endometrioid, Brenner or mesonephroid tumours have been adequately followed up for their true prognosis to be known.

Prognosis in relation to stage

Survival rates in relationship to clinical stage have been recorded only for borderline tumours of the serous type. In two series the 5-year survival rate for patients with IA, IB and IIA tumours was 100 per cent whilst that for patients with IIB tumours varied from 86 to 100 per cent and that for women with stage III neoplasms from 56 to 82 per cent. A 5-year survival rate of 80 per cent was recorded for patients with stage IV neoplasms (11, 13). Aure et al (1) reported 5, 10 and 20 year survivals of, respectively, 96, 94 and 78 per cent for patients with stage IA tumours and 94, 86 and 86 per cent for stage IB tumours. Clearly there is agreement that the prognosis for stage I and IIA tumours is extremely good but accurate data for survival of patients with stage III or IV tumours is lacking, largely because the series quoted have contained only a very few patients whose neoplasm had attained these clinical stages at the time of diagnosis: nevertheless the prognosis for patients with apparently advanced disease is obviously very much better than is that for women with a frankly adenocarcinomatous tumour of the same stage.

Prognostic indices

The development of prognostic indices for women with a tumour of borderline malignancy presents a challenging problem, particularly because clinical stage is a less accurate indications of eventual outcome than is the case in overt adeno-carcinomata. Attempts have been made to grade the degree of epithelial abnormality in borderline tumours, using such features as the degree of multilayering, the amount of epithelial budding, the extent of nuclear atypia and the number of mitotic figures, and such a grading system has proved useful in some hands (20) but not in others (4, 13).
Another approach to the grading of borderline tumours is the quantitative immunohistological assessment of their content of secretory products. Heald, Buckley and Fox (10) found that many ovarian epithelial tumours, whether benign or malignant, contained CEA and whilst semi-quantitative measurement of the tumour content of CEA, using a dilutional technique, failed to reveal any discriminatory differences between benign and malignant serous neoplasms there was a clear cut difference between malignant mucinous tumours, which invariably had a high content of CEA, and benign mucinous neoplasms which either

had a low content of, or stained negatively for, CEA. A measurement of the CEA content of borderline mucinous tumours showed that about 50 per cent had a CEA content similar to that of malignant tumours whilst the remainder had a CEA content more typical of a benign neoplasm. In the borderline group of neoplasms there was no relationship between the CEA content and the degree of epithelial abnormality but it could be postulated that those borderline neoplasms with a high CEA content may be more likely to pursue a malignant course than are those with low CEA levels: unfortunately however, it remains to be proven that this is the case. More recently, and disappointingly, it has been shown that the immunohistochemical demonstration of tumour hCG is of no value in discriminating between benign, borderline and malignant ovarian epithelial neoplasms (14).

Biological nature of borderline tumours

It is clear that epithelial tumours of borderline malignancy form a well defined pathological entity. Their true biological nature remains, however, uncertain. It is tempting to consider these tumours as benign neoplasms which are in the course of becoming malignant but, certainly for the serous tumours, this does not appear to be the case. These neoplasms have a homogenous pattern of epithelial abnormality with no alternation of benign and borderline type epithelia and when they recur still usually show a histologically borderline appearance; even metastases retain this borderline pattern. It appears therefore probable that the borderline serous tumours have been of this nature ab initio and tend to retain this pattern of growth and proliferation indefinitely: it is true that occasional cases become overtly adenocarcinomatous but malignant change can occur in any benign or low grade malignant neoplasm, e.g. a squamous cell carcinoma arising in a mature cystic teratoma or a stromal sarcoma arising in a Müllerian adenosarcoma. The situation with the borderline mucinous tumours is less clear cut for in these it is common to find an admixture of normal and abnormal epithelium, this

possibly suggesting that malignant change is occurring in a
previously benign tumour: nevertheless the natural history
of these tumours indicates that a progression to frank malignancy is unusual and that they retain this borderline pattern
throughout their course.

Borderline tumours, even when in Stage III or IV, still appear to advance in a relatively leisurely fashion and this
adds further strength to the view that these neoplasms do
not evolve into overtly malignant tumours but pursue a course
which is neither fully benign nor frankly malignant, a pattern
of clinical behaviour which is as equivocal as is their histological appearance. It would appear therefore that in biological terms the borderline tumours are not ones which have
been diagnosed in a transitional stage of their evolution
but represent a specific type of tumour of low grade malignancy,
a status which they probably retain throughout their course.

Management of ovarian tumours of borderline malignancy

These neoplasms present a difficult problem of management to
the gynaecologist who has to steer a middle course between
undertreatment of a possibly fatal neoplasm and un unnecessa-
rily rigorous therapeutic regime for a tumour which will not,
in most cases, kill the patient. All the currently available
evidence suggests that the treatment of borderline tumours
is essentially surgical. To consider first those patients in
whom the tumour is confined to the ovaries: if there is bilateral involvement the patient should, irrespective of her
age, be subjected to a bilateral salpingo-oophorectomy and
hysterectomy: the same treatment should be applied to those
women with unilateral tumours who have completed their families. A major problem is the management of a unilateral ovarian borderline tumour in a young woman who wishes to have
children: in such cases it is first necessary to biopsy the
contralateral ovary in order to ensure that the neoplasm is
really unilateral, and if this is proved to be the case it
is probably justifiable to perform a unilateral salpingo-
oophorectomy. Women treated in this fashion should, however,

be advised to complete their families as soon as possible
and then submit themselves to hysterectomy and removal of
the contralateral tube and ovary. There is no evidence that
either adjunct chemotherapy or pelvic radiotherapy is necessary for patients with tumour confined to one or both ovaries (2, 6).

Patients with apparent extraovarian spread at the time of
diagnosis pose an as yet unanswered therapeutic question. The
first stage is certainly hysterectomy and bilateral salpingo-
oophorectomy, probably with omentectomy and certainly with
biopsy of the peritoneal or omental lesions. If the extraovarian lesions are histologically frankly malignant then
the patient should be treated as if she had an overt adenocarcinoma at the same clinical stage: if they show a benign
or borderline histological pattern a case can be made out for
not proceeding to further therapy but for simply following
up the patient with considerable care. In a proportion of such
cases the extraovarian lesions will either not progress or
will regress and under these circumstances no further treatment is warranted: in some patients they will progress and
treatment for adenocarcinoma can then be instituted. Certainly, therapeutic decisions are not a matter of urgency and
time spent in careful observation can not be regarded as
dangerous in view of the indolent course pursued by those
neoplasms which do progress.

REFERENCES

1. Aure, J.C., Hoeg, K. and Kolstad, P. 1971. Clinical and
   histologic studies of ovarian carcinoma: long term follow-
   up of 990 cases. Obstet. Gynecol. 37, 1-9.
2. Creasman, W.T., Park, R., Norris, H., Disaia, P.J. Morrow,
   C.P. and Hreschchyshyn, M. 1982. Stage I borderline ovarian tumors. Obstet. Gynecol. 59, 93-96.
3. Czernobilsky, B. and Morris, W.J. 1979. A histologic study
   of ovarian endometriosis with emphasis on hyperplastic and
   atypical changes. Obstet. Gynecol. 53, 318-323.
4. Fox, H. 1982. Ovarian tumors of borderline malignancy. In:
   Diagnosis and Management of Gynecologic Neoplasms. (Ed.
   C.P. Morrow, J. Bonnar and T. O'Brien) Raven Press, New
   York.
5. Fox, H. and Langley, F.A. 1976. Tumours of the Ovary. Heinemann, London.

6. Guthrie, D., Davy, M.L.J. and Philipe, P.R. 1982. A study of 656 patients with early ovarian cancer. Brit. J. Obstet. Gynaecol. (In press).
7. Hallgrimson, J. and Scully, R.E. 1972. Borderline and malignant Brenner tumors of the ovary: a report of 15 cases. Acta Pathol. Microbiol. Scand. Sect. A. 80, Suppl. 233, 56-66.
8. Hart, W.R. 1977. Ovarian epithelial tumors of borderline malignancy (carcinoma of low malignant potential). Hum. Pathol. 8, 541-549.
9. Hart. W.R. and Norris, H.J. 1973. Borderline and malignant mucinous tumor of the ovary: histologic criteria and clinical behaviour. Cancer 31, 1031-1045.
10. Heald, J., Buckley, C.H. and Fox, H. 1979. An immunohistochemical study of the distribution and carcinoembryonic antigen in epithelial tumours of the ovary. J. Clin. Pathol. 32, 919-926.
11. Julian, C.G. and Woodruff, J.D. 1972. The biological behaviour of low-grade papillary serous carcinoma of the ovary. Obstet. Gynecol. 40, 860-867.
12. Kao, G.F. and Norris, H.J. 1979. Unusual cystadenofibromas: endometrioid, mucinous and clear cell types. Obstet. Gynecol. 54, 729-736.
13. Katzenstein, A.A., Mazur, M.T., Morgan, T.E. and Kao, M. 1978. Proliferative serous tumors of the ovary: histologic features and prognosis. Amer. J. Surg. Pathol. 2, 339-355.
14. Mohabeer, J., Buckley, C.H. and Fox, H. 1982. An immunohistochemical study of the incidence and significance of hCG synthesis by epithelial ovarian neoplasms.
15. Nikrui, N. 1981. Survey of clinical behaviour of patients with borderline epithelial tumor of the ovary. Gynec. Oncol. 12, 107-119.
16. Purola, E. 1963. Serous papillary ovarian tumours: a study of 233 cases with special reference to histological type of tumour and its influence on prognosis. Acta Obstet. Gynecol. Scand. 42, Suppl. 3.
17. Roth, L.M., Czernobilsky, B. and Langley, F.A. 1980. Ovarian endometrioid adenofibromatous and cystadenofibromatous tumors: benign, proliferating and malignant. Cancer 48, 1838-1845.
18. Roth, L.M., Langley, F.A., Fox, H., Wheeler, J. and Czernobilsky, B. 1982. Ovarian clear cell adenofibromatous tumors: benign, of low malignant potential, and associated with invasive clear cell carcinoma.
19. Roth, L.M. and Sternberg, W.R. 1971. Proliferating Brenner tumors. Cancer 27, 687-693.
20. Russell, P. 1979. The pathological assessment of ovarian neoplasms. II. The proliferating "epithelial" tumours. Pathology 11, 5-26.
21. Santesson, I. and Kottmeier, H.L. 1968. General classification of ovarian tumors. In: Ovarian Cancer, UICC Monograph Series, Volume II (Ed. J. Gentil and A.C. Junqueira) pp 1-8. Springer-Verlag, Berlin.
22. Serov, S.F., Scully, R.E. and Sobin, L.H. 1973. International Classification of Tumours No. 9. Histological typing of Ovarian Tumours. World Health Organization, Geneva.

22. NEW DEVELOPMENTS IN THE SURGICAL TREATMENT OF OVARIAN
CANCER

C. Thomas Griffiths

During tha past decade a better understanding of the natural
history of ovarian carcinoma and the availability of adjuvant
therapy have greatly expanded the usefulness of surgical treatment. Newer developments in surgical management include extended surgical staging and surgical cytoreduction.

Surgical staging of early cancers

Erroneous operative staging of putative stage I cancers has
been well demonstrated in the past by the 30-40 percent mortality rate in this group of patients in whom apparently localized tumors were completely excised. The significantly better
survival curve of patients with stage II disease treated by
whole abdominal irradiation compared to that of patients
treated with pelvic irradiation alone suggests that unrecognized or microscopic spread of stage II disease to the upper
abdomen has taken place in a large percentage of cases (1).
Cognizance of early and frequently occult tumor spread to
the right hemidiaphragm, the distal omentum and the para-aortic
lymph nodes distal to the left renal vein has led to careful
examination or biopsy of these areas as routine components
of surgical staging. The incidence of "subclinical" metastases
at these sites, according to the collective series reported
by Piver, is listed in Table 1 (2).

Table 1. Incidence (percent) of subclinical metastases (2)

Site	Stage I	Stage II	
Diaphragm	11.3% (44)*	23% (26)	*() = No. pts. studied
Aortic Nodes	10.3% (58)	10% (10)	
Omentum	3.2% (27)	0% (9)	

Cytologic study of saline recovered after lavage of the peritoneal cavity is necessary for adherence to the current staging system.

Although presumably of ominous import, the prognostic significance of positive cytologic washings has not been clearly
defined (3).

A multi-institutional study of stages I and II ovarian carcinoma conducted by the National Cancer Institute of the United
States has yielded some valuable information and will be
published in the near future. Sixty eight patients, who had
been initially staged at referring hospitals, were subjected
to second staging laparotomies according to standard protocol
at the participating institutions. Gross and microscopic
findings at the second operations resulted in the "upstaging"
of 31 patients. Primary staging errors had been made in 18
percent of stage I patients and in 43 percent of stage II patients. The prognostic information to be derived from the
accurately staged patients will be more valuable than the
data relevant to therapy. Fifty eight patients with encapsul-
ated stages Ia or Ib, grade 1 or 2 tumors were considered
at low risk for recurrence and were randomly allocated to
observation only or to melphalan administration over an 18-
month period. Since no recurrences were observed in either
treatment group, adjuvant therapy is probably not required
for these favorable cases. High risk patients were defined
as those with stages Ia or Ib tumors with perforated capsules
or grade 3 histology, stage Ic tumors, or stage IIa, b or c
tumors without macroscopic residual disease.

Forty nine patients were allocated to an 18-month course of
melphalan and 47 patients to a single peritoneal infusion of
^{32}P chromic phosphate. Only eight recurrences (16 percent)
were observed in the first treatment group and six recurrences
(13 percent) in the second treatment group. Since the results
of the two treatment groups were the same, and other studies
suggest that these two therapeutic regimens are ineffective,
one can assume that the low recurrence rate in these patients,
presumably at high risk, was the result of meticulous surgi-

cal staging and the exclusion of occult stage III cases. The delineation of a group of patients in whom adjuvant therapy is indicated must await analysis of the interaction of the high-risk variables. It may be that among stage I and II patients, who have been meticulously staged, and who have no macroscopic residuum, only those with grade 3 tumors or stage IIb tumors will require adjuvant irradiation or combination chemotherapy.

Surgical cytoreduction

Surgical management of advanced cancer has been palliative and includes diversionary procedures to relieve obstructed gastrointestinal or urinary tracts, techniques to diminish serous effusions and enurosurgical procedures to ablate intractable pain. Although operations of these types are planned to circumvent or alleviate the effect or tumor masses, surgical excision of such masses as a direct means of relief has been rare if the cancer is otherwise inoperable. The concept of operability carries the strong implication of complete tumor excision with a margin of normal tissue; consequently, tumor resection without expectation of complete excision violates the traditional tenets of surgical oncology. In recent years less than complete tumor excision, often termed a "debulking" or "cytoreductive" operation, has been applied to the treatment of Burkitt's lymphoma, testicular germ cell tumors and epithelial carcinomas of the ovary. The validity of surgical cytoreduction has been seriously challenged, and a tendency to extend the concept to sarcomas and gstrointestinal and head and neck carcinomas has arosed vociferous dissension from the exalted ranks of surgical oncologists.

Historical perspective

The widely advertised admonition to remove as much ovarian tumor tissue as possible originated with the ovariotomists of the nineteenth and early twentieth century who were re-

ferring to the excision of adherent primary tumors, rather
than to metastatic disease. On the other hand, beginning in
1916, a number of gynecologic surgeons including Bonney, Graves,
Lynch and Meigs, advocated the removal of primary tumors despite the presence of metastases and the removal of metastatic
implants when possible. In 1934 Meigs suggested that such operative procedures would render the tumor more susceptible to
postoperative irradiation. During the third quarter of the
century Munnell of New York strongly advocated a maximal surgical effort followed by radiation therapy for stage III ovarian cancer and provided retrospective clinical data to support this theses (4).

The theoretic rationale for surgical cytoreduction may be
divided into three possible mechanisms: 1. A direct effect
whereby reduction of tumor burden relieves the host of direct
tumor insult and increases survival time by reversing the
natural course of the disease. 2. The concept of first-order
kinetics is employed in that the rapid exponential decrease
in tumor size by excision permits elimination of the residuum
by adjuvant therapy. 3. Excision of larger tumor masses, insensitive to adjuvant therapy, results in the retention of
gross or microscopic cellular aggregates of relatively greater
sensitivity to adjuvant therapy.

The unique natural history of the epithelial carcinomas of
the ovary suggests that tumor volume has an indirect relationship to the survival time of the host. The epithelial carcinomas are relatively non-invasive and destruction of vital
organs is unusual. With increasing tumor growth, however, there
·is progressive mechanical interference of gastrointestinal
function with disordered small bowel motility as the predominant result (5, 6). The metabolic effects of the enlarging
tumor bulk are no less inimical and the net result of the
mechanical and metabolic tumor effects is chronic protein malnutrition leading to a kwashiorkor-like state and death (6, 7).
Excepting those cases in which hematogenous dissemination has
occurred, the proximity of death appears to be related to the
volume of proliferating tumor within the abdominal cavity.

A number of clinical observations support an inverse relation between postoperative tumor volume and survival in stage III disease, irrespective of the extent of excision or subsequent therapy. Patients with stage III disease and no macroscopic tumor remaining after primary operation have survived significantly longer than patients with residual macroscopic disease (8, 9). The absence of palpable tumor following primary operation has been associated with a better prognosis than when palpable tumor remains (10, 11).

In recent years the diameter of the remaining tumor mass after primary operation has been used to define the extent of residual disease. Clinical data have indicated that patients with residual mass diameters that exceed a specific upper limit have a markedly compromised survival time irrespective of adjuvant therapy. The upper limit has ranged from 1 cm to 3 cm (3, 12, 13, 14, 15, 16). An increment in survival time corresponding to a decrement in residual mass diameter below the specified upper limit has also been noted (12, 13). Patients with residual tumor consisting only of miliary implants (diameter 0.5 cm or less) have had survival times that range between that of patients with larger lesions and that of patients with no residual macroscopic disease. In the following paper van Lindert et al selected a diameter of 0.5 cm or less as their goal in accomplishing surgical cytoreduction (17). Although the concept of first-order kinetics has provided the rationale for the chemotherapy of micrometastases after excision of a primary tumor, it cannot be applied to surgical cytoreduction of ovarian cancer. Since ovarian tumor masses often exceed 1 kg in weight, or 10^{12} cells and optimal surgical cytoreduction would reduce that mass to 1 gram in weight or 10^9 cell, the thesis appears attractive. On the other hand, according to the cytokinetics principles of tumor regression established by Skipper and Schabel and their associates, seven additional three-log "cell-kills" would be required to kill the last cancer cell (18). Obviously, the 1/8th contribution of surgical cytoreduction would be negligible.

The most compelling cytokinetic principle favoring an inverse

relationship between tumor mass size and chemotherapeutic
response has been that of the growth fraction (19). The growth
fraction is defined as the proportion of tumor stem cells that
are actively dividing. Since non-stem cells are destined to
die spontaneously, they are of no importance. Consequently,
the numerator of the growth fraction is the number of cells
in mitotic cycle, whereas the denominator is comprised of
dividing cells and resting cells that retain the potential
to divide (GO phase). Studies of experimental tumor growth
have demonstrated an asymptotic curve that represents two
parameters: exponential growth and a doubling time that increases exponentially. The exponential increase in doubling
time is the result of a decreasing growth fraction, which
means that small tumors (1-5 mg) have a high growth fraction,
whereas larger tumor masses have a low growth fraction. Tumor
masses with a high growth fraction are sensitive to most chemotherapeutic agents and those with a low growth fraction are
proportionately insensitive to chemotherapy. Although these
experiments have been carried out in animals, clinical data
accumulated in the human suggest that the same growth characteristics pertain (20).

A clinical bridge between these experimental data and the
efficacy of chemotherapeutic regimens observed in patients
with ovarian cancer metastases of 5 mm or less can be inferred
from Table 1. Caution must be exercised, however, in equating
tumor mass size with chemotherapeutic sensitivity. As pointed
out by Goldie and Coldman, an innate property of tumors is
a spontaneous mutation rate toward phenotypic drug-resistance
(21). Although the probability of resistance is a function
of the spontaneous mutation rate and the size of the cellular
population, progression to biochemical resistance takes place
rapidly during periods of exponential tumor growth. The Goldie-
Coldman hypothesis suggests that tumors of large size will
be phenotypically resistant to chemotherapy and, therefore,
surgical cytoreduction may be ineffective unless the entire
tumor mass can be removed. The clinical data from the University of California at Los Angeles (UCLA) series in which masses

larger than 10 cm in diameter portended limited survival, despite optimal surgical cytoreduction, are consistent with this
hypothesis (13).

Table 2. Survival time after primary surgical cytoreduction

Mass Size	Pts.	Median Surv. Mos.	No. 5-Yr. Survivors
BHW-1 (12)			
< 1.5 cm	41	22	9
> 1.5 cm	26	11	0
BHW-2 (25)			
< 1.5 cm	13	54	5
> 1.5 cm	3	10	0
MDA (15)			
< 2.0 cm	29	28	-
> 2.0 cm	53	15	-
UCLA (13)			
< 0.5 cm	7	40	1*
0.5-1.5 cm	24	18	-
> 1.5 cm	16	6	0
UTRECHT			
< 0.5 cm	26	> 24	2*
0.5-2.0 cm	7	21	0
> 2.0 cm	20	12	0

* by actuarial table
ABBREV:

BHW   = Boston Hospital for Women
MDA   = M.D. Anderson Hospital
UCLA   = University of California, Los Angeles
UTRECHT = University of Utrecht, The Netherlands

Effect of surgical cytoreduction on survival

Substantive clinical data can be marshalled to support the concept of an inverse relationship between largest residual mass size and survival time as illustrated in the foregoing section. The prime question to be addressed is whether patients who have undergone surgical cytoreduction below a specified size limit fare as well as those patients whose metastatic masses were below that size limit de novo. In a retrospective study from the Boston Hospital for Women (12) approximately half of those patients with a residual mass size below 1.5 cm in diameter had undergone resection of larger metastatic lesions. The survival curve for this group was identical to that of the group in which the largest metastatic lesions were below 1.5 cm at the outset (Figure 1). In a series from the University of California, Los Angeles (UCLA) the survival curve of 14 patients whose residual mass size of 1.5 cm or less had resulted from the excision of metastatic lesions ranging between 1.5 and 10 cm was not significantly different from the survival curve of patients whose preoperative metastases were less than 1.5 cm (13). On the other hand, surgical cytoreduction below the 1.5 cm limit in ten patients whose preoperative metastases were larger than 10 cm resulted in a survival curve that differed little from that of patients who had suboptimal surgical excision. The latter finding is consistent with the Goldie-Coldman hypothesis.

Although it can be argued that the improvement in survival depends more upon limited or less invasive tumor growth than upon extended surgical resection, data from a retrospective series at the M.D. Anderson Hospital (15) as well as the UCLA series (13) tend to negate this assertion. In these studies the survival of patients who required only hysterectomy, bilateral oophorectomy and infracolic omentectomy i.e. those with limited stage III disease, was no better than that of patients who required more extensive cytoreductive procedures. Similarly, in the Boston Hospital for Women series (12) the improvement in survival time of patients who had undergone optimal cytoreduction was shown by multivariate analysis to

be independent of extent of spread or organ involvement, histologic grade or the operation performed.

The answer to the prime question is the affirmative with the
qualification suggested by the UCLA series, that excision of
extremely large masses only partially reverses an unfavorable
prognosis.

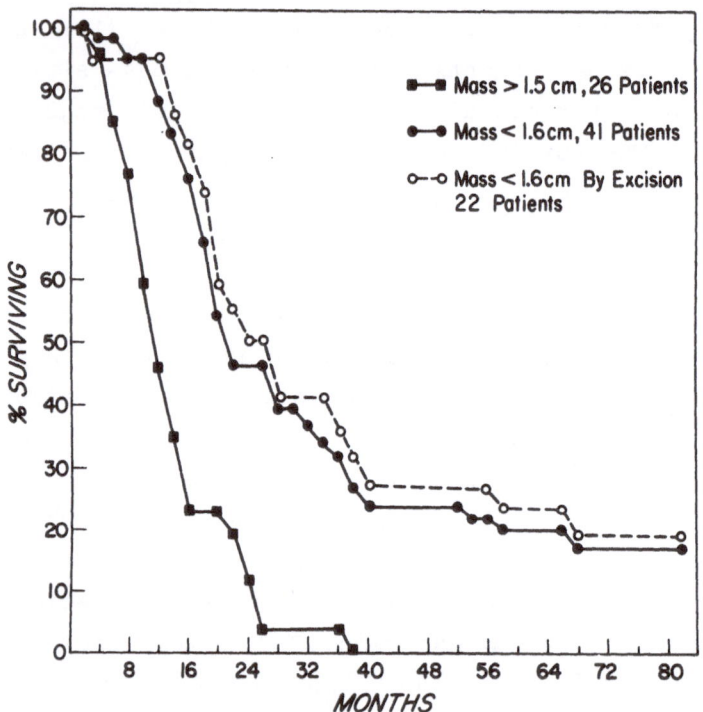

Figure 1. Relation of survival to size of largest residual
metastasis after primary operation for stage III ovarian cancer.

The effect of surgical cytoreduction on sensitivity to chemotherapy

An objective response, defined as a 50 percent or greater
shrinkage of tumor size, has been the usual measure of chemotherapeutic sensitivity. In the treatment of advanced ovarian
cancer the attainment of a complete response confirmed by
multiple intraperitoneal biopsies has been predictive of a
prolongation of survival time well in excess of that observed

in patients with lesser degrees of response (14, 22). The
available evidence with respect to response of residual tumor to chemotherapy after surgical cytoreduction must be derived from seven published series by three institutions in
which the mass size prior to chemotherapy as well as the complete response rate determined by intraperitoneal biopsies
are stated. The institutions and series are as follows: National Cancer Institue (NCI) (14), M.D. Anderson Hospital (MDA)
(15, 23, 24), Sidney Farber Cancer Institute (SFCI) (22), Vanderbilt University (16). The overall objective response rates
to melphalan (14, 15), hexamethylmelamine (23) and cis-platin
(24) ranged around 50 percent irrespective of maximal residual mass size. Similarly, the complete response rates ranged
between 0 and 18 percent with no apparent effect of residual
mass size on these figures. In contrast, three different drug
combinations used at the NCI (14), SFCI (22) and Vanderbilt
University (16) induced objective responses in 100 percent
of patients whose masses were less than 2-3 cm in diameter
and the complete response rate in this group approached 100
percent. The overall response rate and complete response rates
among patients with masses larger than 2 cm approximated those
obtained with single agents. In summary, surgical cytoreduction
enhances tumor sensitivity to effective drugs in combination
but not to those same drugs when used singly. As a corollary
the superiority of drug combinations over single agents is
mainly apparent in patients with minimal residual disease.

Secondary surgical cytoreduction

In many instances the patient initially deemed inoperable
responds favorably to one or more courses of chemotherapy and
is once again subjected to laparotomy for a second attempt
at surgical cytoreduction. This pattern has been fostered by
the medical oncologists' reluctance to seek a second surgical
opinion earlier and by the erroneous belief that chemotherapy
can render an inoperable tumor operable. Without question,
women with advanced ovarian cancer associated with ascites,
pleural effusions and malnutrition must undergo at least one

course of chemotherapy and hyperalimentation prior to the
imposition of yet another surgical insult. On the other hand,
resectability is not dependent upon the size of the tumor,
but, rather, upon the host-tumor interface. In fact, reduction
of mass size by chemotherapy obscures the guidelines for surgical cytoreduction in that even a 5 mm tumor implant imposes
a threat beyond that predicted by the Goldie-Coldman model,
since an increases proportion of resistant cells is the inevitable result of natural selection by previous treatment.
Furthermore, the interdependence of a small residual mass
size and combination chemotherapy in achieving a complete remission indicates that little benefit will be derived from
a secondary surgical cytoreduction, unless the patient is
still eligible for effective combination chemotherapy.
Unfortunately, known drug resistance, or the patient's in-
tolerance to further chemotherapy without strict dose limitation, will often militate against additional chemotherapy.
In the second Boston Hospital for Women series in which the
patients were unselected (25) the tumor-free survival times
of 15 patients in whom primary surgical cytoreduction was
attempted was far better than that of nine patients in whom
definitive operation was delayed until a favorable response
to chemotherapy was obtained. Since the pre-treatment characteristics were more favorable in the latter group, the improved
survival of the primary surgical group was attributed to the
use of combination chemotherapy; fewer than one-half of the
secondary surgical group were eligible. In the series of van
Lindert et al reported herin (17) all patients in this study
received combination chemotherapy, but the survival of patients with primary operation was better than that of patients
who had chemotherapy prior to operation. In the UCLA series
(13) optimal surgical cytoreduction was accomplished in 69
percent of 39 patients who underwent primary operation, but
was possible in only 38 percent of 32 patients subjected to
secondary cytoreductive operations (26).
It has been our opinion that resectability is technically
easier prior to initiation of chemotherapy, since edema at

the interface of the tumor and normal tissue produces cleavage planes which tend to become fibrotic after response to chemotherapy. Hacker et al (13) echoed this subjective observation and also favored primary, as opposed to secondary, surgical cytoreduction. Recently acquired data from our institutions show that surgical cytoreduction after one to four courses of combination chemotherapy (cyclophosphamide/adriamucin/cis-platinum) will result in survival times comparable to that of patients who have undergone primary cytoreduction provided that all macroscopic tumor is removed. Secondary surgical cytoreduction in which any gross disease remained failed to influence survival.

End-results and conclusions

Survival figures from five series on ovarian cancer cytoreduction are recorded by residual mass size in Table 2. Because of the small numbers of patients, differences in the median survival times of patients with small disease are probably not significant. Absolute five-year survival rates are available only for the BHW series (12, 25). If this traditional measure of therapeutic end-results is used, the results of the later series probably represents an improvement. The first series was comprised of primary-care patients in whom a small metastatic mass size was readily attainable in two thirds of the patients. In contrast, the second series was a prospective, though uncontrolled, trial in which selection was only adverse as dictated by patient referral. Despite failure to accomplish optimal primary cytoreduction in three of 16 patients, two stage IV patients, five patients ineligible for combination chemotherapy and two deaths from intercurrent disease, the five-year survival rate was 31 percent. A major revelation, however, lies in the fact that two of the five-year survivors subsequently died of their disease and a third developed recurrence seven years after primary cytoreduction. Only two patients are disease-free after five years.

A few conclusions can be drawn with assurance and a few only tentatively. An inverse relation between maximal residual mass size after primary operation and survival in stage III ovarian cancer is well supported. Histologic grade is a stronger prognostic determinant, but it does not negate the effect of mass size. Surgical resection of all masses larger than 1-2 cm in diameter will establish a status equivalent to the absence of larger metastases de novo. Similarly, secondary surgical cytoreduction may extend survival by providing relief from direct mass-effect.

Optimal surgical cytoreduction enhances the sensitivity of the tumor to chemotherapy by removing masses with a low growth fraction. This effect is inhibited by the emergence of phenotypically drug-resistant clones and is, therefore, negligible unless intensive combination chemotherapy is initiated early in the postoperative period. For the same reason, the combined effect of surgical cytoreduction and intensive chemotherapy is in great part negated by the presence of large metastatic masses at the outset. Ideally, surgical cytoreduction should leave no gross disease or, at the most, implants no larger than 5 mm. Although intensive surgical and chemotherapeutic management extends survival, it is not curative. In all probability the development of chemotherapy sufficient to effect cure will also render surgical cytoreduction obsolete.

References

1. Dembo, A.J., Bush, R.S., Beale, F.A., Bean, H.A., Pringle, J.F., Sturgeon, J. 1979. Ovarian carcinoma: Improved survival following abdominopelvic irradiation in patients with a completed pelvic operation. Am. J. Obstet. Gynecol. 134:793-800.
2. Piver, M.S., Barlow, J.J., Lele, S.B. 1978. Incidence of subclinical metastases in stage I and II ovarian carcinoma. Obstet. Gynecol. 52:100-104.
3. Smith J.P. and Day, T.G. 1979. Review of ovarian cancer at the University of Texas systems cancer center, M.D. Anderson Hospital and Tumor Institute. Am. J. Obstet. Gynecol. 135:984-993.
4. Munnell, E.W. 1967. The changing prognosis and treatment in cancer of the ovary. Am. J. Obstet. Gynecol. 100:790-805.
5. Griffiths, C.T. 1979. The Ovary. In Kistner, R.W. ed. Gynecology Principles and Practice, Chicago. The Year Book Medical Publishers.

6. Griffiths, C.T. and Fuller, A.F, Jr.: Intensive surgical and chemotherapeutic management of advanced ovarian cancer. Surgical Clinics of North America 58:131-142.

7. Fuller, A.F., Jr. and Griffiths, C.T. 1979. Ovarian cancer cachexia - surgical interactions. Gynecol. Oncol. 8: 301-310.

8. Parker, R.T., Parker, C.H. and Wiobanks, G.D. 1970. Cancer of the ovary. Am. J. Obstet. Gynecol. 108:878-888.

9. Aure, J.C., Joag, K. and Kolstad, P. 1971. Clinical and histologic studies of ovarian carcinoma. Obstet. Gynecol. 37:1-9, 1971.

10. Declos, L. and Quinlan, E.J. 1969. Malignant tumors of the ovary managed with postoperative megavoltage irradiation. Radiology 93:659-663.

11. Griffiths, C.T.,Grogan, R.H. and Hall, T.C. 1972. Advanced ovarian cancer: Primary treatment with surgery, radiotherapy and chemotherapy. Cancer 29:1-7.

12. Griffiths, C.T. 1975. Surgical resection of tumor bulk in the primary treatment of ovarian carcinoma. Symposium on ovarian cancer. National Cancer Institute Monographs 42:101-104.

13. Hacker, N.F., Berek, J.S., Lagasse, L.D., Neiberg, R.K. and Llashoff, R.M. Primary cytoreductive surgery for epithelial ovarian cancer. Obstet. Gynecol. (In Press).

14. Young, R.C., Chabner, B.A., Hubbard, W.P., Fisher, R.I., Bener, R.A., Anderson, T., Simon, R.M., Canellos, G.P. and DeVita, V.T. 1978. Advanced ovarian adenocarcinoma. A prospective clinical trial of melphalan (L-PAM) versus combination chemotherapy. N. Eng. J. Med. 299:1261-1266.

15. Wharton, J.T. and Herson, J. 1981. Surgery for common epithelial tumors of the ovary. Cancer 48:582-589.

16. Greco, F.A., Julian, C.G., Richardson, R.C., Burnett, L., Hande, K.R. and Oldham, R.K. 1981. Advanced ovarian cancer: Brief intensive combination chemotherapy and second-look operation. Obstet. Gynecol. 58:199-206.

17. van Lindert, A.C.M., Alsbach, G.P.J., Barents, J. Heintz, A.P.M. and Kooyman, C. 1983. The abdominal radical tumor reduction procedure. In: Heintz, A.P.M., Griffiths, C.T., Trimbos, J.B. eds. Surgery in Gynecological Oncology. Martinus Nijhoff.

18. Griswold, D.P., Jr., Schabel, F.M., Jr., Wilcox, W.S., Simpson-Herron, L. and Skipper, H.E. 1968. Success and failure in the treatment of solid tumors. 1. Effects of cyclophosphamide (NSC 0 26271) on primary and metastatic plasmacytoma in the hamster. Cancer Chemother. Rep. 52: 345-387.

19. Schabel, F.M., Jr. 1969. The use of tumor growth kinetics in planning 'curative' chemotherapy of advanced solid tumors. Cancer Res. 29:2384-2389.

20. Shackney, S.E., McCormack, G.W., Cuchural, G.J., Jr. 1978. Growth rate patterns of solid tumors and their relation to responsiveness to therapy. Am. Intern. Med. 89:107-121.

21. Goldie, J.H. and Coldman, A.J. 1979. A mathematic model for relating the drug sensitivity of tumors to their spontaneous mutation rate. Cancer Treat Rep. 63:1727-1733.

22. Parker, L.M., Griffiths, C.T., Yankee, R.A., Canellos, G.P., Gelman, R., Knapp, R.C., Richman, C.M., Tobias, J.S., Weiner, R.S. and Frei, E. 1980. III: Combination chemotherapy with adriamycin-cyclophosphamide for advanced ovarian carcinoma. Cancer 46:669-674.
23. Wharton, J.T., Rutledge, F., Smith, J.P., Herson, J. and Hodge, M.P. 1979. Hexamethylmelamine: An evaluation of its role in the treatment of ovarian cancer. Am.J. Obstet. Gynecol. 133:833-844.
24. Gershenson, D.M., Wharton, J.T., Herson, T., Edwards, C.L. and Rutledge, F.M. 1981. Single agent cis-platinum therapy for advanced ovarian cancer. Obstet. Gynecol. 58:487-496.
25. Griffiths, C.T., Parker, L.M. and Fuller, A.F. 1979. Role of cytoreductive surgical treatment in themanagement of advanced ovarian cancer. Cancer Treat Rep. 63:235-240.
26. Berek, J.S., Hacker, N.F., Lagasse, L.D., Neiberg, R.K. and Elashoff, R.M. 1983. Survival of patients following secondary cytoreductive surgery in ovarian cancer. Obstet. Gynecol. 61:189-193.

23. THE ROLE OF THE ABDOMINAL RADICAL TUMOR REDUCTION PROCE-
DURE (A.R.Tu.R.) IN THE TREATMENT OF OVARIAN CANCER
A preliminary evaluation of prognostic factors at the Univers-
ity of Utrecht, department of oncological gynecology.

A.C.M. van Lindert, G.P.J. Alsbach, J.W. Barents, A.P.M. Heintz,
C. Kooyman.

Introduction

In the Netherlands about 60 percent of patients treated for
epithelial ovarian cancer are in an advanced stage (F.I.G.O.
III and IV).
This means that the diagnosis of stage III and IV ovarian carcinoma is made in 800 - 900 patients per year.
A number of cytostatic agents like melphalan, cyclophosphamide,
chloroambucil, 5-fluorouracil, hexamethylmelamine, doxorubi-
cine and cis-platin has appeared to be effective in the treatment of ovarian carcinoma. By combining these drugs into new
schemes cytostatic treatment has been accelerated.
A number of chemotherapeutic combinations has been tested to
date. Owing to the introduction of polychemotherapy and with
improvements in preoperative and postoperative management,
debulking surgery can prolong survival and we can hope that
the cure rate will also take a favourable turn.

The aim of the Abdominal Radical Tumor Reduction procedure
(A.R.Tu.R.) is to minimize the tumor size in order that chemotherapy or radiotherapy has its optimal effect.
For patients with small residual tumor masses have more favourable prognoses than patients with large residual tumor
masses.

Material and method

Clinical material

A prospective study of 53 patients with advanced epithelial
carcinoma of the ovary (F.I.G.O. stage III and IV), treated

between 1976 and 1981 at the department of gynecology of the
state University of Utrecht, was undertaken.

Operative staging was performed according the F.I.G.O. staging system. All patients underwent a debulking procedure before starting with polychemotherapy or after two or three
courses of inductive polychemotherapy, depending on the preoperative or intraoperative state of resectability. Each tumor was graded as to degree of differentiation according to
a modified Ewing classification. Borderline tumors were excluded. Patients pretreated with chemotherapy elsewhere (in
most cases single agent) or patients admitted to the hospital
for relapse treatment were excluded.

Between the years of 1976 and 1981 polychemotherapy was given
using Hexa C.A.F. (hexamethylmelamine, cyclophosphamide, metho-
trexaat and 5-fluorouracil), C.H.A.D.$_5$ (cyclophosphamide, hexamethylmelamine, adriamycine and cisplatin) or C.P. (cyclophosphamide and cis-platin).

Microscopic complete remission and macroscopic complete remission were detected by laparoscopy or laparotomy and intraperitoneal biopsy.

Surgery

Special preoperative orders:

A thorough preoperative bowel preparation is very important.
Preoperative initiation of antibiotics is recommended consisting of 1.0 gr. Cephalosporin and Metronidazol 0.5 gr. i.v.
by infusion - one hour before operation and five and twelve
hours after surgery.

Because patients with advanced ovarian cancer are frequently
debilitated and emanciated, hyperalimentation is being used
more often in these patients.

Technique for Surgical Treatment of advanced cancer of the ovary

The abdomen is opened by a vertical incision that extends from
xiphoid to symphysis. The surgical approach then largely depends on the location and volume of the tumor masses.

Omentectomy: In some instances only infracolic omentectomy is
adequate because the gastrocolic ligament is uninvolved. If
tumor inplants are present in the gastrocolic ligament however, total omentectomy (dissection from the stomach) sometimes in combination with splenectomy has to be done.
Removal of the tumor from the diaphragme and liver surfaces.
Total pelvic evacuation of the tumor: It is desirable to incise the posterior peritoneum lateral to and just above the
pelvic brim, as carried out at the start of a radical hysterectomy.
This approach exposes the ovarian vessels and clamping them
early decreases the blood loss.
This procedure permits identification or the ureter, which
can be isolated and left attached to the medial peritoneal
flap. The ovarian vessels running in the infundibular ligament
can be isolated, clamped, cut, tied and double ligated in
toto.
As soon as a similar procedure is carried out on the opposite
side, a considerable amount of blood is diverted from the
ovarian cancer. With the ureter protected from injury, it is
possible by blunt and sharp dissection to incise the peritoneum down to the round ligament and, after it is clamped
and ligated, to continue the incision of the peritoneum lateral to the bladder. If the bladder flap of peritoneum is involved with cancer, the incision in the peritoneum should be
continued to the pubis. The lateral side of the peritoneum
over the bladder can be elevated and dissected by a sharp
and blunt dissection from the bladder, which is then left
denuded. The flap of peritoneum is dissected off the dome
of the bladder and left attached to the lower uterine segment and is removed as an en bloc dissection with the uterus.
Posteriorly, with the ureter under direct vision, the peritoneum medial to the ureter is incised down over the rectum.
This frees up the cul-de-sac from the bowel and leaves it
attached to the back part of the uterus. The entire specimen
can be removed as the hysterectomy is carried out.
The retroperitoneal approach allows easy elevation of the

ascending, descending and sigmoid colon, and by gentle dissection beneath both ureters to the bifurcation of the aorta,
samples of representative pelvic, paraaortic and vena caval
lymph nodes may be removed safely and efficiently.

Bowel resection

Resection and reanastomosis of a portion of intestine are
recommended only if removal of the metastatic site clears the
abdomen of all known tumor more than 0.5 cm diameter. Intestinal resection with excision of multiple segments of bowel
can be associated with prolonged recovery, leading to debili-
tation and delay of postoperative treatment. In many instances,
peritoneal implants, which usually lack deep invasiveness,
can be freed from the muscularis of the bowel wall by sharp
dissection. This technique of "peeling dissection" allows
removal of tumor bulk without actually entering the lumen of
the bowel and therefore reduces postoperative morbidity.

Special postoperative care

Immediately after operation the patient has to be admitted
at an intensive care unit for: monitoring the vital signs,
continuation of the hyperalimentations, and
completion of the short-term antibiotic regimen.

Results

Age

Twenty-three patients were younger than 50 years, 16 patients
were between 50 and 59 years and 14 patients were over age
59. Patients younger than 50 years had a better actuarial
survival than patients over age 49 (Fig. 1).
It could be suggested that the difference in survival is explained by the fact that patients under age 50 tend to have
more effective debulking operations than patients over age
49, possibly partly due to a more favourable histologic grade
(Fig. 2 and 3).

FIG. 1

ACTUARIAL SURVIVAL BY AGE FIGO STAGE III AND IV

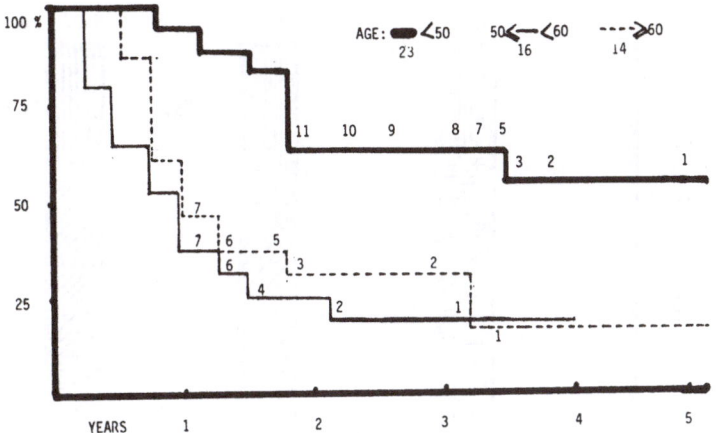

FIG. 2

RESIDUAL TUMOR SIZE BY AGE

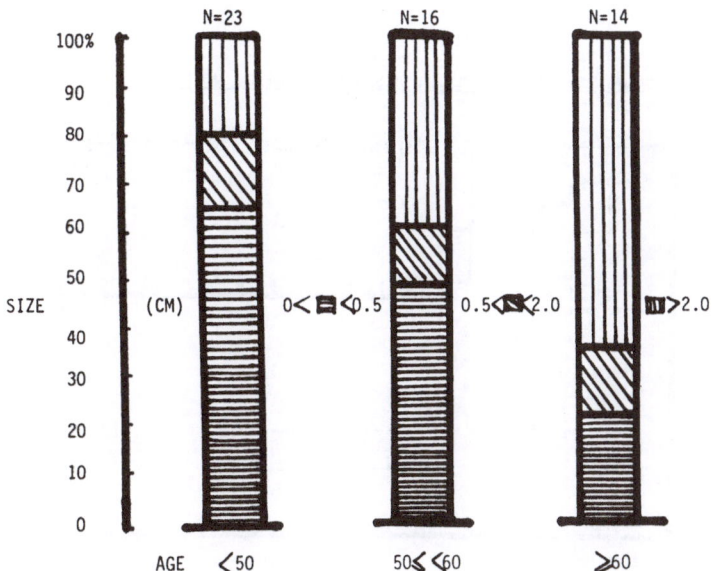

280

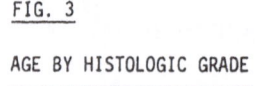

FIG. 3

AGE BY HISTOLOGIC GRADE

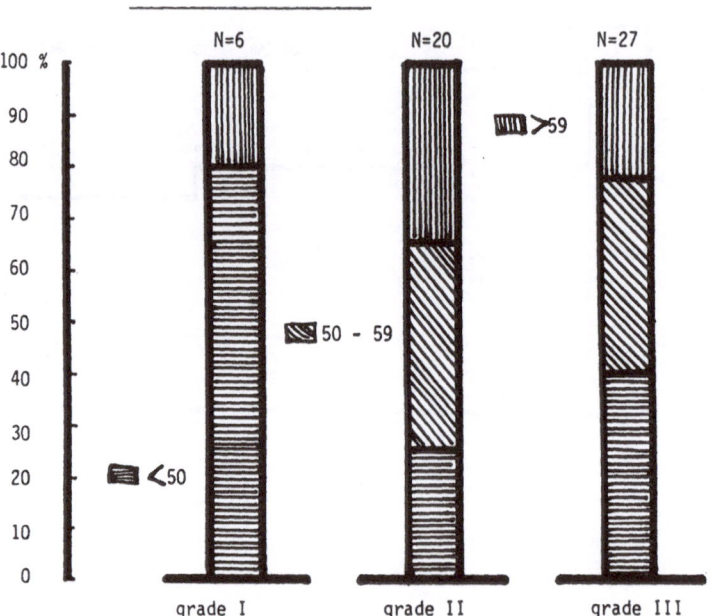

FIG. 4

ACTUARIAL SURVIVAL BY RESIDUAL TUMOR SIZE FIGO STAGE III AND IV

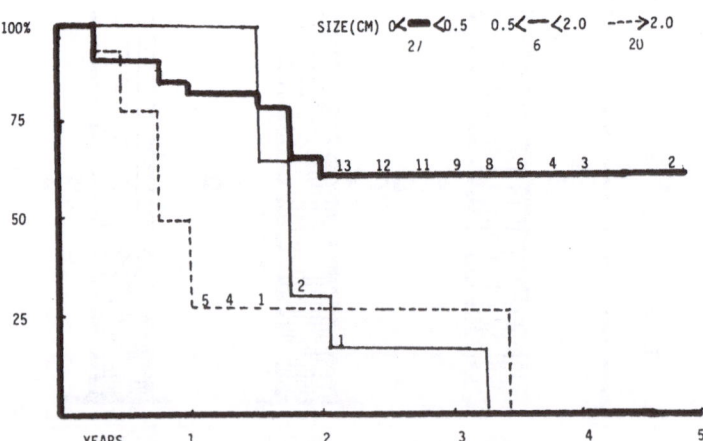

Residual tumor

The largest residual tumor mass after operation was less than
2 cm in 33 patients (62%) and less than 0.5 cm in 26 patients
(49%). Patients survival correlated well with the amount of
residual tumor remaining after debulking procedure. When tumor nodules were absent or less than 0.5 cm in diameter after
the operation (26 patients), the actuarial surviving was significantly better (p = 0.05) than when residual tumor was
between 0.5 cm and 2 cm (6 patients) and more than 2 cm diameter (20 patients), as can be judged from fig. 4 and 5.
Well differentiated tumors seem to be more favourable for
debulking than moderately and poorly differentiated tumors
(Fig. 6).

FIG. 5

ACTUARIAL SURVIVAL BY RESIDUAL TUMOR SIZE FIGO STAGE III AND IV

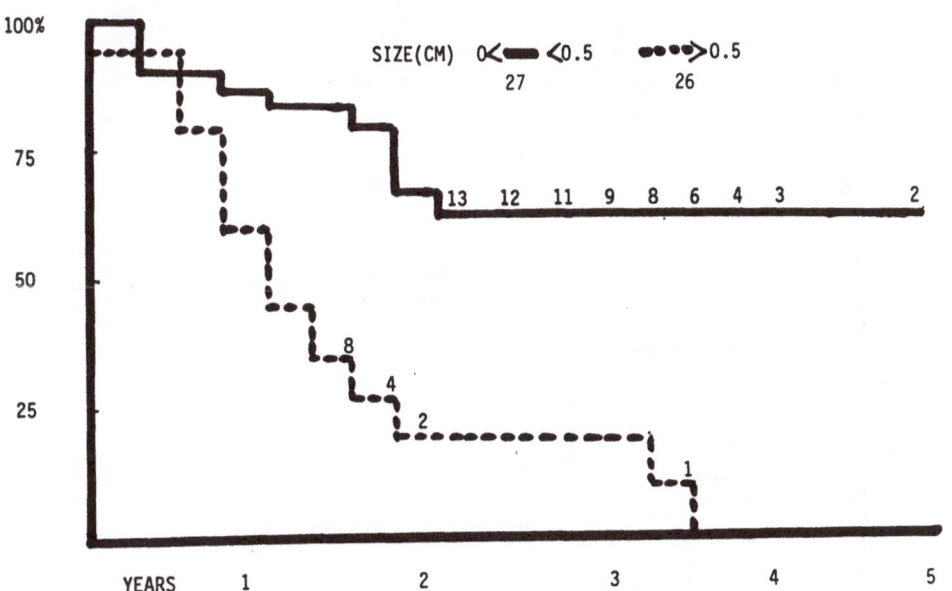

Histologic grade

The degree of differentiation (grade) of the tumor was directly related with the survival rate (Fig. 7, 8 and 9).

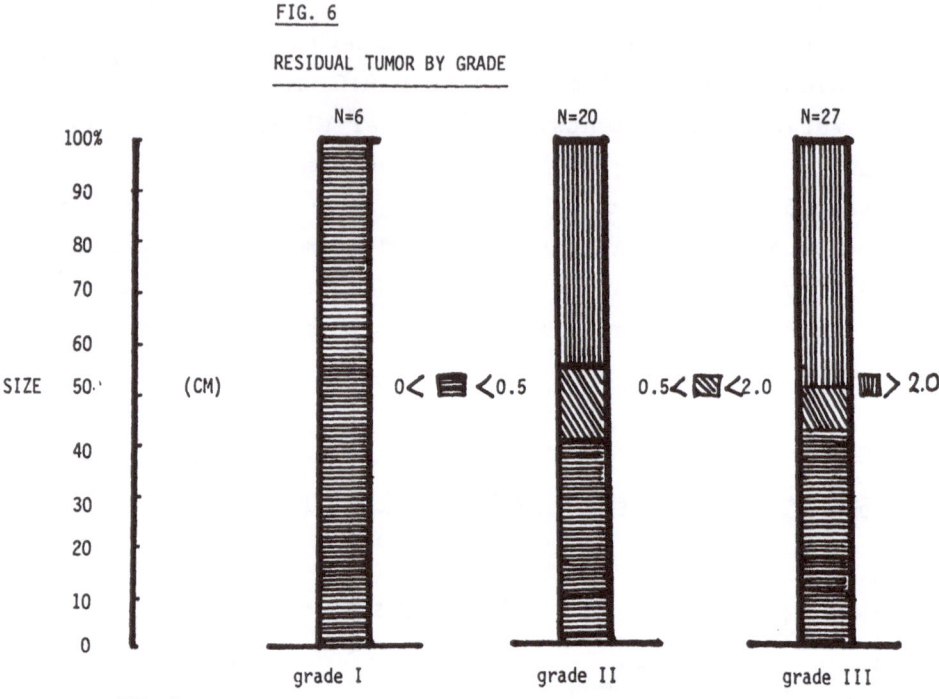

FIG. 6

RESIDUAL TUMOR BY GRADE

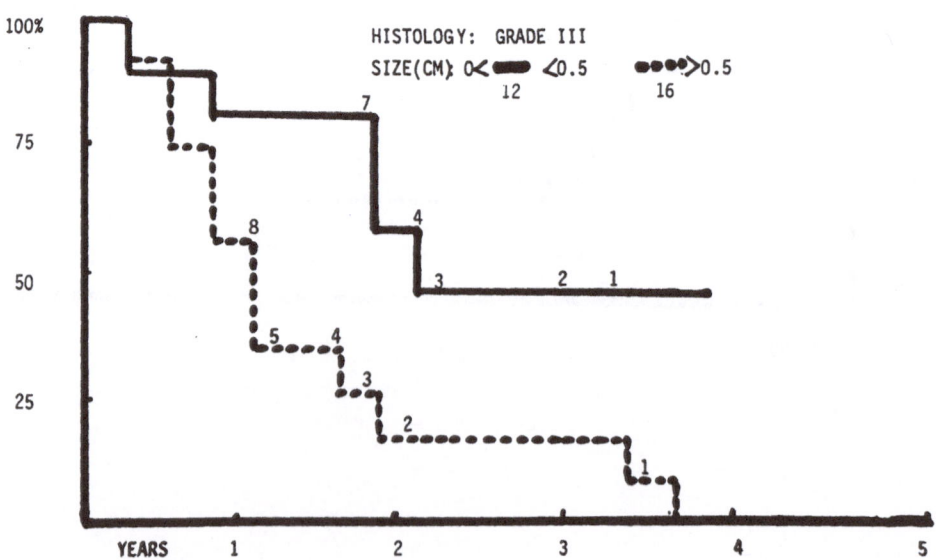

FIG. 7

ACT. SURVIVAL BY HIST. AND RES. TUMOR SIZE FIGO STAGE III AND IV

FIG. 8

ACT. SURVIVAL BY HIST. AND RES. TUMOR SIZE FIGO STAGE III AND IV

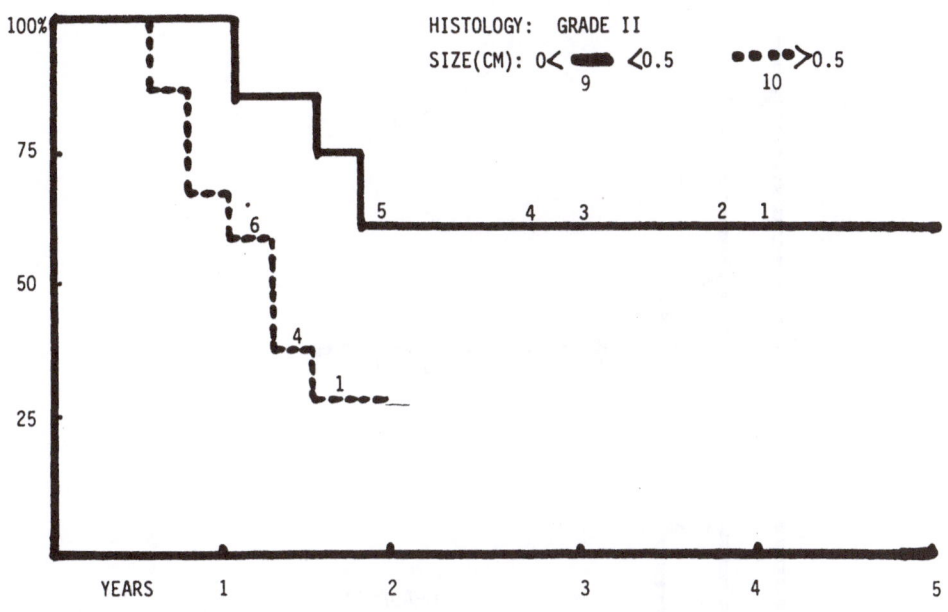

FIG. 9

ACT. SURVIVAL BY HIST. AND RES. TUMOR SIZE FIGO STAGE III AND IV

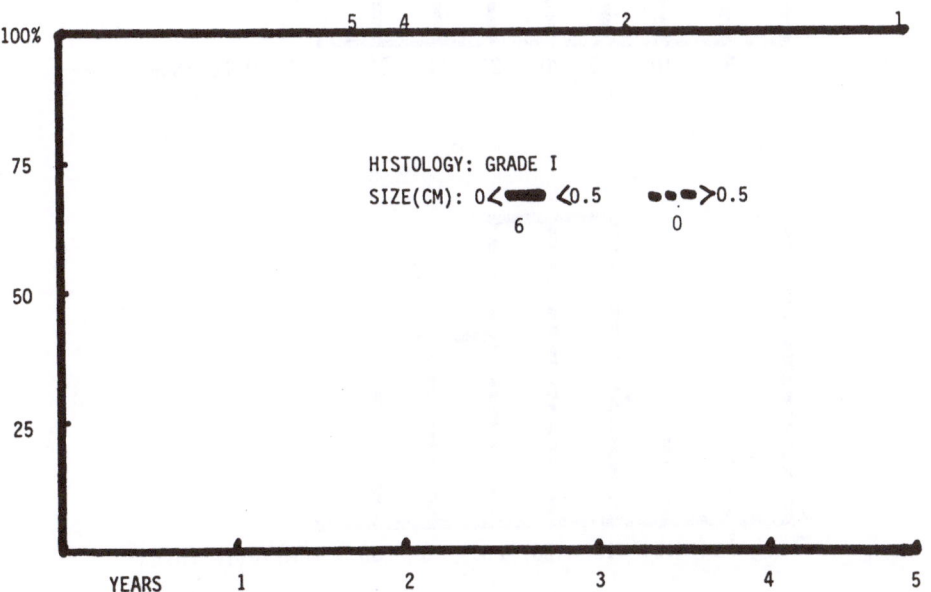

284

FIG. 10

FIGO STAGE III AND IV: MITOTIC INDEX AND HISTOLOGIC GRADE

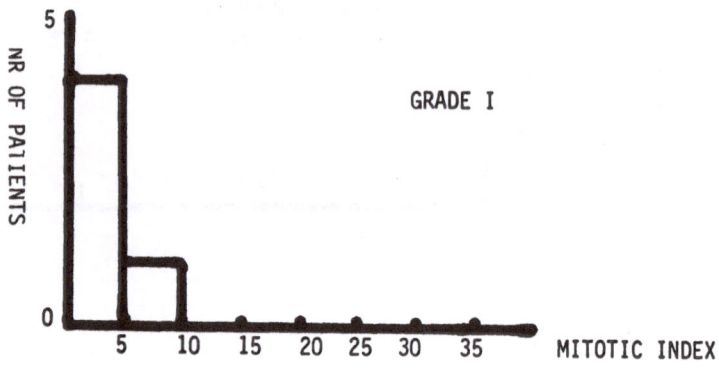

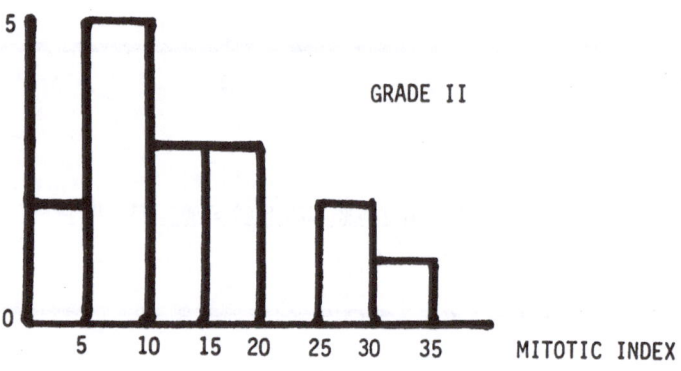

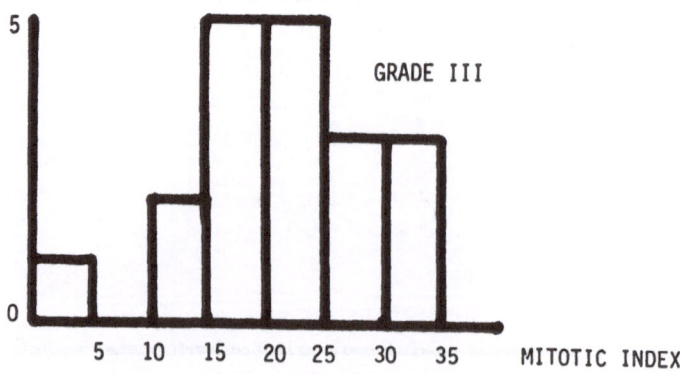

Mitotic index

There is a relation between mitotic index and histological
grade of the tumor tissue before treatment with chemotherapy.
Fig. 10 demonstrates that, the worse the tumor is differentiated the higher the mitotic index will be.

Inductive polychemotherapy before debulking

For patients with an irresectable tumor mass in first instance
or high risk patients for operation at the beginning of the
treatment, two or three courses of inductive polychemotherapy
were given.
In 10 out of 16 patients with inductive polychemotherapy be-
bore debulking, the residual tumor after debulking surgery
was less than 0.5 cm diameter.
Fig. 11 compares the actuarial survival of these 10 patients
with that of 16 patients with residual masses less than 0.5
cm who did not have inductive chemotherapy.

FIG. 11

ACTUARIAL SURVIVAL BY RESIDUAL TUMOR ≤0.5 CM AND INDUCTIVE
POLYCHEMOTHERAPY BEFORE DEBULKING

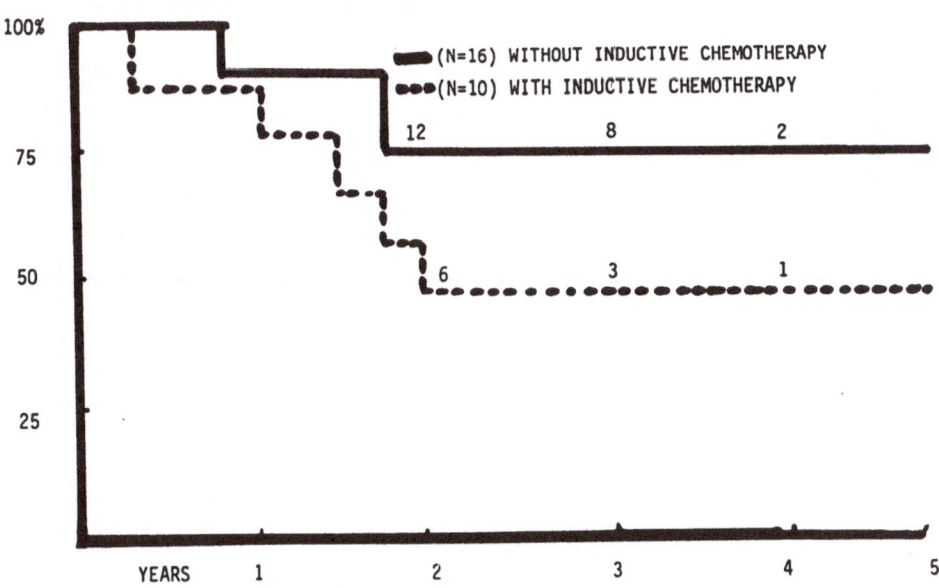

286

Duration of surgery

The duration of the operation is an index of difficulty of
resectability of the tumor mass. Difficulty in resecting the
mass could be possibly caused by the virulence of the cancer
so that polychemotherapy would be less effective in spite of
an optimal debulking.
Fig. 12 gives the results of a small number of patients with
optimal debulking surgery in relation to the duration of surgery. As it can be judged from this figure there is evidence
that a long lasting operation is not useless.

FIG. 12

ACTUARIAL SURVIVAL BY RESIDUAL TUMOR $<$ 0.5 CM AND DURATION OF THE SURGERY

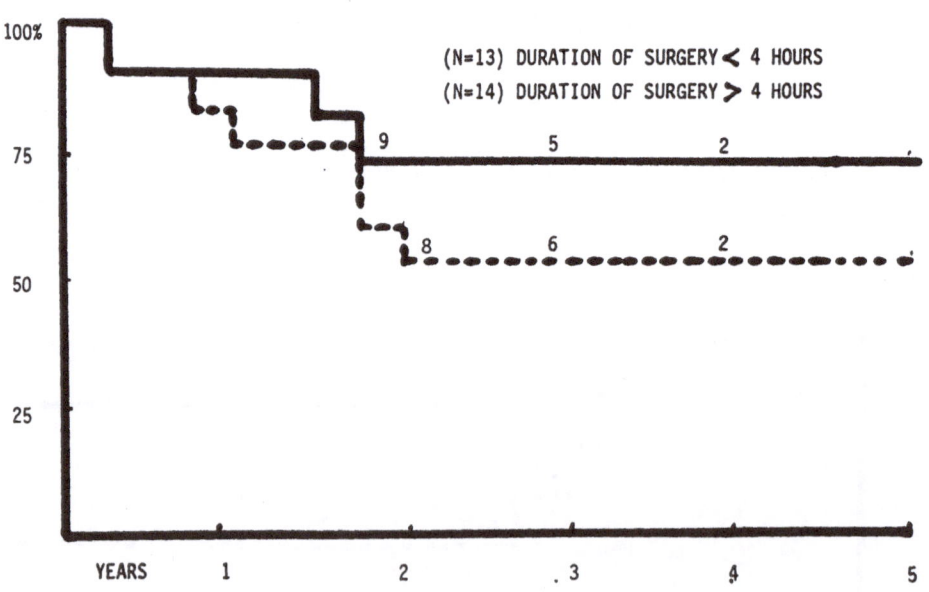

(N=13) DURATION OF SURGERY $<$ 4 HOURS
(N=14) DURATION OF SURGERY $>$ 4 HOURS

Postoperative complications

Table 1 summarizes the postoperative complications in the 53 patients.

TABLE 1

SEVERE POSTOPERATIVE COMPLICATIONS

MORTALITY	3%
HAEMORRHAGIC SHOCK	3%
FISTULAS	5%
SEPSIS	5%

Comment

In the present porspective study we can reconfirm the existance of some prognostic factors such as histologic grade, residual tumor mass, age and mitotic index. In addition a relatively new aspect is the "favourable" diameter of the remnants of tumor tissue left behind at Abdominal Radical Tumor Reduction (called by us A.R.Tu.R.).
The turning point for a change to a better prognosis is in our study 0.5 diameter residual tumor mass. This diameter is smaller than generally accepted (1, 2).
In a recnet (1983) updating of a larger number of patients we can reconfirm our results given in this report.
Studies are in progress to look for possible relationship between the prognostic parameters like age, histologic grade, residual tumor, etc. to calculate a predictive value from these parameters, single or in combination.

References

1. Griffith, C.T. 1975. Surgical resection of Tumor bulk in the primary treatment of ovarian carcinoma. Symposium on ovarian cancer. National Cancer Institute Monographs 42: 101-104.
2. Smith, J.P. and Day, Jr, Th.G. 1979. Review of ovarian cancer at the University of Texas Systems Cancer Centre, M.D. Anderson Hospital and Tumor Institute. Am. J. Obstet. Gynecol. 135:984.

24. EVALUATION OF THE "SECOND-LOOK OPERATION"

Neil B. Rosenshein, M.D., F.A.C.O.G.

Epithelial ovarian cancer places the entire abdominopelvic
cavity at risk. This cavity is lined by a serous membrane,
the peritoneum, which covers the parietes of the abdominopelvic cavity and reflects to cover the various viscera. The
peritoneum is complicated in its arrangement due to rotations
of the gut and fusion of free peritoneal surfaces during fe-
tal development. The result is that the peritoneal cavity is
divided into a greater and lesser peritoneal sac each with
its associated recesses. The para-aortic and pelvic nodes
located outside the peritoneal cavity but within the abdominopelvic cavity are at risk in epithelial ovarian cancer. The
clinical evaluation of an ovarian cancer patient's response
to therapy by an abdominal and pelvic examination is fraught
with difficulties as large volume of tumor can be present
within the abdominopelvic cavity and defy detection. Clinical
evaluation is thus only a crude estimate of complete remission, partial remission, or stabilization of disease as defined in Table I. The importance of determining accurate disease status is so that chemotherapy can be discontinued in
the disease free individual to avoid the long term complications of therapy.

Tumor markers, cul de sac cytology, sonography, computed tomography of the abdomen, laparoscopy and laparotomy have been
advocated in the evaluation of the patient with ovarian cancer.
Surgery in the form of laparotomy continues to be the mainstay for the definitive evaluation of the ovarian cancer patient. Surgery gives an accurate determination of the success
of treatment, the distribution and size of residual tumor

Table I

CRITERIA FOR RESPONSE

COMPLETE REMISSION	- Complete disappearance of all measurable tumor and all clinical evidence of disease.
PARTIAL REMISSION	- 50% or greater decrease in the cross perpendicular product of all measurable tumors lasting a minimum of 30 days.
STABILIZATION	- Any response less than partial remission or no evidence of progression for a minimum of 30 days.

---

and permits the removal of residual tumor. It is important at the end of a planned course of treatment to accurately assess tumor status as prolonged therapy is associated with significant toxicity.

The surgical exploration of those patients who have completed a planned course of therapy without clinical evidence of residual disease (complete remission) and are being considered for termination of chemotherapy is termed the "second-look operation". The "second-look operation" should be restricted to the patient who has had definitive surgical therapy with complete remission of residual tumor after additional therapy; or the patient who receives adjuvant treatment after all apparent disease has been surgically removed. The "second-look operation" has been used to refer to the following other situations:

1. Restaging - The referred patient in whom the initial laparotomy findings are unclear and staging is incomplete.

2. Re-operation - The patient with limited initial surgery who had significant tumor regression with post-operative therapy, so that the patient is now operable.

3. Re-exploration - The patient who develops an isolated
                    resectable recurrence years after hav-
                    ing apparently been tumor free.

4. Re-evaluation - To monitor the patient on chemotherapy,
                    to determine whether the non-palpable
                    disease is responding to chemotherapy
                    or to detect early recurrences.

The "second-look operation" as defined previously has become
an integral part of the management of the epithelial ovarian
cancer patient.

Historical Perspective

The idea of re-operation on the ovarian cancer patient was
reported by Marchetti in 1941. He treated eight patients by
exploratory laparotomy and biopsy followed by radiation and
a second operation (1). Parks in 1945 reported three cases
treated in a similar manner (2).

The concept of re-exploration for patients with visceral malignancy during an asymptomatic phase was pioneered by Wangensteen (3). The re-operation of patients who were asymptomatic
and without clinical evidence of disease six months after
initial surgery was begun in 1949 in patients with colon cancer (4). He and his associates reported on twelve patients
with epithelial ovarian cancer in 1961 with re-operation every six months till the patient was disease free (4). Only one
patient was disease free at the first operation, one patient
underwent seven operations all positive till she died (4).

Reports beginning in 1966 from the M.D. Anderson Hospital and
Tumor Institute detail the beginning of their program of re-
exploration after an interval of treatment. One of the indications cited by Rutledge for re-exploration was "to assist
in evaluating the need for continued treatment" (5). The
timing and indication for the "second-look operation" have
changed at this institution; only those patients who have
received twelve or more chemotherapy cycles are currently
subjected to a "second-look operation" (6). The patient does
not have to be in complete remission to be a candidate for

re-operation (6-8). Wharton in 1981 defined "second-look laparotomy" as a second laparotomy performed after completing
twelve courses of chemotherapy to determine the status of the
disease or its response to chemotherapy and to resect any remaining carcinoma (9).

Tepper et al. in 1971 reported a series of seventeen patients
with advanced ovarian cancer who had an exploratory laparotomy, 3000 rads of radiation, thio-tepa, and re-exploration 4
to 8 weeks after completion of radiation if the clinical response to therapy was satisfactory. Three of the seventeen
patients had no gross residual tumor found (10).

Wallach in 1975 concluded that "second-look operation" should
be performed for all patients with initial non-resectable disease in whom ovaries have been left and a complete clinical
regression is noted on chemotherapy (11).

Current investigators limit the "second-look operation" to
asymptomatic patients with a clinical complete remission who
are being considered for termination of therapy (12-14).

The procedure

Prior to the "second-look operation" the patient should be
meticulously evaluated for disease within the realm of clinical detection. A thorough history and physical examination
should be done with special attention to the vagina, pelvis,
and inguinal nodes. Suspicious areas should be biopsied prior
to surgery. A recent chest x-ray should be reviewed. If the
patient is asymptomatic and the clinical impression is of a
complete remission, the surgeon should proceed with the "second-look operation".

A midline incision long enough to give adequate exposure in
both pelvis and upper abdomen is essential. The first step
is to obtain peritoneal cytology in the following manner. Any
peritoneal fluid that is found is retrieved. The patient is
then placed in a reverse Trendelenburg position and the pelvis is lavaged with a bulb syringe and all fluid is retrieved.
The patient is then placed in a Trendelenburg position and
the right and left gutters are lavaged. Finally the entire

peritoneal cavity is lavaged. All samples should be labelled
and sent separately for cell block. The peritoneal cavity is
then manually and meticulously explored. Special attention
should be paid to the under surface of the diaphragm. Thick-
enings or adhesions are biopsied. Areas of residual disease
left at primary operation are biopsied. The small intestine
is exteriorized and inspected. A transperitoneal incision
is made at the base of the mesentery of the small bowel to explore the retroperitoneal space. All suspicious areas should
be biopsied and a node dissection done. This is important as
Creasman has reported four cases of retroperitoneal disease
at the time of "second-look operation" eventhough there was
no evidence of intra-abdominal residual cancer (15). Residual
infracolic omentum is then removed, further omentectomy should
be done if it appears suspicious. There is currently no information to indicate blind biopsies of the peritoneum adds
to the yield of information about disease status. Residual
ovaries, uterus or cervix that remain should be removed. In
the situation where residual tumor masses are detected they
should be resected "en bloc" if possible, radical surgical
excision should be restricted to those patients in whom removal results in clearing the abdomen of visible tumor.

Results

The effectiveness of the "second-look operation" in detecting
occult disease when applied to the patient with epithelial
ovarian cancer in clinical complete remission is reviewed in
Table II (16-24). Of the 340 patients reported, 44% were found
to have persistent disease. The range was from 17 to 62%. The
range of positive "second-look operations" may reflect the
durability of the response, i.e., those who have a prolonged
clinical complete remission greater than one year will be at
significantly less risk to have occult disease detected at
"second-look laparotomy". Twenty percent of the patients with
a negative "second-look operation" will go on to have a recurrence. The range for recurrence varies from 5 to 28% also
reflects the duration of response prior to laparotomy.

Table II

"Second-look operation" Summary

Study	Patients	Clinical Status	Duration of Rx (months)	Positive Second Look		Recurrences	
Wharton	8	CR	12	5/ 8	(62%)	---	
Soo	25	CR	---	6/ 19	(32%)	---	
Stuart	21	CR	12	6/ 21	(29%)	2/15	(13%)
Curry	27	CR	12	10/ 27	(37%)	3/17	(19%)
Greco	35	CR	6	18/ 35	(51%)	---	
Phillips	21	CR	24	4/ 23	(17%)	1/19	(5%)
Piver	18	CR	23	10/ 18	(56%)	---	
Schwartz	128	CR	---	64/128	(50%)	18/64	(28%)
Mangioni	26	CR	6-12	16/ 26	(62%)	----	(13%)
Hopkins	35	CR	12	12/ 35	(35%)	3/23	
Total	340			151/340	(44)	27/138	(20%)

The validity or the ability of the "second-look operation" to select those individuals having a high probability of persistent ovarian cancer from those who do not depend on the sensitivity and specificity of this procedure. The sensitivity of the "second-lood operation" to give a positive finding when the person tested truly has persistent disease is determined by:

$$\frac{\text{True Positives}}{\text{False Negatives + True Positives}}$$

Using the data from Table I it appears that sensitivity of the test is 83%. The specificity of the "second-look operation" or the ability to give a negative finding when the person treated is free from disease is determind by:

$$\frac{\text{True Negatives}}{\text{False Positives + True Negatives}}$$

The number of false positives can not be determined from the available data; eventhough a certain proportion of cases will be called positive and in fact not be a true positive. Therefore, specificity can not be determined.

Survival after "second-look operation" varies directly with the residual tumor volume (23). The five year survival rate reported by Schwartz and Smith was 72% in the patient with no evidence of disease, 38% for patients with microscopic tumor, and 15% with macroscopic tumor (2 centimeters in diameter) (23). The results of cytoreductive surgery in this group of patients demonstrate a five year survival fo 27% with complete tumor removal, 29% for residual tumor less than 2 centimeters, and 9% for residual tumor greater than 2 centimeters (23).

Wharton and Herson in an analysis of thirty-six patients who have had a "second-look operation" found neither pre-treat-,emt stage, grade, or tumor diameter allows one to determine which patients will survive (9). This may reflect the fact that the analysis was restricted to a small group of selected patients, those who had undergone a "second-look operation". In summary, patients with a clinical complete remission who have a negative "second-look operation" as defined by negative cytology and negative biopsies have an excellent prognosis.

Residual tumor at "second-look laparotomy" significantly compromises patient survival.

Adjunctive Techniques

Computed tomography and laparoscopy will be discussed as adjunctive measures to aid in the evaluation of the patient who is to undergo "second-look operation". Computerized tomography (CT) is a non-invasive means of evaluating the pelvic and abdominal contents. The CT scan offers a relatively high degree of resolution and the ability to evaluate the entire peritoneal cavity (25-26). These features suggest its usefulness as a diagnostic tool in the assessment of response to therapy. The author has evaluated this technique as an adjunct to "second-look operation". The results are summarized in Table III. The first group of eighteen patients studied had three false negatives, the second group of thirteen patients had only one false negative but three false positives.

The overall sensitivity of the CT scan was 56% and specificity was 86%. While the specificity, the ability to give a negative finding in the patient free from disease is acceptable, CT lacks the sensitivity to detect the patient with persistent disease.

A negative CT scan is certainly a positive indication to proceed with a "second-look operation".

Laparoscopy has long been used to evaluate the status of the peritoneal cavity (27). It is accepted by most investigators that the use of laparoscopy is restricted because of the limited evaluation of the peritoneal cavity (28). In addition to that limitation there is the morbidity associated with doing the procedure, of particular concern is bowel perforation which is reported in one series to occur in 8% of patients (28). Laparoscopy has been reported to detect 15 to 40% of patients with persistent disease (22, 29-32). The majority of positive findings are related to cytologic washings (22, 29-32). Subsequent "second-look laparotomy" detected 20 to 45% of patients with a negative laparoscopy had persistent tumor.

Table III

Second-Look Operation versus Computed Tomography

	True Negative	False Negative	True Positive	False Positive
Group I (18 patients)	12	3	3	–
Group II (13 patients)	7	1	2	3
Total	19	4	5	3
	31			

While laparoscopy can make the determination of persistent disease it is associated with complications and limitations. It is the authors approach to combine a thorough clinical assessment with a CT scan. If the impression on both assessments is of a clinical complete remission then a "second-look operation" is undertaken. If the CT scan is positive a laparoscopy precedes the "second-look operation". If the laparoscopy is negative, i.e., no visualized tumor, surgery proceeds. If tumor is visualized a decision then has to be made regarding the appropriateness of further surgery (Fig. 1).

Summary

The "second-look operation" should be restricted to those patients with a clinical complete remission, and are being considered for termination of therapy. Several points can be made regarding the "second-look operation". Approximately 44% of patients with a clinical complete remission will have detectabel disease at "second-look operation", and in addition 20% will recur. The longer the duration of the complete clinical response the less frequent a positive "second-look operation" will be, and the greater the chance of survival.
The importance of this procedure is its high degree of sensitivity (83%) permits therapy to be discontinued in the disease free patient, or to be modified or re-instituted in the patient with persistent disease. Cessation of therapy is important to the patient with a complete response because of the toxicity associated with prolonged therapy.

References

1. Marchetti, A.A. 1941. Ovarian cancer: Clinicopathologic evaluation. New York State J. Med. 41:23.
2. Parks, T.J. 1945. Carcinoma of the ovary treated postoperatively with deep x-ray. Report of three cases. Am. J. Obstet. Gynecol. 49:676.
3. Wangensteen, O.H., Lewis, F.J., Tongen, L.A. August 1951. The "second-look" in cancer surgery. Lancet 303.
4. Santoro, B.T., Griffen, W.O., Wangensteen, O.H. 1961. The second-look procedure in the management of ovarian malignancies and pseudomyxoma peritonei. Surgery 50:354.

5. Rutledge, F. and Burns, B.C. 1966. Chemotherapy for advanced ovarian cancer. Am. J. Obstet. Gynecol. 96:761.
6. Schwartz, P.E. 1981. Surgical management of ovarian cancer. Arch. Surg. 116:99.
7. Smith, J.P., Delgado, G., Rutledge, F. 1976. Second-look operation in ovarian carcinoma: Postchemotherapy. Cancer 38:1438.
8. Smith, J.P., Rutledge, F., Wharton, J.T. 1972. Chemotherapy of ovarian cancer: New approaches to treatment. Cancer 30: 1565.
9. Wharton, J.T. and Herson, J. 1981. Surgery for common epithelial tumors of the ovary. Cancer 48:582.
10. Tepper, E., Sanfilippo, L.J., Gray, J. et al. 1971. Second-look surgery after radiation therapy for advanced stages of cancer of the ovary. Am. J. Roentgenol. 112:755.
11. Wallach, R.C., Kabakow, B., Jerez, E., Blinick, G. 1975. The importance of second-look surgical procedures in the staging and treatment of ovarian carcinoma. Semin. Oncol. 2:243.
12. Lewis, J.L., Griffiths, T., Morrow, C., Wharton, T. 1978. Managing ovarian cancer: the second-look operation. Contemp. Obstet. Gynecol. 12:137.
13. Castaldo, T.W. 1981. The value of a second-look laparotomy in patients with ovarian cancer in Gynecologic Oncology: Controversies in Cancer Treatment, Ed. Ballon, S.C., G.K. Hall and Co., pp. 335-344. Boston.
14. Schwartz, P.E. 1981. The value of a second look laparotomy in patients with ovarian cancer in Gynecologic Oncology: Controversies in Cancer Treatment, Ed. Ballon, S.C., G.K. Hall and Co., pp. 345-353, Boston.
15. Creasman, W.T., Abu-Ghazaleh, S., Schmidt, H.J. 1978. Retroperitoneal metastatic spread of ovarian cancer. Gynecol. Oncol. 6:447.
16. Wharton, J., Rutledge, F., Smith, J. et al. 1979. Hexamethylmelamine: An evaluation of its role in the treatment of ovarian cancer. Am. J. Obstet. Gynecol. 133:833.
17. Soo, I.S.C., Khoo, K., Whitaker, S. 1981. Evaluation of ovarian cancer by second-look laparotomy after treatment. Aust. N.Z. J. Surg. 51:30.
18. Stuart, G.C.E., Jeffries, M., Stuart, J.L. et al. 1982. The changing role of "second-look" laparotomy in the mamagement of epithelial carcinoma of the ovary. Am. J. Obstet. Gynecol. 142:612.
19. Curry, S., Zembo, M., Nahhas, W. et al. 1981. Second-look laparotomy for ovarian cancer. Gynecol. Oncol. 11:114.
20. Greco, F.A., Julian, C.G., Richardson, R. et al. 1981. Advanced ovarian cancer: Brief intensive combination chemotherapy and second-look operation. Obstet. Gynecol. 58: 199.
21. Phillips, B., Buchsbaum, H.J., Lifshitz, S. 1979. Reexploration after treatment for ovarian carcinoma. Gynecol. Oncol. 8:339.
22. Piver, S., Lele, S., Barlow, J. et al. 1980. Second-look laparoscopy prior to proposed second-look laparotomy. Obstet. Gynecol. 55-571.

23. Schwartz, P. and Smith, J.P. 1980. Second-look operations in ovarian cancer. Am. J. Obstet. Gynecol. 138:1124.
24. Mangioni, C., Mattioli, G., Natale, N. 1975. The "second-look" operation in long-term therapy of ovarian malignancies, in Diagnosis and Treatment of Ovarian Neoplastic Alterations, Ed. Day Watteville, H., Excerpta Medica, pp. 153, Amsterdam.
25. Stephens, D.H., Williamson, D., Sheedy, P.F. et al. 1977. Computed tomography of the retroperitoneal space. Radiol. Clin. N. Amer. 15:377.
26. Redman, H.C. 1977. Computer tomography of the pelvis. Radiol. Clin. N. Amer. 15:441.
27. Rosenoff, S.H., Young, R.C., Anderson, T. et al. 1975. Peritoneoscopy: A valuable staging tool in ovarian carcinoma. Ann. Intern. Med. 83:37.
28. Berek, J.S., Griffiths, T., Leventhal, J.M. 1981. Laparoscopy for second-look evaluation in ovarian cancer. Obstet. Gynecol. 58:192.
29. Rosenoff, S.J., DeVita, V.T., Hubbard, S. et al. 1975. Peritoneoscopy in the staging and follow-up of ovarian cancer. Semin. Oncol. 2:223.
30. Mangioni, C., Bolis, G., Molteni, P. et al. 1979. Indications, advantages and limitations of laparoscopy in ovarian cancer. Gynecol. Oncol. 7-47.
31. Smith, W.G., Day, T.G., Smith, J.P. 1977. The use of laparoscopy to determine the results of chemotherapy for ovarian cancer. J. Reprod. Med. 18:257.
32. Spinelli, P., Luini, A., Pizzetti, P. et al. 1976. Laparoscopy in staging and restaging of 95 patients with ovarian carcinoma. Tumori 62:493.

25. NUTRITIONAL SUPPORT IN GYNECOLOGIC CANCER

C. Thomas Griffiths

The cachexia of progressive neoplastic disease has long been
recognized as an inhibitor of aggressive therapy as well as
a contributor to the eventual demise of the host. Nutritional
depletion associated with localized disease is rarely apparent
clinically, but has become appreciated during the past decade.
Complications of intensive chemotherapeutic, radiotherapeutic
and surgical treatment, particularly when used in combination,
have been most common among patients with unrecognized nutritional deprivation. In addition, the availability of nutritional support by either enteral or parenteral hyperalimentation
has provided an impetus to the identification of these patients. Questions to be answered include: 1. Can nutritional
support reverse the adverse nutritional effects of cancer?
2. Can nutritional support improve the response to chemotherapy, radiotherapy or surgery? 3. Can nutritional support improve the tolerance to these therapeutic modalities?
An answer to the first question requires an understanding of
the process of cachexia as it develops with each tumor-host
relationship. Adverse nutritional effects may be: 1. mechanical 2. metabolic 3. paraneoplastic.
Mechanical effects result from direct interference of the
tumor mass or masses with gastrointestinal function. Among
the gynecologic cancers ovarian carcinoma and those endometrial
carcinomas that implant on peritoneal surfaces are prime ex-
amples. Disordered small bowel motility secondary to tumor
implantation and interference with neural transmission through
the myenteric plexus makes carcinomatous ileus a prominent
feature of advanced disease, and often simulates partial small
bowel obstruction. The pressure effect of ascites not only

distends the abdomen, but limits gastric capacity and leads
to premature satiety.

The metabolic effects of the tumor are related to the consumption of host substrate and the catabolic products resulting
therefrom. Although the role of the tumor as a parasite has
been well demonstrated. In addition, the energy consumption
of the tumor increases with tumor volume and tumors in excess
of 1.4 kg (equivalent to most stage III ovarian carcinomas)
may consume 50 percent of the intake of the patient at rest.
In the oxygen-poor microenvironment of the tumor, energy is
derived by anaerobic glycolysis (Embden-Myerhof pathway),
which is not only an inefficient energy source, but also leads
to an accumulation of lactic acid. The energy-dependent con-
version of the excess lactic acid into glucose in the liver
(Cori cycle) further depletes energy stores. The predominant
catabolic effect of the tumor on the host is protein deficiency.
With an increasing demand for glucose and amino acids, proteolysis of skeletal muscle protein maintains the pool of
free amino acids necessary for glyconeogenesis and visceral
protein synthesis by the liver. The translocation of skeletal
to visceral protein by way of the alanine cycle is further
exaggerated by the additional requirement for visceral protein imposed by ascites formation. Although the energy required for the reduction of lactate and for gluconeogenesis
may be supplied by lipolysis, fat cannot be converted to glucose. Replacement of both glucose and biosynthetic interme-
diates sequestered by the tumor cell must be provided from
protein stores. Unlike fat, protein is a functional energy
store and proteolysis is represented by a corresponding loss
of functioning tissue. Patients do not die from loss of fat,
but fat patients can die from loss of functional protein.
Paraneoplastic effects result in anorexia and in an aversion
to certain foods. Elevated levels of circulating lactic acid
may be responsible in part for anorexia, and as yet uniden-
tified products of tumor catabolism change taste thresholds
to make sugar and meat unpalatable. Finally, the tumor may
also inhibit the normal host response to starvation. During

prolonged periods of decreased food intake adaptation from
the oxidation of glucose to the use of ketones as an energy
source minimizes the breakdown of protein to amino acids
for gluconeogenesis. The cancer patient, however, does not
adapt in this manner and protein loss continues, resembling
the behavior of a patient with severe sepsis.

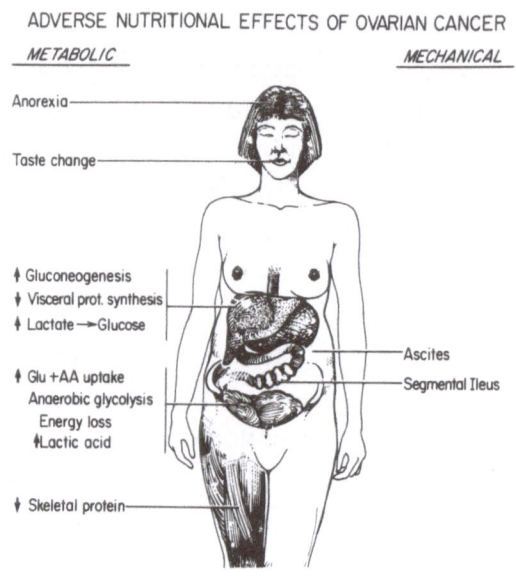

ADVERSE NUTRITIONAL EFFECTS OF OVARIAN CANCER

METABOLIC   *MECHANICAL*

Having considered the adverse effect of the tumor on the
body's economy, one must consider the effect of therapy, particularly when its adverse effects become additive to those
of the tumor. Metabolic response of the host to a surgical
wound is consonant with those induced by tumor as follows:
anorexia, weight loss, increased metabolic rate, lactic
acidosis, decreased glucose tolerance and increased gluconeogenesis. Many patients with recurrent or advanced gynecologic cancer will be in a borderline state of nutritional
compensation which may be clinically inapparent. Increased

metabolic demands and a further reduction in nutrient availability imposed by an extensive operation are likely to tip
the balance. Nutritional decompensation, the final phase of
the cancer cachexia syndrome, results from the inability of
depleted skeletal muscle stores to keep pace with the amino
acid requirement for gluconeogenesis and wound healing. As
a consequence of limited amino acid availability, wound healing is impaired and visceral protein synthesis sharply cur-
tailed. A subsequent fall in serum albumin is accompanied
by a rapid increase in extracellular fluid and even ascites.
Pulmonary function is restricted by fluid accumulation and
the inadequacy of depleted respiratory musculature. Although
not as dramatic as an extensive operation, the super-impos-
ition of rigorous combination chemotherapy on a nutritionally
depleted patient will also accelerate the cachectic process
and death may be forestalled only by early cessation of tumor growth. In addition to anorexia and weight loss, intensive chemotherapy compounds a nutritional deficit by inter-
fering with protein synthesis and intracellular enzyme function and with the tumor shares an inhibition of cellular and
humoral immunity.

As assessment of the direct effect of nutritional support,
particularly total parenteral nutrition (TPN), in reversing
the nutritional deficits imposed by neoplasia has been difficult to separate from the concurrent effect of anticancer
therapy. As a result of a number of studies recently summarized in the review article by Brennan (2) the effect of TPN on
tumor-bearing patients has been to increase weight, blood
glucose and insulin, plasma amino acids and nitrogen balance,
and gluconeogenesis from amino acids has been inhibited. Most
of these effects also have been observed in the starved or
injured patient. In addition, a return of skin-test responsiveness to recall antigens has been observed in more than
50 percent of anergic patients with cancer after TPN.

In general, the effect of nutritional support on enhancing
tolerance of cancer therapy has been reported as favorable,
but the evidence is inconclusive. Patients undergoing ope-

rations for esophageal and gastric cancers, as well as advanced ovarian carcinomas, have shown a decrease in complications and mortality when supported by TPN. Postoperative weight loss, serum albumin levels and alanine gluconeogenesis in the cancer patient have been favorably affected by the use of preoperative and postoperative TPN. Similar metabolic effects have been noted among patients undergoing chemotherapy and irradiation, but a significant difference in tolerance to these therapeutic modalities based upon nutritional support has not been confirmed.

Although early uncontrolled studies suggested an improved response rate to chemotherapy among patients concurrently undergoing TPN, a number of prospective trials have failed to support these observations. Data relevant to gynecologic cancers has been scanty. Indications for nutritional support in patients with gynecologic cancer should be the same as those for other malignancies. The nutritional state of the patient, the disease process and the proposed therapy are taken into account in determining the need for nutritional support as well as the means whereby it will be delivered. A number of studies have indicated that enteral nutrition has been as effective as parenteral nutrition and has carried fewer complications, providing the gastrointestinal tract is intact. Patients with gynecologic cancers, particularly those of the cervix and vulva, are best treated by high protein oral preparations or even elemental diets in the presence of radiation enteritis. Anorexia and premature satiety may be overcome by the use of small feeding tubes and constant drips. Patients with intra-abdominal disease, particularly ovarian carcinoma, tend to have sufficient impairment of small bowel function that parenteral nutrition is indicated. Patients with ovarian carcinoma without serous effusions, who are less than ten percent below ideal body weight and whose serum albumins are greater than 3.5 g/ml, can be maintained postoperatively with peripheral amino acid solutions alone. On the other hand, patients with ascites, moderate to severe gastrointestinal symptoms, serum albumins below 3.5 g/ml, greater than ten per-

cent weight loss, and anergy on skin testing with recall antigens are best treated with preoperative and postoperative TPN.
A number of nutritional indices which measure skeletal muscle
mass and estimate the functional capacity of visceral proteins
have been used as guidelines as described by Blackburn and
associates (1).
TPN solutions have been standardized and contain 200-250 grams
of glucose per litre and 23-50 grams of crystalline amino
acids per litre. Standard electrolytes are addes according
to patient requirements with the addition of small amounts
of calcium, magnesium and phosphate daily. Multivitamins,
vitamin K and trace metal solutions are other daily additives
and intravenous fat is provided once weekly to prevent essential fatty acid deficiency. Metabolic complications continue
to be hypophosphatemia and non-ketonic hyperglycemia. The
subclavian route is preferred, although it is somewhat more
difficult to place a line in that location than by way of
jugular vein. The earlier complications of sepsis have been
almost completely overcome by appropriate aseptic management.
In conclusion, it must be emphasized that routine nutritional
support of the patient with cancer is unjustified unless effective primary therapy is available. When aggressive surgical
and chemotherapeutic management result in complete remissions
in the majority of patients and yet are associated with inten-
sification of nutritional morbidity, nutritional support, including TPN, is strongly recommended until the host can re-
cover from the side effects of treatment. As stated by Brennan, "No patient need die of malnutrition because of a non-
functioning gastrointestinal tract during aggressive effective antineoplastic therapy."

References

1. Blackburn, G.L., Bistrian, B.R., Maini, B.S., Schlamm, M.T.,
   and Smith, M.F. 1977. Nutritional and metabolic assessment
   of the hospitalized patient. J. Parenteral and Enteral Nutrition. 1:11-22.
2. Brennan, M.F. 1981. Total parenteral nutrition in the cancer patient. N. Engl. J. Med. 305:375-382.

3. Burt, M.E., Gorschboth, C.M. and Brennan, M.F. 1982. A controlled prospective randomized trial evaluating the metabolic effects of enteral and parenteral nutrition in the cancer patient. Cancer 49:1092-1108.
4. Copeland, E.M., Daly, T.M., Ota, D.M. and Dudrick, S.J. 1979. Nutrition cancer and hyperalimentation. Cancer 43: 1208-2216.
5. Fuller, A.F., Jr. and Griffiths, C.T. 1979. Ovarian cancer cachexia - surgical interactions. Gynecol. Oncol. 8:301-310.

26. PSYCHOLOGICAL ASPECTS OF GYNAECOLOGICAL ONCOLOGY SURGERY

Gerjanne Bos, clinical psychologist

Introduction

The diagnosis of cancer constitutes a psychological crisis
for the patient (1) Patients with cancer frequently report increased levels of anxiety, depression, anger and guilt. In
addition, they are faced with overwhelming feelings of loss
due to disappearance of good health, the possibility of death
and loss of control, self-esteem, employment and social status.
Patients with cancer are stigmatised by society: the word and
the disease cancer have profound impact and evoke powerful
emotional reactions . The myth that cancer is contabious (2)
is still persistent and further isolates many patients.
In gynaecology we have to deal with different sites of cancer:
the vulva, vagina, cervix, endometrium, tubes and ovaries. In
contrast with many other countries, breast cancer in the Netherlands does not belong to gynaecological oncology.
Gynaecological cancers are unique in that they are particularly catastrophic due to the direct impact they have on essential
components of the woman's identity, her genital organs (3, 4).
The most fundamental effect of gynaecological oncology surgery
is the severe blow to the patient's self-esteem and her femi-
nine identity.
Other aspects are also important. For instance, the fact that
genital organs have a connotation leading to feelings such as
shame, embarrassment and ignorance. Another relevant aspect
is that genital cancer may symbolize dramatic retribution for
real or fancied sexual transgressions such as masturbation,
induced abortion, contraceptive practices, or unsanctioned

sexual partners (5). As a special source of problems between
patients and their partners I would like to mention magazine
reports linking genital cancer with promiscuity or a bad hy-
gienic situation. They accuse each other as being the cause
of the disease.

The patient with genital cancer

Because of the differing sites and types, each cancer has its
own specific consequences, in terms of both threatening life
and of disfigurement. Therefore one cannot consider the special
cancer patient. Moreover, reactions to surgery vary considerably from patient to patient and are largely influenced by
the woman's characteristic defense mechanisms, personality
history, life stage and family size (4) and I think by her
female role too. Needless to say that pre- and post-surgical
information and support also play a very important role (6).
In summary, the specific cancer patient does not exist, yet
there are many problems which to a smaller or larger extent
occur in all patients.

Psychological aspects of medical care and follow-up

Pre-operative period

The diagnosis of cancer by a positive Pap-smear followed by
a positive biopsy, can be extremely confusing, especially for
those patients who have had their regular controls. They are
astohished: "I recently had a negative smear!". They do not
believe it and are convinced that a mistake was made and say:
"I am always so clean of body! Why me? It is not fair!" It
comes very unexpected for them: "I am healthy and all of a
sudden ..... cancer!" It comes as a blow, as a world-shaking
event. They report feeling shocked, terrified, numb, panicky
or stunned. The patient and the family too, are faced with a
crisis situation. Simply hearing the word cancer often pre-
vents a patient from assimilating the complete diagnosis, indicated treatment and prognosis. Women say they appreciate
that their husbands accompany them, when they are told the
diagnosis.

The husband is in a better position to share from the beginning the emotions involved, which is of great importance for
their relation. Expression of strong emotions is reported from
extreme crying, for hours, to not crying at all verbalised as:
"I felt icy, frosty, I have not shed a tear over it!" They cannot understand the situation they are in, and are completely
desperate! All the while, time goes on and nearly all patients
want to be treated as soon as possible, the sooner the better.
They want to get rid of the cancer rapidly preferring operation.
They want to remove everything that is "dirty". It is a time
of panic and hurry, patients report extreme restlessness, often
resulting in a typical reaction: cleaning of the complete
house. On the other hand practical matters require their attention; family and children have to be informed, often child-
care must be arranged. Patients seem to be most concerned
about their small children, stating: "My husband will manage
to survive, he will find another woman". Many patients do not
seem to be able to share their sorrows, as they say: "I only
asked my husband to find a "good" mother for the children".
And if patients try to speak about their anxiety over dying,
their husbands often are inclined to blow these remarks away,
saying: "Everything will be all right", or, "Do not talk about
it", or even worse: "Do not make a fuss". Maybe they try to
spare each other, but every time I hear this I am shocked about
the inability of human to communicate and to share feelings
in such a situation.

Hospitalization

Patients often react to the prospect of an operation with anxiety. There is the common fear of death from surgery or anaesthesia and fear of pain or mutilations. The patients' anxiety about their impending surgery is often revealed in vivid
dreams and nightmares and they frequently visualize their mu-
tilated bodies, their death or their funeral (7).
After the turbulent time at home for most of them, being in
the hospital bed, is the first time they are really alone with
their body and soul. One patient told about her last night before surgery: how she touched the still intact, smooth skin

of her abdomen and that, for the first time, she cried.

Doctor-patient relation

The relation with the physician is very important. Most patients need assurance that he or she is a competent surgeon. In fact, studies have shown that, aside from technical competence, the most important characteristic to patients is compassion. For some patients, lack of warmth and failure to demonstrate real concent by the surgeon are a justifiable basis for changing physicians (7).

Patients are more relaxed when everything is explained and when they are well informed. They mention that trusting the surgeon is very, very important because: "You have to give yourself completely" and "You have to surrender". In order to relieve anxiety, to feel safe, they honour their surgeon as a hero!.

Once the surgery is over and patients realize that they have come through, the process of coping with the injury to the body begins. In the beginning their concerns are about purely medical and bodily matters like: pain, problems with urine and catheters. But also these accents on physical situations can lead to psychological problems, e.g. older patients especially have to overcome their resistance to touch themselves on that "queer" place and ask me why they could not have the cancer in another place!

Post-operative period

Frequently I feel very sorry for patients, for the life they lived before cancer was diagnosed. After this life-changing event they are regretting that they had not enjoyed life, that they had received little love.

A 65-year old lady told me: "I wished I could live my life again. I do not want to go home to my husband; he is severe and cold. I only want to leave hospital to see my grandchildren"!

So I realize that sometimes we make the faulty assumption that, once the patient is discharged, the family will take good care of her and that she will receive the attention and support she needs at home. In reality, some patients fear their release

from the hospital nearly as much as their admission to it. But,
even if the home-situation is not so negative and sad, difficulties are overwhelming and often unavoidable.

Patients miss the protection of the hospital. Everybody was
nice, they got much attention from nurses and doctors and at
home they have to do it all alone and nobody has sufficient
understanding of the situation.

They report feeling isolated, isolated from others and isolated
from themselves. A 20-year old girl with ovarian cancer told
me, that now, back to work again, she had completely lost contact with everybody around her. She could no longer laugh at
jokes; she could not talk and behave as she did before within
her peer group and, what troubled her most, she had lost contact with her own personality. She had become a stranger to
herself and even her body was strange to her: "It is not my
body any longer, it feels hostile!" She was so desolate and
lonely, I only could hold her in my arms.

After discharge depressive feelings are found in over 50% of
the patients (8); it is a time of mourning, so intense and
complex, that we wonder how they manage. They mourn about the
mutilation, about the loss of uterus, ovaries, vagina or clitoris, and even about the change in colour of their labia.
They mourn over the loss of menstruation and fertility; when
there is a childwish this can even lead to extreme reactions.
They worry about changes in sexuality, about a dry painful
or shortened vagina.

In summary, patients mourn about female organs and functions,
which from the first day of their life determined their being
exclusively female, and which socialized them to femininity,
to a female role.

Patient-doctor relation

Many women no longer feel as if they are female. That makes
them sad, angry and resentful. These resentful feelings are
also directed towards their formerly beloved surgeon: their
image of him or her changes drastically. I did not feel at
ease when they mentioned this. But I think it can be inter-
preted in the following way: before operation there was panic

and everything was done in a hurry; the patient wanted to be
operated very quickly to be rid of the cancer and whe thanked
God and the surgeon that she was still alive. But after the
operation many doubts emerged: "Was it necessary to remove the
uterus? In the mirror I saw that it was such a small spot on
my cervix". "In the newspaper I read that a hysterectomy is
nowadays more fashion than necessity". "Was such a big operation really indicated, since I heard that the removed tissue
proved to be clean"? "Was it wise to be in such a hurry, why
not a baby first"?. In that stage they are holding their physician responsable for all their misery. At first I could only
explain this behaviour as the well-known agressive phase in
the mourning process. But htis explanation was not completely
satisfactory. From patients in the psychotherapy group I learned that before they really know they have cancer, they undergo operation and are rid of the cancer! That is why we should
take into account that these patients have only had CANCER FOR
A FORTNIGHT. They want to forget the cancer on an emotional
level, and are only mourning in fragments. And realising that,
I now carefully ask them, why the doctor shortened the vagina,
or removed the uterus. After some silence and hesitation, the
answer is: "Because of the cancer"? And I again: "Could it be
that it is still too painful for you to accept that you have
had cancer; Do think it over and let us talk about it another
time". And after a week patients reveal that they are more con-
scious of the fact that the cancer is the cause of the mutilation and also become aware that this is rather difficult to
accept and makes them sad. In this way agressive feelings can
be replaced by feelings of grief and the way may be opened to
work through the mourning process.

Coping with cancer

The psychological aspects of cancer and especially how patients
cope with cancer, is a poorly developed field in The Netherlands. Research data about coping with cancer, mainly comes
from the U.S.A. where psychosocial oncology is at least decades
ahead in a few centers (9). Surgeons in this rapidly and enorm-

ously developed field (10), realising that treatment sometimes
has to be as formidable as the disease itself, can try to
ignore the psychological aspects (10), or, realising that
somatic interventions have psychological consequences, may
handle in accordance with this reality.
Therefore it is up to the medical profession to make use of
the knowledge and experience of social workers and psychologists in favour of the well-being of these patients.

Psychotherapy

Until now psychotherapy was mostly applied to persons with
emotional problems stemming from character defects, irrealis-
tic fears, incapability ot solve problems, sexual inadequacies
or relational problems. Psychotherapy however, can also serve
as a life-investment, to learn to live in harmony with one-
self. In fact, the main goal of psychotherapeutic intervention
is to improve the quality of life.
Therefore, the active participation of patients is needed and
interventions are aimed at throwing overboard harmful ballast,
such as guilt and shame.
Psychotherapy is aimed to converse:
- passivity into activity
- helplessness into responsability
- dependence into individuality
- insecurity into assertiveness
- self-disgust into self-esteem (possibly the most essential
                             ingredient for human happiness)
- restlessness into harmony
Would that not be of great help to cancer patients, too?

Problems in psychotherapy

There are many problems in this field, such as: misunderstan-
ding, prejudice, resistance. The more serious criticism concerns psychologists who only try to measure mental states,
whereas the results of pshychotherapeutic interventions are
difficult to evaluate. As to measuring in cancer patients, I
think it is only fair to measure patients psychologically in

a treatment program, evaluating primarily psychotherapeutic results, just as is done in a medical setting. Another problem is that many measuring scales are developed for psychiatric patients or for patients with sexual inadequacies based upon coital frequencies, length of foreplay (12) etcetera. We should not bother cancer patients with scales of these type and besides that, asking for quantity does not reveal anything about quality!

In the meantime the patient is overwhelmed with other problems, and does not know how to solve them.

Our concern must not be limited to prolonging survival and collecting more data on patients, or to quote De Vita, Director of the National Cancer Institute of the United states (7): "Instead of only assessing, measuring, registrating, we have to help our patients to adjust to the emotional trauma of cancer and its treatment. We are obliged to make further efforts to help this return to life be a quality experience".

It is my experience that patients with cancer have less resistance and are more open for psychoterapy than the traditional psychotherapy clients. Due to their high motivation, they learn very quickly. Especially remarkable are the rapid changes in behaviour: taking more initiatives and responsability and becoming more assertive, creating their own happiness and working on their own harmony.

The effect of cancer and its treatment on the quality of life is often underestimated; there is an immense price paid in physical discomfort and in psychological and social trauma. Therefore De Lise et al (13) conclude: "If psychological and social intervention is needed and is not provided in a timely and appropriate manner, cancer treatment can never be considered a success regardless of the medical results".

References

1. Capone, M.A., Good, R.S., Westie, K.S., Jacobson, A.F. 1980. Psychological Rehabilitation of Gynecologic Oncology Patients. Arch. Phys. Med. Rehabil. 61, 128.
2. Sontag, S. 1979. Illness as Metaphor. A. Lane, London.
3. Dennerstein, L., Wood, C, Burrows, G. 1977. Sexual response following hysterectomy and oophorectomy. J. Obstet. Gynec.

49, 92.

4. Derogatis, L.D. 1980. Breast and Gynecologic Cancers. In: Vaeth, J.M., Blomberg, R.C., Adler, L. (eds): Frontiers of Radiat. Ther. Onc., Basel, S. Karger, AG, 14, 1.

5. Donahue, V.C and Knapp, R.C. 1977. Sexual rehabilitation of gynecologic cancer patients. Obstet. Gynec. 49:118.

6. Reading, A.E. 1981. Psychological preparation for surgery: patient recall of information. J. Psychosom. Research, 25, 57.

7. DeVita, V.T. 1980. In: Coping with Cancer. A Resource for Health Professional. Nat. Cancer Inst., Bethesda.

8. Trimbos, C.J. 1981. Het verwerken van kanker. T. Kanker, 4, 3.

9. Cassileth, B.R. 1979. The Cancer Patient, Social and Medical Aspects of Care. Lea & Febiger, London.

10. Abitol, M.M., Davenport, J.H. 1974. Sexual dysfunction after therapy for cervical carcinoma. Am. J. Obstet. Gynecol. 119:181.

11. Bindemann, S. 1982. Psychotherapeutic Interventions: Treatment and evaluation of treatment. Proceedings of the Second EORTC Quality of Life Workshop, Odense, 11.

12. DeLisa, J.,Miller, R.M., Melnick, R.R., Mikulic, M.A. 1982. Rehabilitation of the Cancer Patient. In: Cancer, Principles & Practice of Oncology.
Eds.: DeVita, V.T., Hellman, S., Rosenberg, S.A., Lippincott, Philadelphia. 1730.

27. THE ROLE OF THE SOCIAL WORKER IN GYNAECOLOGICAL ONCOLOGY

Elise van Kleef, Winy Doff, Marion Kreyenbroek

Introduction

In the womens clinic at the University Hospital in Amsterdam
stress is layed in both teaching and in practice on the importance of providing "total care". Just after World War II
our hospital recognized the important implications of psycho-
social factors in illness and the process of healing and began to attract social nurses to the clinic. It is to the credit
of professor Kloosterman, head of our women's clinic, that
during his professorship not only the first medical social
workers came into service, but also that he cleared the way
to multidisciplinar, cooperation.

Social work in the department of gynaecology

A pleasant atmosphere on the ward is of utmost importance to
patients and all of the staff. Every thursday morning from
9.30 to 11 o'clock we provide an opportunity for all the ward
patients to talk in an open group and invite them without restriction, to talk about the feelings, frustrations and problems caused by being in the hospital. Everybody is offered
the opportunity to complain. The position of being dependant
normally discourages one from making complaints, so we have
to encourage them. In our experience, patients have many complaints about our hospital system, when given the opportunity.
This open discussion is designed to encourage the patients towards independence. For example we discuss how to pose questions
to the medical staff, how to cope with feelings of dependence
towards the nursing staff; in short, numerous problems and
experiences which accompany a hospital admission are discussed.
Once a week there is a multidisciplinary case meeting in which

all patients are presented. Senior and junior medical staff,
ward sister, staff nurses and social workers are present at
this meeting. If desired someone from outside or other dis-
cipline is invited.

In this meeting an extensive discussion on type of illness,
course and treatment in a pure medical sense is followed by
a discussion about relevant psycho-social aspects. In a much
narrower context we consult each other about that information
and those feelings which are specific to individual care.

In addition there is a weekly staff meeting on the gynaecological ward, intended for senior nursing and medical staff and
medical social workers. The meeting, which opens with a discussion of points raised by the open patient group, is intended
to discuss the problems within the team, exchange information
about developments within the various disciplines and to plan
for the future.

Social work and the oncological patient

Our experience in the gynaecology department has led us to
develop the following procedure with oncological patients.
First contact: When a woman hears from her doctor that it will
be necessary to take her into hospital and there is the possibility of an AVRUEL operation, one of us is called in.

We find it important that the doctor draws in the social worker
directly when the patient is informed about the diagnosis and
treatment, to exclude misunderstandings in what is, and what
is not said, and to provide immediate support.

At this very first confrontation, when women have just heard
they have cancer, it becomes clear what a tremendous shock this
diagnosis causes.

Recurring remarks are:

"I keep thinking they made some mistake" and: "It is like a
dream, this is not really happening to me", "It is as if I
were part in a film", "I look at myself, but see another person than the one I was yesterday or a week ago". Such negative
feelings characterize the acute critical situation in which
the woman in question finds herself. After the first shock she

would rather talk about practical arrangements to be made and express her worries about husband and children than ask crucial questions like: "what exactly is going to happen to me?" But during this first consultation the fear of dying and certainly the fear of having to leave behind her loved ones, do show through, however vaguely. Practical problems arising from the planned admission can be discussed and help can be offered. We tell the women that it is always possible to phone us during the days she is waiting for admission and offer to resume the contact after discharge.

Furthermore we find it essential to patient (and partner if present), that before admission a second opportunity is provided to talk with the doctor. When a woman is sent for treatment by another medical centre, we introduce ourselves on the ward.

After operation we find that the immediate physical circumstances of the patient take all their energy and the attention, support and caring of doctors and nursing staff during this period are of main importance. The social workers are also part of this team. It is certainly possible that the emotional needs of the patient, in coming to terms with her illness, can be most effectively met by somebody not directly involved in medical and nursing procedures. For example we regularly find that patients with cancer try to "keep smiling" when visited by family and friends, to avoid causing any more worry. However, there is a clear need to express feelings of worry and fear and sometimes to let tears flow. This is possible and exceptable towards a trusted disinterested professional who knows the situation and the hospital. To add to the support given to close family by the medical and nursing staff, the medical social worker is available throughout the admission period.

Groupwork after radical gynaecologic surgery

In the recovery period, we raise the possibility of participation in the patient discussion groups and invite the patient to enlist for the first available group. We also offer to introduce her to an ex-patient who is, or has been in a discussion

group, to talk about her motivation and experiences with this
group. Of course the patient is free to say yes or no. Often,
however, patients feel very stimulated after such a visit, because in this way they can see with their own eyes how a fellow-
sufferer has come out of the battle.
Of course there is always at the time of admission the opportunity to consult, with or without partner, doctor, nurse or
social worker. Experience has shown that this possibility of
extensive consultation proves very important, also at the
time of discharge.
The final discussion, includes the doctor, medical social worker, the patient and possibly her partner. We can give guidelines as to what the patient may and may not do, what sort of
sexual problems may occur and other important points for them
in their situation.

Premises in these patient discussion groups

All members of the group have had radical surgery. There is
no selection according to age; we have seen women in the age
group 25 to 62 years. Having or lacking a partner, children,
or work is of no importance in entering the group.
We work with 2 social workers per group of at least 6 and at
the most 8 women. Every fortnight we assemble in the hospital
for a discussion lasting about two hours. The number of group
meetings varies from 8 to 12. The social workers will not pass
irrelevant individual information to staff members of the hospital; of course it is important to share general aspects.

The importance of a patient discussion group

In our contacts with patients we repeatedly have found that
in the period after discharge women meet with several physical
and psychological problems. Psychological problems include
feeling very insecure and in doubt about themselves, feelings
of deep loneliness, not being a part of their direct surround-
ings, and depressions. Also there are many sexual problems. An
AVRUEL operation always affects a woman's sexuality. The predominant problem is fear of coitus. The vagina is shorter and

dry. It requires endless patience and practice to finally let
the partner enter. Coitus may remain painful for a long time
and for this reason some of the women and their partners
conclude that in their relationship sex belongs to the
past.

Single young women do not know what to do. They have difficulty in beginning a new relationship because:
- they cannot have children
- they are already experiencing the menopause
- they have had cancer.
The extent to which the woman herself is capable of coping with
her new situation also depends on our ways of informing her
about a state of stability yet to be found. In order to help,
we must know how the woman experiences sex.
As soon as the members of a particular group have become more
or less familiar with each other they talk about sex problems
without any reservations and help each other with things that
for many were till then too intimate to talk about. Many women
have severe problems with urinating. With every new group this
is the first subject to be aired.
All women to a differing degree are troubled by the fact that
they do not feel any urge before urinating, which can lead to
embarassing situations. Hearing the problems of others, they
recognize their own and obviously feel relieved to talk about
them openly.
Apart from the relief brought by recognition, the women also
find support with one another. Helped by that support and relief they turn out to be capable of finding creative solutions
for their shared problems.
We do not in any way want to suggest that all these women have
had troubles in the same manner or degree, but we have found
it necessary to develop special care for these patients. Our
experience has proved the importance of these groups. Indeed
we find it prerequisite to the use of radical surgery. We believe that the quality of life after an AVRUEL operation depends not only on the medical success, but largely on the degree of success the patient has in physically and emotionally
overcoming her illness.

Reference

Olson, M. 1981. Intervention by a social work team (a study
of the social work team at the womens clinic of Wilhelmina
Gasthuis, Amsterdam, Holland), Manpower Monograph 15, Syracuse
University, New York

Subject Index